1990

*Lovesickness in the Middle Ages*

University of Pennsylvannia Press
MIDDLE AGES SERIES
Edited by EDWARD PETERS
Henry Charles Lea Professor
of Medieval History
University of Pennsylvania

A complete listing of the books in this series
appears at the back of this volume

# LOVESICKNESS
## in the
# MIDDLE AGES
## The *Viaticum* and Its
## Commentaries

---

## MARY FRANCES WACK

*upp*

UNIVERSITY OF PENNSYLVANIA PRESS

*Philadelphia*

Chapter 6, "The Measure of Pleasure: Peter of Spain on Men, Women, and Lovesickness," is a revised version of an article appearing in *Viator* 17 (1986): 173–96, copyright © 1986 by the University of California Press.

Library of Congress Cataloging-in-Publication Data

Wack, Mary Frances.
    Lovesickness in the Middle Ages : the Viaticum and its
commentaries / Mary Frances Wack.
        p.    cm. — (Middle Ages series)
    Bibliography: p.
    Includes index.
    ISBN 0-8122-8142-X
    1. Lovesickness.    2. Constantine, the African, ca. 1020–1087.
Viaticum.    3. Medicine, Medieval.    4. Lovesickness in literature.
5. Literature, Medieval—History and criticism.    I. Title.
II. Series.
RC543.W33    1990
362.2—dc20                                                    89-22450
                                                                 CIP

# CONTENTS

List of Figures    vii
Acknowledgments    ix
Introduction    xi

PART I

## LOVESICKNESS IN THE MIDDLE AGES

1  Pathology and Passion: Lovesickness in Antiquity and the Early
   Middle Ages    3
2  Constantine's *Viaticum*    31
3  "Noble" Love: Gerard of Berry's *Glosses on the Viaticum*    51
4  What Part of the Body Does Love Afflict? Giles' *Gloss on the
   Viaticum*    74
5  Peter of Spain: *Questions on the Viaticum*    83
6  The Measure of Pleasure: Peter of Spain on Men, Women, and
   Lovesickness    109
7  Is Love Curable by Herbs? Bona Fortuna's *Treatise on the Viaticum*    126
8  Recreating a Context for the Lover's Malady    146

PART 2

## THE TEXTS

Constantine the African, *Viaticum* I.20    179
Gerard of Berry, *Glosule super Viaticum*    194
Giles, *Glose super Viaticum*    206
Peter of Spain, *Questiones super Viaticum* (Version A)    212
Peter of Spain, *Questiones super Viaticum* (Version B)    230
Bona Fortuna, *Tractatus super Viaticum*    252

Notes    267
Bibliography of Works Cited    315
Index    339

# FIGURES

1.1 Bronze statuette of emaciated man   4

1.2 Antiochus and Stratonice   16–17

1.3 Amnon and Thamar   20

1.4 The Bride of Canticles   23

1.5 The Crucifixion   26

2.1 Portrait of a medieval physician   33

2.2 Doctor treating a patient   36

2.3 Coitus   42

2.4 Vinous therapy in a garden   43

2.5 Bathing   44

2.6 Music and sleep   45

3.1 Medical master and students   53

3.2 Cerebral localization of the inward wits   57

3.3 "Disease woman"   60

3.4 Marriage   67

3.5 Wine, women, and games   68

3.6 Chess   69

3.7 The poet-lover kneels before his lady   71

3.8 Bed-ridden man wounded by love   73

4.1 Dialectic   77

4.2 Tavern scene   80

5.1 "Caput phantasticum" with internal senses   91

5.2 King René, Love, and Desire   95

5.3 Ages of man   99

5.4 Diagram of elements, qualities, seasons, ages, and humors   100

5.5 God of Love shoots lover with arrow of beauty   103

6.1 A lady dying from love   111

6.2 Woman occupied with work and children   115

6.3 Couple embracing   119

6.4 Jan Steen, "The Doctor's Visit"   124

7.1 Practical medicine    128

7.2 Taking the pulse    137

7.3 Jan Steen, "The Doctor's Visit" (1663)    138

7.4 Purgation    140

7.5 Basil    141

7.6 Litigation    143

7.7 Traveler refreshed with wine    144

8.1 *Gravoire* with lovers    148

8.2 A young man lies with his mother    155

8.3 Virgin and Child    156

8.4 Siege of the Castle of Love    161

8.5 A sorceress acts as go-between    163

8.6 Vergil hoisted and Vergil's revenge    165

8.7 Husband beating his wife with a stick    168

8.8 Parade shield with chivalric lover    170

8.9 Pietà Roettgen    172

# ACKNOWLEDGMENTS

It is a pleasure to acknowledge the many people who have aided me during my work on lovesickness. The generosity of the Dean of Graduate Research and the English Department Gift Fund at Stanford University enabled me to enjoy the research help of Carolyn Anderson, Susan Aronstein, and Thomas Moser, Jr. Nearly every section of this book has benefited from Steven Kruger's unfailingly generous attention. I take it as a mark of the subject's interest that so many students volunteered to help with the project, including Dorothea Anagnastopoulos, William Clune, Lenore Kitts, Ian McCarthy, Julie Richardson and Rebecca Sammel.

I would like to thank all my colleagues whose conversations, criticisms, and responses to inquiries have helped me chart my course through some unexplored interdisciplinary waters. If at any point I have run aground, the fault is mine, not theirs. I am particularly grateful to Theodore Andersson, George Brown, Luke Demaitre, Patrick Ford, Hester Gelber, Barbara Gelpi, Arthur Groos, Gundolf Keil, Marsh McCall, Michael McVaugh, Jody Maxmin, Robert Polhemus, David Riggs, Richard Rouse, Susan Treggiari and Linda Voigts for their encouragement in whatever form it took, whether listening to work in progress, commenting on drafts, offering expert opinion in areas outside my own, or providing moral support. Deepest thanks of all go to Monica Green, who generously spent time tracking down and transcribing *Viaticum* manuscripts in Europe for me and who, in her careful readings of various drafts, has served as both Socratic gadfly and Socratic midwife.

This book could not have been completed without support for research and writing from Pew Foundation funds at Stanford, an NEH Summer Stipend, an ACLS grant for recent recipients of the Ph.D., and a stimulating year at the Stanford Humanities Center. The Gift Fund of the English Department has enabled me to include illustrations, and the interlibrary loan division of Green library at Stanford has materially expedited my research. The heroic efforts of Sonia Moss in the summer of 1988 enabled the timely completion of the manuscript.

For permission to quote from unpublished manuscripts I am indebted to the following: The Master and Fellows of Gonville and Caius College, Cambridge; The Dean and Chapter of Durham; Trustees of the British Museum; The Master and Fellows, Trinity College, Cambridge; The Master and Fellows, St. John's College, Cambridge; Leonard E. Boyle, O.P., Prefect, The Vatican Library; Wissenschaftliche Allgemeinbibliothek, Erfurt; Biblioteca Nacional, Madrid; Bayerische Staatsbibliothek, Munich; The Bodleian Library, Oxford; Corpus Christi College, Oxford; Bibliothèque Nationale, Paris; Bibliothèque Municipale, Rouen; Burgerbibliothek, Bern; British Library Board. I am grateful to the University of California Press for permission to publish a revised version of an article that first appeared in *Viator* 17 (1986) as "The Measure of Pleasure: Peter of Spain on Men, Women, and Lovesickness."

My deepest obligation is to Randy Lagier, who patiently bore with my slaving over a hot computer, who provided material and spiritual comfort as needed, and who, in the last long weeks, cheered me toward the finish line.

# INTRODUCTION

Several years ago, as the result of publicity about my research, I received numerous letters and phone calls. Some wrote to say that they suffered from lovesickness and wanted to sign on as research assistants to learn more about their illness. Others described their symptoms so that I could make phone diagnoses of their conditions. One lawyer asked me to testify as an expert witness for the defense in a murder trial ("insanity by reason of lovesickness"). Several said that they had endured obsessive, unrequited love for as long as forty years. Therapists working with "love addiction" thought that my research (in the garbled form in which it was reported) was a historical prologue to their own. My fifteen minutes of media fame made it clear that lovesickness is still a reality for many people in American culture.

The symptoms are familiar. You can't sleep because your mind races with fantasies. During the day you can't concentrate on what you're doing. Food loses its appeal. Maybe you desire "forbidden fruit"—a hopeless fantasy but not any the less compelling. Or perhaps the person you long for is so superior to you in looks, wit, charm, intelligence, and social connections that even hoping for an affair with such a paragon seems absurd. You swing between fits of crying and depression and manic elation. Sometimes just the thought of the person makes your heart pound, or makes you suddenly catch your breath. You're miserable, and yet you almost welcome the misery, because "you have to suffer for true love."

In the Middle Ages, were these symptoms of erotic preoccupation to persist, threatening breakdown from insomnia, weakness, and depression, a knowledgeable observer would have labelled them "lovesickness," or in Chaucer's phrase, "the loveris maladye / Of Hereos."[1] The disease of love, according to medieval physicians, is a disorder of the mind and body, closely related to melancholia and potentially fatal if not treated. In their view, however, lovesickness did not afflict everyone alike: the sufferer was typically thought to be a noble man.

The patient's high status meant that he—or his family—could afford professional medical care from a university-educated doctor, unlike the vast majority of the population who depended on village empirics, if anyone at all, for their medical needs. The university physicians were trained to recognize symptoms of love. By interpreting signs in the patient's body and behavior (for example, by testing his pulse to see if it changed dramatically when the beloved was mentioned) the doctor could diagnose the malady even if the patient were unwilling to reveal its source. He would then prescribe a regimen designed to restore the body's strength and to distract the mind from its obsession. Baths, good food, wine, and sleep insured the return of physical vigor, while therapeutic intercourse, business affairs, legal difficulties, real or concocted, and various types of sports and games, like riding or chess, distracted the mind from its fantasies. If left untreated, however, the disease of love could degenerate into melancholia, thought to be even more difficult to cure than lovesickness.

There is no simple way to correlate the medieval understanding of lovesickness with contemporary views of love and its disorders. Now that love has become an acceptable topic of research in behavioral and social sciences, the classifications of love and its disorders have proliferated bewilderingly as researchers attempt ever finer discriminations among them. At the moment there is no common conceptual vocabulary for talking about the range of behaviors, feelings, and attitudes called "love." Where one sees sickness, another sees romance. Medieval lovesickness shares features with depression (appetite loss, insomnia, dysphoria, inability to concentrate), with "limerance," a modern form of lovesickness (cardiorespiratory symptoms), with "melancholia," "addictive love," "infatuation," "romantic love," "empty love," and "eros."[2]

While I am not suggesting that medieval lovesickness is the precursor of any particular modern concept, the texts in this volume do contain suggestive historical antecedents for a number of problems central to current inquiries into love. For example, biomedical research has suggested that unusual levels of neurotransmitters may be involved in the uncontrollable emotional highs and lows in the initial stages of romantic love.[3] Medieval physicians would have agreed in principle, since, in the tradition of Galenic medicine, they believed that an imbalance of material substances in the body (humors) led to lovesickness. And though they debated whether the disease afflicted the brain, the heart, or the generative organs, they usually concluded that the malady was located in the brain.

Medieval physicians' interest in the processes of sexual desire as they affect lovesickness anticipates a recent call not only for research "that connects the psychophysiology of sexual arousal to the psychology of love" but also for greater "attention to the environmental and demographic context within which love unfolds."[4] As I have already noted, the lover's malady was generally considered a class-specific ailment in the Middle Ages. This social restriction implies that the doctors recognized the influence of social context on the origin and course of the disease. The manifestations of lovesickness, including idealization of the love object, preoccupation, depression, insomnia, erratic moods, and social withdrawal, are meaningful *as symptoms of illness* only within a system of shared beliefs and symbolic conventions. Even bodily symptoms bear social meanings.[5] As a team of medical anthropologists explains: "Everywhere and in all periods it is the individual who is sick, but he is sick in the eyes of his society, in relation to it, and in keeping with the modalities fixed by it. The language of the sick thus takes shape within the language expressing the relations beween the individual and society."[6]

Between the fifth and fifteenth centuries society changed dramatically, the relations of individuals to society altered, and the store of medical texts describing the disordered relation of a lover to his social surroundings expanded significantly. These developments support the theory that diseases like lovesickness are culturally constructed, and raise questions that have not yet been fully answered. Why was there an apparent upsurge in European interest in the disease of love in the twelfth century? How does lovesickness differ from and interact with "courtly love"?[7] Given the differences between the lover's malady and "courtly love," how did symptoms of illness become culturally valued signs of romantic love? Despite their differences, do they have a common psychological origin or common social context? Drawing upon the evidence that the physicians provide, this book offers detailed answers to these questions.

To understand the significance of Constantine the African's chapter on lovesickness in the *Viaticum*, we must consider the state of medical learning in Europe in the early Middle Ages. After the disintegration of the Roman Empire, which entailed the loss of Greek and Latin medical works and the decline of learned medicine as a secular discipline, the medical tradition of lovesickness largely disappeared from European culture. It was not until a North African named Constantine (d. ca. 1087) brought a cargo of Arabic medical texts to southern Italy in the late eleventh century that the disease of love became an important part of medieval culture. The chapter on lovesickness from one of Constantine's translations known as the *Viaticum* (originally a handbook for travellers without access to medical care) was the most widely-read text on the subject until a translation of the *Canon medicinae* of the Arabic physician Avicenna entered medical curricula in the late thirteenth century. Constantine's chapter on love thus achieved currency at the same time that the conventions of idealized, "courtly" love took shape in vernacular literature. When medicine, together with law and theology, became one of the three higher faculties of the medieval university around 1200, the *Viaticum* became an authoritative text in medical curricula. It bequeathed a conceptual framework for lovesickness that held firm for four centuries, and as a result it gradually acquired a body of expository commentaries that grew out of academic physicians' lectures on the text. The *Viaticum* commentaries are the earliest corpus of European medical writing that attempts to integrate a view of erotic love that is Greek and Arabic in origin into medieval Christian culture. These manuscripts are thus a prime source for tracing the reciprocal influences of medicine and culture on medieval views of passionate love.

Medieval documents on lovesickness have, with few exceptions, remained disappointingly inaccessible, either buried in manuscripts difficult to decipher, or locked away in rare and inadequate Renaissance printings. Because the medieval medical tradition of lovesickness is of major importance for the development of love conventions, and ultimately for the ideology of romantic love, the primary sources deserve to be better known. When it is argued that "a culture's sexual discourse plays a critical role in the shaping of identity," or indeed that medieval medical discourse on sexuality enabled the West to develop an *ars erotica*, readers will need the original documents at hand.[8] This volume makes available to modern readers for the first time editions and translations of the chapter on love in the *Viaticum* and of the commentaries on it by Gerard of Berry, Egidius, Peter of Spain, and Bona Fortuna.

In addressing the problem of reconstructing alien cultures, the anthropologist Clifford Geertz has compared ethnography with reading a manuscript: "Doing ethnography is like trying to read (in the sense of 'construct a reading of') a manuscript—foreign, faded, full of ellipses, incoherencies, suspicious emendations, and tendentious commentaries, but written not in conventionalized graphs of sound but in transient examples of shaped behavior."[9] Reversing the comparison, one could say that constructing a reading of these manuscript chapters on love means doing ethnography—seeing through the "conventionalized graphs of sound" to the shaped behavior they encode. The task is not a simple one. The manuscripts are, in fact, plagued by fading, ellipses, and incoherencies. Their discussions of lovesickness are couched in the scholastic jargon of the medieval universities and rest on the foundations of Galenic humoral medicine, a system whose terminology is now largely forgotten. The difficulty of the texts calls for explicit and extensive interpretation.

The first part of this volume, which seeks to reconstruct both the forms and the meanings of the lover's malady in the Middle Ages, consists of eight chapters. The middle chapters, which treat the medical texts individually, are framed chronologically and thematically by the first chapter, on notions of lovesickness that predate the arrival of Constantine and Arabic medicine, and by the last chapter, on the social and psychological context of the lover's malady in the later Middle Ages. These two chapters offer "before" and "after" pictures, so to speak, by which the influence of the medical idea of love on medieval culture may be gauged. What appears in the first chapter as a history of ideas and texts becomes in the last a social and psychological interpretation of the lover's malady as a form of behavior in late medieval culture. What we can only document as a literary fantasy of love in the early twelfth century becomes a well-attested social reality by the fourteenth. The last chapter draws together the testimony of medical, literary, artistic, and religious sources to show how the medical notion of lovesickness influenced the transformation of "courtly love" from literary convention to social practice.

The middle chapters of the first part analyze, in chronological order, the sections on love in the *Viaticum* (chapter 2) and in the commentaries written by Gerard of Berry, Egidius, Peter of Spain, and Bona Fortuna (chapters three through seven).[10] The commentaries embody the lectures of medical professors who, like their modern counterparts, were pressed by exigencies of time and space.[11] The continuity of attention to lovesickness—it might, after all, simply have been skipped in the lectures—suggests that its study was impelled by intellectual and social needs that can be reconstructed.

The commentaries span the thirteenth century, a period that also saw the expansion and transformation of courtly literature, the influx of Aristotelian texts, and the rise of the universities. In the ways the commentators filled what they perceived as gaps in Constantine's account of morbid erotic love, or debated what seemed problematic, we find specific indices of cultural concerns. Moreover, because medicine was a separate faculty of the medieval university, with its own disciplinary traditions and professional and practical concerns, the medical texts on love embody a distinctive vision of their subject. They are theoretical yet also pragmatic; tinged with material determinism; and in their recommendation of therapeutic intercourse, at variance with official Church morality. At the same time, by virtue of their institutional setting and their authors' "cultural literacy," the medical texts are also permeated by clerical assumptions, not all of them consciously articulated, about love and women. These are texts in which multiple voices can be heard, not all of them in harmony.[12]

In offering my own commentary on the medical texts, I take several lines of approach. When I focus on the letter of the text, I turn first for clarification to medieval medicine and to scholastic natural philosophy. Other types of discourse (literary, theological) are brought to bear as needed. But since some of the most interesting questions about medieval lovesickness cannot be answered within the framework of medieval science, I have also drawn upon semiotics, anthropology, feminist theory and psychoanalysis to develop the social and psychological implications of medical discourse.

The second part of this volume offers working editions and translations of the *Viaticum's* chapter on love and of its four commentaries.

This book also makes available a rich body of visual material that can help us to understand the lover's malady in its cultural setting. Some of these materials, such as diagrams of the inner wits, the doctrine of the humors, and materia medica, convey complicated information quickly and schematically. Therapies for lovesickness aimed to restore the normal rhythms of daily life through diet, exercise, restoration of mental tranquillity, and reintegration into the social group. Such regimens are illustrated in the health handbooks known as *Tacuinum sanitatis*.[13] Since nearly all the cures for lovesickness are depicted in these handbooks for preserving health, the pictures suggest the kinds of situations patients and readers would have associated with the physicians' therapeutic recommendations. They also suggest how familiar the medical doctrines were, how un-exotic and unspecialized. At the same time, the illustrations serve as a bridge between medicine and literature. The depiction of men and women strolling in gardens in the health handbooks, for example, parallels illustrations of literary gardens modeled on the garden of Love in the *Romance of the Rose*. Other illustrations, taken from literary and biblical texts, show how visual representations reinforce the written texts concerning lovesickness. Medieval depictions of Amnon and Thamar, the Bride of Canticles, and Antiochus and Stratonice indicate that languishing lovers were fully imaginable to both artist and audience; such figures provided a frame of reference for the widespread assimilation of university-based teaching on lovesickness.

# PART ONE

§§§§§§

# *Lovesickness in the Middle Ages*

# PATHOLOGY AND PASSION
## Lovesickness in Antiquity and the Early Middle Ages

Passionate love . . . [is] a fragile crest where death and regeneration vie for dominance.

Julia Kristeva[1]

As antiquity gave way to the Middle Ages, an unknown poet in fifth-century Vandal Africa told the story of a young man named Perdica. Sent to study in Athens as a boy, Perdica made offerings to all the gods except Venus and Cupid when, years later, he set out for home. The journey was exhausting, and he and his companions turned off the road into a shady grove cooled by a stream to rest during the midday heat. After they had eaten, Perdica fell asleep. Piqued, the neglected Cupid pierced "the youth's breast with a savage dart." With that an image appeared to Perdica in a dream; he fell in love with it. The next day, as he crossed the threshold of home, he saw in the figure who greeted him the woman of his dreams—his mother.

Perdica spent that night tormented by incestuous desire. Unable to sleep, fearful, racked with sighs, he begged Love for peace. Should he reveal his love to his mother? Oedipus at least had entered his mother's bed unknowingly. By daybreak his limbs were weakened, and he refused food. His worried mother called in the city's physicians, but they could find nothing. The oldest and most experienced of them, Hippocrates, was also puzzled by the symptoms. Yet he too found no physical cause for Perdica's malady. But as he took the youth's pulse, his mother entered the room. His pulse, which had been slow and regular, suddenly raced; Hippocrates had discovered Perdica's secret. "The cause is near, mother; the gifts of medicine reach an end. Here there is suffering of the mind; I am useless. May the gods grant the rest." With that Hippocrates relinquished the case.

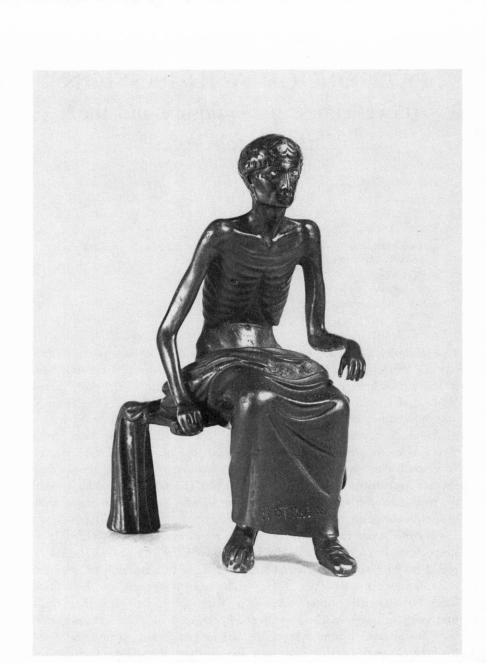

*Figure 1.1.* Bronze statuette of an emaciated man (Roman, 1st c. C.E.). "Perdik" is inscribed on the bottom of the robe, between the legs. The left wrist is held up for the physician to check the pulse. Byzantine Visual Resources, © 1988, Dumbarton Oaks, Washington, D.C. (47.22).

The mother's attempts to comfort her son were in vain; torn by love and shame, he sickened even further. Pallor suffused his body. His emaciation progressed so far that his eyes were hollow, his nose stood out sharply, his wasted arms revealed their tendons, and his ribs protruded (Figure 1.1). Searching for a quicker way to die than this slow wasting, he resolved on death by hanging.

The miniature epic entitled *Perdica's Malady* (*Aegritudo Perdicae*) at once chronicles the youth's fatal passion for his mother and epitomizes a number of themes implicit in the lover's malady in the European Middle Ages.[2] At the root of lovesickness lies an unfulfilled, sometimes unspeakable desire that may be incestuous or otherwise socially unacceptable. Yet the mind and body are such close partners that bodily symptoms reveal what the patient represses. Sighing, sleeplessness, and wasting from refusal to eat betray the mind's effort to master its overwhelming passion. The clever physician can interpret these signs and penetrate to the cause of the malady. Medicine, however, treats the body, a commixture of elements. Its remedies cannot transgress so far against social norms as to prescribe incestuous love.

Ancient literature and medicine agreed in their descriptions, if not their evaluations, of eros experienced as illness.[3] Like other aspects of classical culture, the concept of an erotic malady passed into the European Middle Ages, but it did so by a double route. A few Greek medical works survived the cultural breakup of the Roman empire to be translated into Latin, read, and recopied in Europe between the sixth and eleventh centuries. Though these texts were carefully preserved by the efforts of monastic scribes, they did not generate further medical discussion in the West on the lover's malady. In contrast, a greater number of Greek medical works was translated into Arabic and stimulated extensive discussion of the disease of love in Arabic medicine. When the eleventh-century African merchant Constantine shipped a cargo of Arabic medical works to Italy, he brought with him a richer stock of medical ideas about love than were hitherto available. The first part of this chapter surveys ancient and Byzantine discussions of lovesickness that were available in the West before Constantine's arrival in order to show that the *Viaticum's* teaching on lovesickness represented a new, fuller way of conceptualizing the lover's malady and of interpreting and controlling erotic behavior.[4]

Medical views of love were not the only source, however, of the European understanding of lovesickness. Ideas about passionate love from the Bible and Biblical commentary, and from classical and vernacular literature formed a "horizon of expectations" for Constantine's first readers. The following sections of the chapter trace the representations of lovesickness through these sources in order to account for the eager reception given to the *Viaticum's* chapter on love. The Biblical notion of "love languor" and stories that recounted episodes of lovesickness, such as those of Amnon and Thamar, and Antiochus and Stratonice, helped prepare the way for the medical doctrines of passionate love reintroduced in the eleventh and twelfth centuries.

Although some of the texts discussed below have been studied by specialists in the history of lovesickness, to my knowledge no one has yet examined the ensemble to explain why Christian Europe was able to incorporate Greco-Roman and Arabic doctrines on the lover's malady and its cures into high medieval culture. Nor have these sources been fully explored for what they can tell us about the social and interpersonal relationships underlying pathological love, about the lived experience behind the doctors' dispassionate prose.[5]

## Medical Texts of Antiquity

Despite the encomiums to Eros in Plato's *Symposium*, the Greeks and Romans mistrusted passionate love. Cultural ideals of rationality and self-control were threatened by erotic love, which overthrew reasonable governance of the body and the mind and challenged the basic structures of society. The poetry of Sappho and Ovid describes love's physical and psychological disruptions, while the tragic stories of Medea, Hippolytus, and Phaedra dramatize the threat love poses to social order. "When desire is doubled it becomes love; when love is doubled it turns into madness." The Greek saying characterizes love intensified beyond proper measure as a form of madness.[6] It was the madness of love that drove Sappho to leap to her death, and love that robbed Lucretius of reason—so, at least, went the legends.

Ancient medicine, however, offers little systematic discussion of love, and what there is comes relatively late.[7] Not until the fourth century of the common era does love appear as a separate classification of mental disease. Before then it is associated with mania, melancholy, phrenesis (frenzy), and other mental illnesses. Nonetheless, the ancient tradition is important for the lover's malady in the Middle Ages for several reasons. In Arabic and European medical works from the eleventh century onwards, lovesickness remained associated with melancholy and mania, either as a subtype of the former, or as a precursor to both conditions. Chaucer's Arcite, for example, fares in his changeable moods "Nat oonly lik the loveris maladye / Of hereos, but rather lyk manye, / Engendred of humour malencolik."[8] In addition, the symptoms and therapies for lovesickness were largely drawn from ancient recommendations for mania and melancholy.

Moreover, mania and melancholy were the center of an ancient problematic that we have seen in *Perdica's Malady* and that resurfaced in the Christian Middle Ages. Mania and melancholy pose fundamental questions about the relations of soul and body and about the domains of medicine and ethics. These maladies, which affect body and soul alike, were the foci for medical and philosophical discussion of "diseases of the soul." Can there be, properly speaking, any such thing, or are diseases only of the body? What is the role of moral suasion or logotherapy, the ancient counterpart to Freud's "talking cure," in curing a patient of the fixed ideas or of the "profound anger" of melancholy? What is the patient's responsibility for disorders of his soul? What can the physician treat, and what must he cede to the moral philosopher?

Ancient writers gave a variety of answers to these questions, as can be seen in the detailed recent studies of J. Pigeaud.[9] His conclusion, that ancient medicine and philosophy defined their respective domains of competence in dynamic interchange with one another, foreshadows medieval developments. The disease of love, which afflicts both the body and the spirit of a patient caught in a matrix of social and ethical relationships, lay in a cultural zone intersected by the discourses of medicine, literature, natural philosophy, mysticism, pastoral theology, and didactic literature. When Christian Europe began to study the Aristotelianized science of Islam first introduced through Constantine's medical translations, the boundaries of medicine, philosophy, and now moral theology had to be redrawn.[10] In this site of contestation priest and physician vied for professional territory, and that struggle left its mark on medieval attitudes toward the lover's malady.

Lovesickness first becomes a significant part of medical tradition in the writings of Galen (ca. 130–200).[11] His detailed accounts of his medical practice in Rome document cases in which he detected love through its symptoms and cured those suffering from this "passion of the soul." These descriptions were later codified by Byzantine and Arabic medical writers before being reintroduced to Italy in the eleventh century by Constantine the African. Moreover, Galen's lengthy report of the lovesickness of Justus' wife gives us the earliest medical account of woman's psychological and somatic responses to love.

Galen's references to love (he has no specialized term for morbid love) suggest that its diagnosis and treatment were controversial in the medical community of his time. In a commentary on Hippocrates' *Prognostics*, which was translated into Latin by Constantine the African from an Arabic version, Galen disputes the notion held by some that love is a divine illness.[12] Rather, he argues, those who grow sick or pale, who are sleepless or fevered from love, are stricken with the human emotion of sorrow and not by anything divine. His clear distinction between medical and theological views of lovesickness characterizes the medical tradition as a whole. That does not mean, however, that the Platonic inclination to view love born of the sight of beauty as a divine madness ceased to influence the development of medical tradition, or failed to shape Islamic and Christian understandings of passionate love. As we shall see, the somatic perspective of medieval physicians and the transcendent view of the theologians engaged each other in varying ways throughout the high and late Middle Ages.

Galen's appraisal of lovesickness steers a middle course between the transcendent view of love as a divine illness held by his rivals and a crudely somatic understanding of the malady. A commentary on Hippocrates' *Epidemics* gives him the opportunity to describe his treatment of the lovesick in detail, and is worth summarizing at some length:

> I know men and women who burned in hot love. Depression and lack of sleep overcame them. Then, one day, as a result of their love-sorrows they became fevered. The physicians who were treating them sought to heal their bodies by forbidding them to bathe, by ordering rest and a good regimen. But as we took over their treatment and recognized that their suffering consisted of love-sorrow, then we applied ourselves to their cure without revealing to them, much less to others, what we had discovered. We ordered them to take frequent baths, to drink wine, to ride, and to see and hear everything pleasurable. Thus we directed their thoughts toward these things. . . . For if continual love-sorrow oppresses someone, his condition then assumes forms that are difficult to cure. For many it is also good to stimulate anger over an injustice, or to rouse love of competing and of achieving victory over another, according to the inclination of each for a particular sport. . . . One must call forth excitement, wake joy in competition, and counter the desire to quarrel and fight with others by saying to them that these diversions will comfort and heal them. They should imagine that the hounds and the hunt or the horses or the wrestling boys or the quails or the cocks or other things that interest them and that they love are their own. Preoccupation with such things is best for them. After I had explored the conditions of many mentally ill people ("seelisch Kranken") and healed them of their illnesses, so that they were completely healthy again, my friends requested me to write a book containing the prognoses I had learned to recognize in these patients.[13]

This account makes it clear that Galen classified love not as an affliction of the body, as did his unsuccessful rivals, but as a passion of the soul. It should be noted, however, that in Galenic medicine the operations of the soul are a function of the body's humoral composition, so that his view of love is ultimately somatic.[14] But even though he codified Hippocratic humoral theory into a form that provided the basic framework for Byzantine, Arabic, and medieval European medicine, Galen does not specify the humoral basis of lovesickness; that would be a medieval contribution to the disease.

In addition to denying that love is a divine illness or an affliction of the body, Galen also rejects the existence of a characteristic "lover's pulse." In a story in the *Prognostics*, he recounts in circumstantial detail how he, like the physician Erasistratos, diagnosed a case of morbid love.[15] The wife of Justus (who may have been a senator or a wealthy Roman or Pergamene) suffered from insomnia without fever, and refused to answer the physician's questions. Galen decided that she was suffering either from a melancholic depression or from a secret worry. Further inquiry revealed that there was no bodily illness, and that her trouble was psychological. By means of the pulse test—noting under what circumstances her pulse became disturbed and irregular—Galen was able to detect her secret passion for the dancer Pylades. Unfortunately, Galen omits to tell what cure he prescribed.

This story has been termed "a great first in the history of medicine" because a *woman* suffers from the sickness of love.[16] It is even more noteworthy because surviving sources indicate that it was a thousand years before the medical community again pursued the question of women's lovesickness. No literary persona such as Phaedra or Medea, she is a female patient who requires Galen's diagnostic skill as much as any man in the grip of lovesickness. Gourevitch suggests that a woman figures in Galen's story because the gradual emancipation of women in Rome granted them a new erotic equality: they could take the initiative in love. Although the appearance in history of woman as a loving subject is significant, Galen's story points less to her emancipation than to its precariousness. Though Galen gives no explicit etiology, the narrative itself, in its emphasis on the woman's embarrassment and secrecy, implies that a socially problematic relationship is involved. In fact, it is doubly problematic because it involves both the threat of female adultery and the crossing of very strong class barriers, especially if her husband was of senatorial rank.[17] A liaison between a freeborn woman and a dancer/pantomime, who was probably either a freedman or a slave, was liable to legal penalties and was in any case disreputable. The lovesickness of Justus' wife signifies that her erotic emancipation had not gone so far that she could express her desire, which threatened domestic and social order, without encoding it in somatic illness. Her "liberty" to suffer from love expresses itself in the repressive form of illness.

For Galen, then, love is not a distinct disease, but one of a number of psychological conditions that can powerfully affect the body. As shown by the pulse story, embedded in a work on prognostics, his interest in love is primarily semeiological and diagnostic. Love is a practical, not a theoretical problem. Indeed, his reports of curing patients of the lover's malady underscore that it *was* a problem that called for medical intervention.

Though physicians in the following centuries organized their remarks on love under a separate heading, implying its status as a distinct disease, they offered no real advances over Galen. Oribasius' chapter on love, together with those of Caelius Aurelianus and Paul of Aegina, may be taken as examples of the most sophisticated teaching on the disease of love available in Europe when Constantine arrived. Oribasius (326–403), physician to Julian the Apostate, devotes a chapter to lovers in his medical compilation, the *Synopsis* (or *Conspectus ad Eustathum*), but like Galen he offers no specific etiology.[18] In the eighth book, on diseases of the nervous system, he catalogues symptoms and cures that were to become standard items in Islamic and European medical treatises for those "who are consumed by love." The physician may recognize such patients because they are sorrowful and suffer from insomnia. Their eyes are hollow and they do not weep; they are like those who are filled with toil.[19] Their eyelids move more frequently than any other part of the body.

Oribasius protests, as Galen did, against those physicians who fail to recognize the nature of the malady, and who forbid the patients to take therapeutic baths or who restrict their diets. Rather, the physician should prescribe just the opposite: baths, wine, listening to amusing stories or speeches, and striving against adversaries all have their use in curing lovers. Although Oribasius, drawing upon the work of Rufus of Ephesus (b. after 50 C.E.), the greatest physician of the late Empire next to Galen, recommends therapeutic intercourse for melancholy, he fails to mention it in his chapter on lovers. As we shall see, however, once this cure entered discourse on morbid love, it became controversial and served as a test case for competing professional and cultural values.

The *Synopsis* proved influential in both western and eastern medical traditions. In the West, our concern here, it was translated into Latin twice around the sixth century, and is preserved in a dozen or so early manuscripts and fragments.[20] Given that some of the surviving manuscripts are in a script used at Montecassino and surrounding areas in the eleventh century, perhaps the incomparable library under Desiderius (abbot 1058–87) contained an Oribasius manuscript that Constantine might have consulted.[21]

In order to understand European developments of lovesickness after Oribasius, we must briefly trace its course in the East. As we have seen, there was no consensus in ancient medicine on love's nature or status as a disease; Galen and Oribasius speak of lovers, not of a disease called "love." Galen's works indicate that the medical community considered illness-producing love to be related to both mania (the "divine madness" of Plato) and melancholy. When Arabic physicians translated and synthesized ancient and Byzantine medicine, they reorganized the discussions of love. Lovesickness became a separate diagnostic category with symptoms drawn from mania and melancholy, as well as from Oribasius' and Paul of Aegina's chapters on lovers. Therapeutic intercourse, which Rufus of Ephesus had advocated for melancholy, became a prominent cure for love. We find in al-Rāzī (b. 865), for example, that "the cure for love is frequent coitus."[22] The earliest of the better known medical works to complete this synthesis of symptoms and therapies was the *Zad al-musāfir* of ibn al-Jazzār, which served as the source for Constantine's *Viaticum*.[23]

This integration did not occur in the West. In contrast, a major work available to the early Middle Ages differed significantly both from Galen's views on love and from the Arabic synthesis introduced by Constantine. *On Acute and Chronic Diseases*, a translation of Soranus' (2nd c. C.E.) lost treatise by Caelius Aurelianus (5th c. C.E.), was recommended by Cassiodorus (ca. 490–ca. 583) as basic medical reading.[24] Caelius Aurelianus' departure from the classical and Arabic tradition on the question of therapeutic intercourse underscores the significance of Christian Europe's later acceptance of the cure. His discussion of melancholy, however, elucidates in part the psychological dynamics underlying lovesickness.

In the section of his compendium on chronic diseases Caelius Aurelianus quotes Plato on the types of mania, among which is one called *eroticon*. Mania may result from, among other things, love (*amor nimia*) or the drinking of love philters (potions intended to make the drinker fall in love), and is most frequent in young and middle-aged men. The symptoms of mania include many of those that reappear in Byzantine and Islamic accounts of lovesickness: unhappiness, mental anxiety, tossing in sleep, frequent blinking of the eyes, and disturbances of the pulse. "When mania lays hold of the mind, it manifests itself now in anger, now in merriment, now in sadness or futility, and now, as some relate, in an overpowering fear of things which are quite harmless" (539).

Although Caelius Aurelianus' symptoms for mania correspond to the later discussions of the signs of lovesickness, his therapies are much at variance with what later came to be the standard remedies for love. He rejects purgatives because they injure the body, and dismisses drunkenness, music, and love, on the grounds that they all increase madness rather than allay it. Though his rejection of therapeutic intercourse is based on medical rather than moral grounds, it foreshadows the split between medieval physicians and priests on this issue.[25]

> Some physicians hold that love is a proper remedy for insanity, on the grounds that it frees the patient's mind from the agitation caused by madness and thus purifies it. They are not aware of the obvious truth that in many cases love is the very cause of madness. . . . Nor should we disdain the view of those who have actually called love a form of insanity because

of the similarity of the symptoms which the victims show. And surely it is absurd and wrong to recommend, of all remedies for the disease, the very thing that you are trying to treat; not to mention the fact that it is impossible to get an insane person to fall in love, for, since he is bereft of reason, he cannot properly appreciate beauty. . . . Moreover, even if the patient falls in love, there is considerable doubt as to which course is preferable, to forbid coitus or to permit it. When the patient sees the object of his desire, he will become even madder if venery is forbidden him. On the other hand, if permitted, it will harm him; for it not only deprives the body of strength but also agitates the soul (557–59).

In Caelius Aurelianus' Platonic formulation, an insane person cannot fall in love because he cannot form a rational appreciation of beauty. In the *Viaticum* and other medieval medical texts on love, in contrast, it is precisely the sight of beauty that drives the soul mad and plunges it into lovesickness. And since the divine is absolute beauty, this cause was a meeting ground for medical and theological views of passionate or ecstatic love. On the other hand, Caelius' rejection of therapeutic coitus, evidence of the ascetic strain in late antique culture that early medieval Christianity nurtured into hypertrophic forms, prefigures the later ecclesiastical condemnations of the cure.[26]

Although Caelius Aurelianus rejects one of the most famous cures for mania and melancholy, his discussion of the latter disease is important for its observations of melancholics' behavior. He notes that "Cicero speaks of black bile in the sense of profound anger; and when Hercules is stirred to mighty wrath, Virgil says 'and thereupon the wrath of Hercules burned furiously with black bile'; for those suffering from melancholy seem always to be downcast and prone to anger and are practically never cheerful and relaxed" (561).[27] In focusing on the symptomatic complex of black bile/melancholy and wrath, Caelius Aurelianus touches upon a contemporary natural philosophical problem of importance for the interpretation of lovesickness.

The pseudo-Aristotelian *Problem* 30, part of a series of medical and natural philosophical questions assembled in Alexandria between the fourth and seventh centuries, explains that melancholic men, who may, despite the debilitating effects of the humor, attain great accomplishments ("melancholic genius"), are nonetheless "easily moved to anger and desire."[28] The medieval scholar David of Dinant copied a Latin summary of *Problem* 30 into his notebooks (*Quaternuli*) sometime before 1210, when they were condemned by the Bishop of Paris as containing heretical matter. He explains that black bile, *colera nigra*, is "smoky," *fumosa*, and its effects are similar to those of wine. And just as wine stimulates lechery (*luxuria*), so many *melan-*

*cholici* are *luxuriosi* because lechery arises from "fumosity" or smokiness. Those who are endowed from birth with a great quantity of hot black bile become mad (*maniaci*), intellectually outstanding (*boni ingenii ad discendum*), amorous, and quickly moved to anger or other emotions (*anime affectus*).[29] In *Problem* 30, then, we have the same complex of symptoms as in Caelius Aurelianus, with this difference, that in the pseudo-Aristotelian problem they are given a humoral origin. The trio of depression, love, and anger evident in these two works emerges so often in descriptions of melancholy and lovesickness (in both medical and literary sources) that it will become a central issue in my interpretation of the disease's social context.

The fate of Caelius Aurelianus' treatise is emblematic of the general fragmentation of late antique culture as it passed into the early Middle Ages. Despite Cassiodorus' endorsement, the parts on acute and chronic disease were separated and epitomized, and were probably scarce at all times.[30] The section on acute diseases circulated under the title *Aurelius* and that on chronic diseases, where mania is listed, under the title *Esculapius*.[31] Much of the theoretical discussion was excised, leaving mainly practical information. The sections on love in the mania chapter appear not to have survived this reorganization.

Thus we can explain the silence of the seventh-century encyclopedist Isidore of Seville on the topic of the lover's malady in his fourth book, on medicine. Though he drew from Caelius Aurelianus for many of his etymologies, he did so by way of the *Esculapius*, which seems not to have contained any statements about love.[32] Nonetheless, in another part of the *Etymologies*, the most influential encyclopedia of learning until it was superseded in the thirteenth century, Isidore says that "love beyond all measure among the ancients was called womanly love" (*femineus amor*; XI.2.24).[33] This comment, coupled with the silence on love in the medical chapter, well illustrates the complex inheritance of medieval views of passionate love; ancient ideas on eros were transmitted through encyclopedias and literary and philosophical works, as well as through medical texts on love. Even more important, Isidore's remark underscores the puzzling paradox, to which I return in the last chapter, of medicine's silence about women's lovesickness. For passionate love to be "womanly love" meant that ancient and medieval culture saw excessive love as characteristic of women, yet women are with few exceptions absent from medical accounts of love. "Womanly love" befell men, who were the subjects of medical discourse. Nevertheless, though women by and large remained outside medical discussions of lovesickness, the notion of "womanly love" held by the masculine world of learning (clerical culture in its broadest sense) significantly influenced the lover's malady in the later Middle Ages.

While Isidore composed the most widely-read encyclopedia of the early Middle Ages in Visigothic Spain, in Alexandria a younger contemporary, Paul of Aegina (fl. ca. 640), compiled an epitome of Greek medicine for physicians who would not read the prolix ancient writers like Galen. Translated into Latin in the tenth century (one manuscript in Beneventan script, now at Montecassino, dates from the late eleventh century) Paul gives the fullest and most systematic account of love among those works available to the West before Constantine's arrival.[34] The Latin translation begins: "There is nothing inconsistent in adding *cupidines* to the diseases (*passionibus*) of the brain, since they are certain cares," which are then defined as a passion of the soul (*passio anime*). The symptoms and therapies follow Oribasius and Galen. For all its relative fullness, however, Paul's chapter on lovers seems meager compared to the Arabic discussions translated in the eleventh and twelfth centuries. He offers no humoral causality; his interest centers instead on semeiology and therapy.

Before Constantine began to translate, then, Europeans had access to only a few medical treatises that discussed the disease of love. If the medical works surveyed above are theoretically unsophisticated in their exposition of love compared to later works, they do tell us one important thing about lovesickness in antiquity and the early Middle Ages, namely, that it was seen as a practical problem requiring diagnosis and therapy, but not necessarily elaborate theoretical explanation. Nonetheless, it is doubtful that the medical view of the lover's malady was a commonplace even in the circles of monastic culture with the best access to ancient texts. Indeed, the corpus of pre-Salernitan medicine shows a strikingly reduced coverage of mental illnesses compared to earlier and later periods. When the care of the soul passed into the hands of the clergy, mental disturbances became a less important part of secular medicine than they had in antiquity.

## Lovesickness in Classical Literature

If Galen omitted to record his remedies for Justus' wife, Ovid, in contrast, offered a panoply of cures for love. In the Middle Ages his poetry was read and memorized in grammar schools and quoted from Provence to Iceland. Alexander Neckham (d. 1217), for example, enjoined scholars who aspired to liberal education to be especially familiar with Ovid's "little book on the remedy for love."[35] (Though Sappho, who was considered the pre-eminent diagnostician of the symptoms of morbid love in the ancient world, "takes from the attendant circumstances of life and from truth itself the emotional experiences which accompany erotically passionate madness," according to Longinus, her poetry was unknown in the Middle Ages.)[36]

The *magister amoris* Ovid taught that sickness could be an artful strategy in the game of love, and that unwanted love could be cured by his remedies. The twelfth-century resurgence of interest in his poetry—an *aetas Ovidiana*—meant that the medical views of love just beginning to circulate in the translations of Constantine and Gerard of Cremona (d. 1187) could draw upon his poetic authority for acceptance. In fact, readers of Constantine's chapter on lovesickness sometimes jotted down lines from Ovid in the margins of their manuscripts. One such early thirteenth-century reader noted: "Ovid gives the cure for this sort of disease in the *Remedies for Love* when he says: 'Sunt fora sunt leges quod tuearis amore' " (a misremembered quotation of line 151: "There are courts, there are laws, there are friends for you to protect").[37] The mutual reinforcement of the Roman doctor of love and the medieval physicians continued into the thirteenth century when the *Viaticum* commentators Egidius and Peter of Spain (d. 1277 as Pope John XXI) quoted Ovid in their analyses of lovesickness.[38]

In a reciprocal development, the early thirteenth-century Old French translator of Ovid's *Art of Love* (*Ars amatoria*) glossed his ancient author in light of contemporary behavior of the lovesick. He justifies the utility of his work for young lovers who out of despair "hang themselves . . . kill themselves by the sword, or by fire or by water" or who "go mad" because of love. "No one can know the sickness of love as well as the one who has tried it."[39] In his view, Ovid offers a how-to manual for those who want to play the game of love—and win. Moreover, the translator's naturalism is a match for that of contemporary physicians who were recommending therapeutic intercourse despite its prohibition by the Church: "He wants to prove that it is not a sin for a man and a woman to go to bed with each other, for it is a natural thing, and nature bestows it, nor is it an artificial thing."[40] Ovid's erotic poetry thus proved a locus for interchange between medical and literary views of love, and its authority no doubt contributed to the swift acceptance of the Arabic medical tradition.

Ovid's poetry bequeathed a grab-bag of symptoms, strategies, and cures to medieval readers; ancient narratives, in contrast, depicted something closer to case histories of lovesickness. Of the narrative depictions of languishing lovers inherited by the Middle Ages, the story of Antiochus and Stratonice, recounted by Valerius Maximus (fl. early 1st c. C.E.), Plutarch (d. ca. 126 C.E.) and others, enjoyed great popularity down to modern times.[41] If we see in the youth's passion for his stepmother a desire for a maternal figure, the story becomes, in effect, an Oedipal comedy, the counterpart to the tragic outcome of *Perdica's Malady*. The story's main lines run as follows. Antiochus, son of king Seleucis, is "seized by infinite love" for his stepmother Stratonice. Because he refuses to reveal his passion, he falls

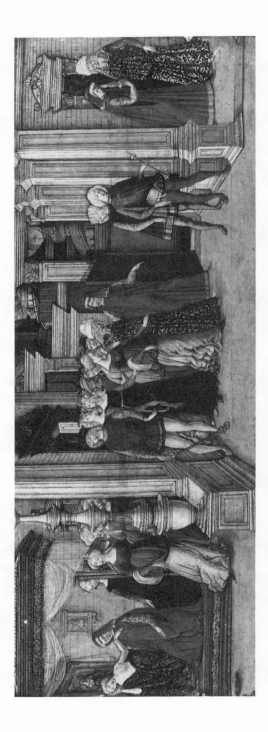

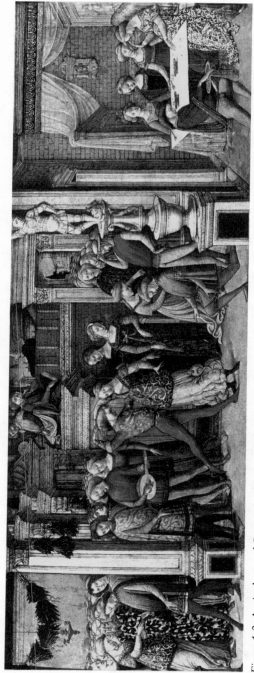

*Figure 1.2.* Antiochus and Stratonice. Two panels narrating Antiochus' lovesickness and cure, by a fifteenth-century Sienese painter known as the Master of the Stratonice Panels. Henry E. Huntington Library and Art Gallery, San Marino, California.

deathly ill. One day as the physician Erasistratus sits by the patient, Stratonice enters. The doctor notices how Antiochus blushes, how his breathing quickens, and how his pulse races. When she leaves, he pales, his breathing and pulse slow. In Figure 1.2 the pulse test is depicted at the far left of the first panel. On the right side of the same panel, just as in the literary versions, Erasistratus announces the youth's malady to the king. Seleucis' love for his son is so great that he hands over "his most dear wife" to him. The second panel shows the wedding festivities and the recovered Antiochus dancing exuberantly in the central scene.

How congenial such a story was to the Western imagination—in compensation for the daily tragedy of renounced desire for the mother?—is shown by the theme's immense popularity in art, in rhetorical exercises, and in literature.[42] Nor did its popularity wane in the Christian Middle Ages. Rodulphus Tortarius (d. ca. 1122), a monk of Fleury, composed a poetic version of Valerius Maximus' *Facta et dicta memorabilium* that contains an account of Antiochus' lovesickness.[43] The signs of love—wasting, blushing, pallor, and erratic breathing—as well as the pulse test figure prominently in his swift retelling of the classical tale. The number of fourteenth-century commentaries on Valerius Maximus indicates that he was studied intensively in the later Middle Ages.[44] Boccaccio's teacher, for example, the monk Dionigi da Borgo San Sepulcro (d. 1340), explains in his commentary the physiological reasons for the accuracy of the pulse test—another example of the crossover between the medical and literary traditions of lovesickness.[45]

This fantasy of Oedipal desire, whose detection and cure lay in the physician's hands, thus formed part of the European matrix of ideas soon to receive the new medical teachings on lovesickness. As we have seen, *Perdica's Malady* does not disguise the incestuous yearning at all, and, significantly, has a tragic outcome. Though the circulation of the poem in the Middle Ages was limited (only one manuscript survives), the story itself was known. Fulgentius and all three Vatican Mythographers mention Perdica's incestuous lovesickness, but allegorize it as a story of agriculture: Perdica's mother is the earth, and he a farmer.[46] The motif appears to have been familiar from art as well as from literary sources. The bronze statuette in Figure 1.1 was recovered near Soissons, France, suggesting that representations of the theme travelled with imperial culture.

## Lovesickness in Christian Sources

To a far greater degree than secular literature, Biblical texts permeated the minds and imaginations of medieval people. As Leclercq says: "The words of the sacred text never failed to produce a strong impression on the mind. The biblical words did not become trite; people never got used to them."[47] Biblical passages on lovesickness are thus of the utmost importance for understanding the medieval views of passionate love that conditioned the reception and use of the medical discussions of lovesickness. The two key texts in this development were the story of Amnon and Thamar in 2 Samuel 13 (2 Kings in the Vulgate) and the refrain in Canticles, "for I am sick with love" (Cant. 2.5, 5.8).

The biblical episode of Amnon's love for his sister Thamar both portrayed the reality of lovesickness and, in its narrative details, offered a vision of the disease that overlapped with those of medicine and secular literature. Like Valerius Maximus and the author of the *Aegritudo Perdicae*, the biblical writer dramatizes how unsatisfied desire expresses itself somatically in the symptoms of lovesickness. The resolution of the story, however, differs significantly from the secular narratives.

> And it came to pass after this, that Amnon the son of David loved the sister of Absalom son of David, who was very beautiful, and her name was Thamar.
>
> 2 And he was exceedingly fond of her, so that he fell sick for the love of her: for as she was a virgin, he thought it hard to do any thing dishonestly with her.
>
> 3 Now Amnon had a friend, named Jonadab the son of Semmaa the brother of David, a very wise man:
>
> 4 And he said to him: "Why dost thou grow so lean from day to day, O son of the king? why dost thou not tell me the reason of it? And Amnon said to him: I am in love with Thamar the sister of my brother Absalom.
>
> 5 And Jonadab said to him: Lie down upon thy bed, and feign thyself sick: and when thy father shall come to visit thee, say to him: Let my sister Thamar, I pray thee, come to me, to give me to eat, and to make me a mess, that I may eat it at her hand.
>
> 6 So Amnon lay down, and made as if he were sick . . .
>
> (2 Kings 13.1–6; RSV 2 Samuel)

Thamar comes to minister to her sick brother. "And when she had presented him the meat, he took hold of her, and said: Come lie with me, my sister. She answered him: Do not so, my brother, do not force me: for no such thing must be done in Israel. Do not thou this folly." Thamar pleads in vain. "But he would not hearken to her prayers, but being stronger overpowered her and lay with her" (Figure 1.3).[48]

> Then Amnon hated her with an exceeding great hatred: so that the hatred wherewith he hated her was greater than the love with which he had loved her before. And Amnon said to her: Arise, and get thee gone. (13.15)

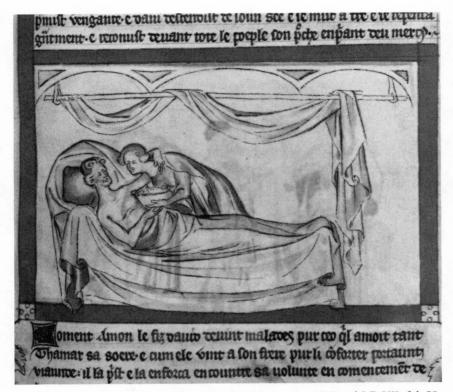

*Figure 1.3.* Amnon and Thamar. London, British Library, MS Royal 2 B. VII, fol. 58.

Amnon's lovesickness is both real and feigned. It is real enough to cause his friend to remark on his loss of weight; Amnon's body involuntarily betrays him. At the same time, he uses his illness as a ploy to obtain his desires. For monastic readers who, as Leclercq says, imaginatively recreated what they read or heard, "giving very sharp relief to images and feelings," Amnon's illness gave an ambiguous picture of lovesickness, as both the physical consequence of immense thwarted desire, and as the deceptive pretext—as in Ovid—to accomplish illicit desire.[49]

The most striking element of the story is Amnon's sudden hate for the woman he loved to the point of sickness. In the terse style of much biblical narrative, the writer does not explain why the reversal occurred, only reports it. In portraying the sudden shift of Amnon's love to hate, did the author perceive a psychological pattern similar to the melancholic anger noted above in Caelius Aurelianus? A medieval interpretation of the passage, at any rate, indicates that it was understood to represent a common pattern of behavior. The illustrated *Bible moralisée* declares that Amnon represents the lecherous rich (*divites luxuriosi*) who wish to accomplish their every will and desire with women.[50] In explaining Amnon's sudden hate, however, the moralized Bible's message is less clear; its ambiguities can be read as projections of cultural fears about women and sexuality. According to the textual gloss, when the lecherous rich cannot have their way with women, they resort to gifts or blandishments (*dono vel simulatione verborum*). The accompanying illustration, however, suggests violence rather than successful seduction, as a woman raises her arms in self-defense against the man pressing himself upon her. Her right hand pushes his head away while her left is drawn back as though to strike him. In the next scene, Amnon, "who hated and despised [Thamar]," casts her from his bed; she leaves "crying and howling" (*flendo et ululando*). Amnon, according to the gloss, signifies the lecherous rich man, who, after he has taken his pleasure with a woman, casts her from him, unaware up to this point that she was intent on gulling him (*illam a se mox expellit se ignorans adhuc per illam esse decipiendum*). Amnon's anger—or that of the lecherous rich—becomes righteous anger, and in a stunning reversal of the literal meaning of the Biblical story, Thamar emerges as the evildoer and Amnon the victim. The medieval reading of the story thus reverses the agency of sexuality and power: male anger is motivated and justified by the threat of female deceit. Blaming the victim is one way of lessening the tension of ambivalent feelings, whether Amnon's or those of any man with the means to achieve his desires.

Although the medieval moralized Bible ignores the question of family relations, it may be significant that Amnon's violent ambivalence directs itself toward his half-sister. As a sibling, she figures the self, but as a woman and potential wife (see v. 13) she figures the mother. His pathological love suggests the narcissistic, ambivalent feelings that Freud claims are at the root of melancholia.[51]

The story of Amnon and Thamar, says Baldwin, bishop of Canterbury (d. 1190), exemplifies incestuous or shameful love, which brings with it suffering and the anxiety of sorrow. This vain love, this shameful love is not only a languor, but a vice of the soul and death.[52] But, he continues, there is a holy love that is languor itself. It suffers anxiously—*amore langueo*—but this languor is a virtue, health, and medicine. Baldwin's contrast between the mortiferous love of Amnon and Thamar and salvific languor introduces the second important biblical tradition for lovesickness in the Middle Ages, exegesis on the Song of Songs.

The most frequently commented book of the Bible in the early Middle Ages, the Song of Songs attracted great interest in the eleventh and twelfth centuries.[53] Desiderius of Montecassino, Constantine's abbot, had a manuscript copied for the library which contained commentaries on that book by Origen, Gregory, "the doctor of desire," and Berengar.[54] Constantine's chapter on love thus entered European intellectual life and attracted its own commentaries when interest in the spiritual languor ("for I am sick with love") of the Song of Songs was at its height.

Exegetes, following Origen, interpreted the Song of Songs as an allegory of the soul's desire for God, the absent Beloved (Figure 1.4). The tropological reading insists on the real experience of love-suffering, and provides a language for the subjective experience of unsatisfiable desire. If the physicians describe lovers' suffering from the outside, so to speak, in the categories of learned discourse, the commentaries in the Song of Songs give us a glimpse into the lived reality of the love Baldwin calls "languor and the passion of an unwell mind."[55] Because the vocabulary of love and lovesickness from the Song was a prime resource for the development of medieval love lyric,[56] it too served as a meeting point for sacred, secular, and medical ideas about love.

Origen sets forth what remained a central interpretative problem not only with the Song, but with the vernacular literature of love as well: the essential ambiguity of love.[57] Just as Scripture uses the same terms for the members of the outer man and the inner man, so too the same words may be used for carnal and spiritual love. "Just as there is one love, known as carnal and also known as Cupid by the poets, according to which the lover sows in the flesh; so also is there another, a spiritual love, by which the inner man who loves sows in the spirit."[58] The soul is moved by spiritual love "when, having clearly beheld the beauty and fairness of the Word of God, it falls deeply in love with His loveliness and receives from the Word Himself a certain dart and wound of love" (199).

The ambiguity of the word "love" is compounded by the reversal of value given to the "wound of love" or love-languor. As Origen says, this wound is not deadly, but rather "health-bestowing"; the wound of love is the "wound of salvation" (199–200). Just as Christ's passion led to the triumph of the resurrection, so in this interpretation of Canticles, love-suffering becomes salvific. But as salutary as the love wound may be, ambiguity nonetheless persists. Origen continues: the wicked one can inflict wounds of cupidity with his darts, wounds so subtle that the "soul scarcely perceives that she has been pierced and wounded by them" (198–99). How then can one distinguish between health-giving and death-dealing love?

The signs of love that Origen lists are no clear guide, because they apply equally well to spiritual and carnal lovers. The lover yearns and longs by day and night, can speak of nothing but the beloved, will hear of nothing else, and can think of nothing else. He desires and hopes for the beloved

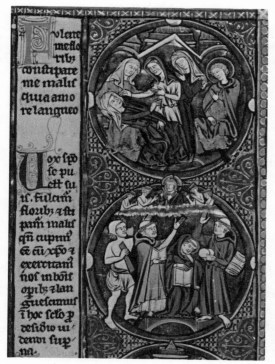

*Figure 1.4.* The Bride of Canticles languishes with love. *Bible moralisée.* Paris, Bibliothèque Nationale, MS lat. 11560, fol. 72r.

alone (198). An anonymous twelfth-century commentator compares the manifestations of languorous desire to "impatient love," which day and night beats at the doors of prostitutes.[59] In fact, the parallelism between sacred and secular love was felt so strongly that the medical *signa amoris* came to be applied to mystical love. For example, Richard of St. Victor (d. 1173) describes identical symptoms for successive stages of both carnal and spiritual passionate love.[60]

Twelfth-century commentators on the Song of Songs attempted to clarify how physical illness could signify spiritual love. In the early thirteenth century, when Constantine's *Viaticum*, accompanied by Gerard of Berry's gloss, was readily available in the universities, Parisian theologians adopted the new, more technical medical discussions of lovesickness to illuminate the workings of mystical rapture. William of Auvergne, bishop of Paris (1228–49) and theologian at the university, remarks to his students in an explanation of rapture: "You ought to remember some things which you experience continually. You see that love is a certain *raptus*, just like that which is called *morbus eros*, which is a violent and most intense illness, in which someone who loves is in such rapture that it barely permits him to think of anyone besides the woman he loves in this way."[61] The remark suggests that love as a medically defined illness was both common knowledge and common experience. Indeed, William's colleague, William of Auxerre, noted that many are driven mad by *amor morbus* when they cannot obtain what they love.[62] By the time of Hugh of St. Cher's popular *De doctrina cordis* (around 1235), the semiotics of lovesickness had so penetrated mystical writing that Hugh was able to borrow the signs of love wholesale from the medical chapters on lovesickness by Constantine the African and Gerard of Berry.[63] Later writers continued to borrow from the medical tradition to elaborate the signs of spiritual love. Medical teachings on lovesickness were thus easily assimilated to religious discourse about passionate love, which powerfully validated the accuracy of the physicians' descriptions.[64]

## The Crucified Christ, Model of Love and Suffering

Christ, the Bridegroom of tropological readings of the Song, suffers the sickness of love as much as the Bride herself does. The era in which the African merchant Constantine entered the monastery of Montecassino witnessed a new emphasis on Christ as a loving savior. More than a Judge and King, Christ was seen rather as "the sweet lover of mankind."[65] He took on and suffered in mortal human flesh out of his great love for humankind. With this shift in theological emphasis, affective attachment to the Cross and Passion also grew. The Cross became an object of intensely emotional devotion, as worshippers reciprocated the loving sacrifice of the Passion with their own compassion. Like the tropological reading of the Song, the Cross mediates between the eternal and the historic, transcendent divinity and subjective individual experience.[66]

Loving compassion for the wounded, suffering body of Christ, under the guidance of the active religious imagination described by Leclercq, could express itself in images of unabashed eroticism. Rupert of Deutz (d. 1129) reports a dream in which he worshiped the Cross. The crucified Christ seemed to return his gaze and accept his salutation. Yet he wanted closer union with his Savior. Rushing to the altar, he embraced and kissed the image. "I held him, I embraced him, I kissed him for a long time. I sensed how seriously he accepted this gesture of love when, while kissing, he himself opened his mouth that I might kiss more deeply."[67] Clearly, Rupert says, this signified the fulfillment of what the beloved of the Song says: "Who shall give thee to me for my brother (i.e., husband), sucking the breasts of my mother, that I might find thee without, and kiss thee, and now no man may despise me?" (8.1) There is much to dwell on in the passage: the remarkable flexibility of gender identity—both Rupert and Christ simultaneously occupy male and female roles; the overt eroticism of their union; Rupert's interpretation of his passionate experience through the Song; and the association of eros and nurturing suggested by the verse from the Song.

Rupert's vision, though perhaps more vividly represented than others, is part of a medieval tradition of affective piety in which experiences of spiritual union were represented through images and gestures of loving behavior.[68] Figure 1.5, which has a number of analogues in medieval art, shows how the Cross could unite divine and human passions of love. The human witnesses depicted in Crucifixion scenes serve as sources of affective identification for the audience.[69] Mary Magdalen, the most carnal of lovers, here passionately embraces the Cross and kisses Christ's wounded feet at the center of the composition. "The power of a visual image to evoke love in the viewer is at its height in the figure of the Magdalen."[70] We may assume that scenes and experiences like this had important implications for the fate of the lover's malady in the Middle Ages. Veneration of the the Cross and identification with Christ's Passion—*imitatio Christi*—forged a bond, in medieval consciousness, between love and suffering. Suffering, moreover, was not weakness, but the ultimate act of love. Since Christ's Passion was taken as a model for affective experience, this strain of affective piety deliberately cultivated "lovesickness." We find, for example, that in the thirteenth century a Dominican friar, contemplating the Redemption, was "rapt in love of God . . . and languished for love, lying for three days without eating or drinking." And in imitation of the bride of the Song of Songs, the thirteenth-century mystic Julian of Mt. Cornillon suffered the sickness of love, which her sisters mistook for physical illness.[71] Given the ambiguity of the symptoms of lovesickness, is it farfetched to think that the theologians' analogy between the two loves, earthly and spiritual, was partially responsible for the ennobling of lovesickness found in vernacular literature?

In any event, the potential for confusion between *morbus eros* and *passio caritatis* was an uncertainty ripe for exploration by vernacular poets of love from Gottfried to Chaucer. Gottfried von Strassburg (d. ca. 1210) boldly melds Christian and erotic suffering into a "eucharistic poetics" in the prologue to his story of Tristan and Isolde: "Today we still love to hear of their tender devotion, sweet and ever fresh, their joy, their sorrow, their anguish, and their ecstasy. . . . Their life, their death are our bread. Thus lives their life, thus lives their death. Thus they live still and yet are dead, and their death is the bread of the living."[72] By the fourteenth century this development came full circle. The parallel between sacred and secular lovesickness

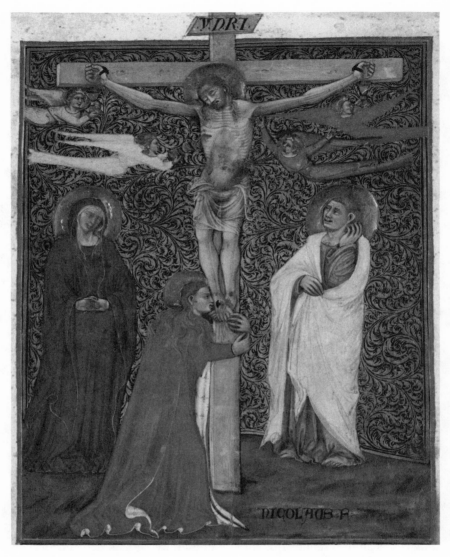

*Figure 1.5*. The Crucifixion. Miniature from a missal by Niccolò da Bologna, active ca. 1369–ca. 1402. Embracing and/or kissing the Cross occurs in numerous devotional paintings. The Cleveland Museum of Art, Gift of J. H. Wade, CMA 24.1013.

then lay so ready to hand that a sermon on the text *quia amore langueo* describes Christ's passion "under the seven secular signs of love-longing."[73]

## Popular Lore

The Tristan story reminds us that there were other, less easily traceable, European notions of lovesickness to which the new medical learning could be assimilated. Love potions and love magic were part of the stock in trade of unrequited lovers in the earlier Middle Ages, as we know from penitentials, canon law, saints' lives, and literature. Guibert of Nogent's (d. ca. 1125) parents were unspelled by an enchantress, and a love potion figures prominently in the *Life* of Christina of Markyate, a twelfth-century recluse.[74] It was commonly thought that through natural or supernatural means—herbs and charms or diabolic aid—one could "turn men's minds to love or hate," states that were sometimes so extreme that they seemed to be diseased.[75] As we shall see, this magically-caused love came to be viewed as a form of *amor hereos* or lovesickness in the later Middle Ages. In the late eleventh and twelfth centuries, however, indigenous tales of love magic and love madness offered material that could be elaborated through the medical doctrines on lovesickness.

The story of the "wasting sickness" of the Irish hero Cú Chulainn is a case in point that is worth closer examination for its similarity to the constellation of anger, love, and sickness that we have seen in the story of Amnon and Thamar and in the ancient discussions of melancholy. Preserved in a manuscript of the twelfth century, it is a native story of love-madness dating from the ninth or tenth century onto which was grafted the learned tradition of lovesickness.[76] Although the narrative suffers from interpolations and dislocations, it nonetheless yields a coherent vision of the dynamics among love, anger, and power in the Middle Ages.

During an assembly of the Ulstermen, during which each man was assigned "his triumph and his prowess," a wondrously beautiful flock of birds settled on the lake; every woman coveted a pair. Ethne Ingubai, wife of Cú Chulainn, claimed them if they were to be caught. Angered by the "whores of the Ulaid" (Ulstermen), as he calls the women who requested him to get the birds, the hero Cú Chulainn nonetheless killed the birds and distributed them to every woman except his wife. Cú Chulainn perceived his wife's anger, though she denied it; he told her not to be angry and promised her the most beautiful birds. When two birds appeared, which his wife counseled him not to touch, he shot anyway and for the first time in his life missed his mark. Downcast, Cú Chulainn sat against a stone. Two women came toward him, laughed at him, and horsewhipped him. "And they continued for a long time, each of them in turn coming still to him to beat him, so that he was almost dead."

Cú Chulainn took to his bed, where he remained for a year "in sickness and in weakness," without speaking to anyone. One day an emissary from the Otherworld arrived with the message that Cú Chulainn was desired there both as the lover of Fand and as a warrior. The prospect of adventure having restored his spirits, he sent for his wife (now called Emer), saying: "They are fairy women who have visited and destroyed me." His friend Loeg recited a poem to restore him: "It is great idleness for a warrior to lie in sleep of wasting sickness, for it shows demons (gloss: women), folk from Tenmag Trogaige (gloss: from Mag Mell), and they have injured (?) thee, they have confined thee, they tortured thee in the toils of women's wantonness." When his wife Emer arrived, she reproached him: "'Shame for thee,' said she, 'to lie for love of a woman, for long lying will make thee sick.'"

The story continues, narrating the jealousy of his wife and how she finally triumphed over Fand, Cú Chulainn's madness at the loss of Fand, and the draughts of forgetfulness finally given to the hero of Ulster and his wife. Let us return, however, to the opening episode with Cú Chulainn and his wife. His anger has a number of objects—the women of Ulster, the fact that he missed his cast at a feast where all were "assigned their prowess"— but his wife's anger plays an important part in his eventual lovesickness. Though she denies anger, she has been slighted before all Ulster, and Cú Chulainn's repeated enjoinders not to be angry indicate her real emotion. When the pair of birds arrives, he then disregards her advice not to touch them.

Though only his despondency after missing his cast is mentioned, we may suspect that his state is more complex than that. His emotion is compounded of humiliation, anger, and knowledge of his wife's own anger, shame, and accurate prediction regarding the birds. The Otherworldly vision thus arrives at a moment of great emotional turmoil.

The women who beat him nearly to death and cause his long wasting may be seen as doubles for his wife: they punish him as he fears or imagines she would, should she give vent to her wrath.[77] His sickness embodies fear of his wife's vengeance, distanced and enacted by the women of the Sídhe. Later in the story she shows exactly how capable she is of violent revenge for an insult to her honor, so that Cú Chulainn has good reason to fear her as well as love her. And since a hero like Cú Chulainn cannot show fear, he experiences it somatically as external punishment and sickness. Loeg's poem attributes Cú Chulainn's sickness to the "toils of women's wantonness." Recalling Cú Chulainn's epithet "whores of the Ulaid," does Loeg refer to the otherworldly Fand or to his wife? If we accept that Fand may function psychologically as a double for Cú Chulainn's wife, then his passionate affair with Fand in the Otherworld can be seen as a fantasy of reconciliation with his wife.

A story from Odo of Cluny's (d. 944) *Collations*, in which a man is whipped by demonic women, suggests the plausibility of this interpretation of Cú Chulainn's wasting sickness. A certain Hukbert of Sens, given to the sin of luxury, saw two women standing by him one night who were not the ones who usually came to him. He realized that they were phantasms. Other people rushed up, but he alone saw the women. He took refuge in the church, but it too was full of phantasmic women, among whom sat one as queen. She ordered them to seize him and whip him. His repentance came too late, and he was given into their power. He fell to the ground, where they whipped him as he screamed out what he saw and felt. After this went on for a time, the women disappeared and those outside saw the troop cross over the bridge. The man died a short time later.[78]

Whether the story reflects Hukbert's experience of madness or Odo's fictional skills, in either case it is the combination of transgression against women with their fearsome vengeance that parallels the psychological dynamic of Cú Chulainn's story. In both stories anxiety over relationships with women unleashes fantasies of their revenge so powerful that they result in illness or death. Such fantasies are collective; in them women tend to become demonized, and love madness becomes the result of love magic.

That lovesickness can be a somaticized form of fear and of anger toward women will be discussed at greater length in chapter eight. For the present, the story of Cú Chulainn shows that early European vernacular traditions of lovesickness offered parallels to the poetry of Ovid and to the learned doctrines of the physicians. Like the other forms of literary and medical discourse surveyed in this chapter, such native stories both conditioned the reception of the new teachings on lovesickness and were themselves enriched by it.

In addition to vernacular literature, penitentials, legal codes, witchcraft treatises and sermons partially document popular as well as learned beliefs in the debilitating powers of love.[79] Thomas of Chobham (fl. 1200–33), for example, lists a number of remedies for "insane love" in his penitential manual for confessors. "For many fall into insane love such that they can hardly be turned from their error. This love is moreover a disease (*morbus*) not only of the mind but also of the body, since the marrows are swollen, the veins disordered, [and] every bodily sense weakened."[80]

Popular lore by its nature is nonetheless difficult to document; the polymorphous variations on the theme of "insane love" in non–learned tradition cannot be fully traced in a study such as this. In contrast, as the documents surveyed in this chapter have shown, the more stable written tradition of learned medicine enjoyed a continuous but limited presence in Europe between the fall of the Roman empire and the revival of scientific learning in the eleventh century. These medical works, however, offer only sketchy analyses of the disease of love, and their limitations suggest why Constantine's chapter on love enjoyed the success it did. Having been granted the status of a separate disease in Islamic medical handbooks, lovesickness reentered the West in the Cassinese monk's latinized version accompanied by a comparatively full theoretical and practical discussion of its causes, symptoms, consequences, and cures.

Yet the success of the medical view of the lover's malady, as shown by the adoption of Constantine's description of lovesickness in a variety of disciplines, rested on a broader basis than that of developments in medical writing alone. The Bible, exegetical and mystical writings, classical literature, vernacular stories, and popular beliefs all agreed with the doctors' diagnosis that passion could breed sickness of body and mind. Such unanimity was a powerful argument for the disease's reality and hastened the acceptance of the Arabic doctrines on lovesickness. "The discovery of love" has been used to characterize the revolution in sensibility that swept through European culture in the late eleventh and twelfth centuries. In this supersaturated mix of texts, ideas, and behaviors, the conception of love in the *Viaticum* and other medical texts, couched in a more precise technical vocabulary, crystallized new ways of interpreting and controlling erotic behavior.[81] If we see the conventions of courtliness as ideals for controlling erotic and aggressive behavior, then it is easy to understand why there was such an affinity between lovesickness and "courtly love" in vernacular literature of the high and late Middle Ages. Both offered techniques for constraining and yet indulging in potentially disruptive erotic impulses.

# §§ 2 §§

# CONSTANTINE'S *VIATICUM*

And *Palladius* the physician was asked about love and said: "Love is a disease which is generated in the brain, when the thoughts are allowed to dwell on one subject and the loved person is constantly brought to mind and the gaze is continually fixed on him."[1]

The generations on either side of 1100 found themselves in a rapidly changing world that for us, in retrospect, marks the watershed between the early and the high Middle Ages. Agricultural improvements transformed the material basis of society. Population expanded and its mobility increased. Norman conquests in the Mediterranean and the first Crusade opened new lands for travel and production. New trade routes and improved communications followed. In short, the social world widened dramatically and its relation to the natural world altered in significant ways. The twelfth century witnessed not just altered physical relations with the natural world, but the emergence of the *idea* of nature.[2]

Several generations of scholars have now documented how nature and human nature were rethought in light of the newly-available Arabic texts from Montecassino and Toledo and how this new understanding found expression in, for example, philosophical and literary works associated with Chartres.[3] The Arabic medical texts that Constantine translated stimulated a new emphasis on the materiality of the human organism, its mutable composition from the elements. In Nemesius' *On the Nature of Man*, which Constantine's patron Alphanus (d. 1085) translated, we learn: "Since man consists of a body, and since every body is composed of the four elements, it is necessary that the affections, which parallel the elements, undergo in man the division, mutation, and flux which belong to the body alone." Or, as the Archpoet says: "Factus de materia levis elementi / Folio sum similis de quo ludunt venti" (Made of matter of a light element, I am like a leaf the winds play with).[4] The materiality of the human organism raised new questions about the relations between body and soul, for which people turned to treatises such as Qustā ibn Lūqā's *De anima et spiritu discrimine* ("On the Distinction between Soul and Spirit," often attributed to Constantine) or the works on the soul (*De anima*) of Aristotle and Avicenna.[5]

At the same time, the rise of literacy changed intellectual and religious life. The reform movements of the late eleventh and twelfth centuries, the emphasis on affective, interior experience and its need for reformation, the rise of the universities and the spread of heresies all grew out of (as well as contributed to) new conceptual vocabularies introduced and spread by scribal culture.[6]

The discovery of the self together with the perception of the need for interior, spiritual reform lent new importance to love in religious and intellectual life. Human nature increasingly came to be seen as a loving nature.[7] Love impelled the quest for perfection and the ascent to God, as Bernard continually and movingly proclaimed in his sermons on *Canticles*. Vernacular poetry offered a secular counterpart: a vision of a love that promised a heightened sense of self in both joy and sorrow, and the occasion and means for moral improvement. At this time, too, the Church promoted an ideal of marriage that on the one hand emphasized equality between men and women, but on the other portrayed women's subjugation.[8]

Constantine the African and his translations are poised at the beginning of this cultural shift. Quickly carried to nearby Salerno, and across Europe to Chartres, Germany and England, these texts provided one of the foundations for the renewal of intellectual life in the twelfth century. The influx of Arabic medicine, derived in large part from the works of Hippocrates and Galen, formed the core of medical instruction for centuries and offered a critical impetus for the development of both practical and theoretical medicine in Europe. Through the *Viaticum* Constantine gave Western physicians, patients, and readers a theoretical framework and a technical vocabulary with which to discuss passionate love. This vocabulary and accompanying theory were admittedly not well developed, yet nonetheless were far more accessible than earlier translations of Greek medical works on lovesickness.

We know for certain little more about Constantine than that he was born in Africa and entered the abbey of Montecassino while Desiderius was abbot (1058–87); 1087 is conventionally accepted as his date of death (Figure 2.1). Peter the Deacon's *Illustrious Men of Montecassino* (*De viris illustris cassinensis*, after 1144) and the *Chronicle of Montecassino* are the earliest and best sources for Constantine's life and writings.[9] Two other legends survive,

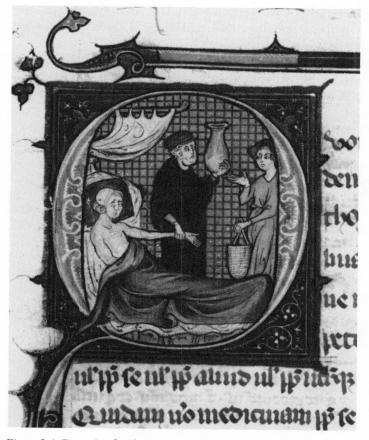

*Figure 2.1.* Portrait of a physician, perhaps meant to be Constantine the African, in the opening initial of the *Viaticum*. Vatican, Biblioteca Apostolica, MS Pal. lat. 1149, fol. 125r.

one apparently from thirteenth-century Salerno, the other from fourteenth-century Montpellier, both from centers of medical learning in active engagement with his work.[10]

According to Peter the Deacon, Constantine was born in Carthage. He traveled to Babylon, where he learned all the arts and sciences, as well as the medicine of the Chaldees, Arabs, Persians, and Saracens. He left Babylon for India, and after acquiring the arts of the Indians, travelled to Ethiopia and Egypt. When he returned to Africa after spending thirty-nine years in study, his countrymen, envious of his accomplishments, tried to kill him. He fled secretly to Salerno, where he disguised himself as a poor man. The brother of the King of Babylon recognized him and led him before Duke Robert Guiscard, the Norman ruler of Salerno, who received him with great honor. Constantine then went to Montecassino, where Abbot Desiderius received him into the community, and where he completed his many translations of Arabic medical texts into Latin.

In the Salernitan legend, Constantine is a merchant who, upon learning of the paucity of European medical works, determined to make good that lack. As he sailed from North Africa to Salerno, laden with books, a storm off Cape Palinuro damaged some of the precious cargo. However, Constantine made it safely to Salerno and there, after converting to Christianity, began his program of translation.[11] In these legends Constantine is figured as a culture hero, transferring the advanced medical science of Islam to a relatively backward Europe—a *translatio studii* in the most literal sense.

Whatever the truth behind the circumstantial narratives of the legends—they tell us more about how later generations saw Constantine than about the man himself—we know that Constantine was at first befriended by Alphanus, the archbishop of Salerno (1058–85) to whom Constantine dedicated his *De stomacho*.[12] Alphanus at some point sent him to his friend Desiderius, Abbot of Montecassino, to whom in turn Constantine dedicated his translation of ʿAlī ibn al-ʿAbbās al-Majūsī's (d. 994) *Kitāb al-Malakī* known as the *Pantechne* or *Pantegni*. If he was not a Christian already, his conversion probably dates from this time.[13]

Montecassino was then in its golden age. Situated at the crossroads of European, Islamic, and Greek cultures, pivotal in both papal and imperial politics, the abbey was an ideal place for bringing the North African's gifts to the West to fullest fruition. The scriptorium was flourishing, and Constantine had pupils who stimulated his translations and compositions.[14] His prologues and dedications portray him as a man for whom knowledge was always part of a living dialogue. We know most about his students Johannes Afflacius and Atto, both of whom continued his translation project. Atto was chaplain to the Empress Agnes, wife of Henry III and mother of Henry IV, and reworked Constantine's texts, though whether from Latin into the vernacular or in the form of Latin paraphrases is not entirely clear.[15] Johannes Afflacius Saracenus finished Constantine's version of ʿAlī ibn al-ʿAbbās' *Kitāb al-Malakī* (*Pantegni*) as well as composed several treatises of his own.[16] In addition, he may have been the one to retranslate the *Viaticum's* chapter on lovesickness from the Arabic, in effect creating a second edition that circulated under the name of *Liber de heros morbo*.[17]

## Arabic Sources

The *Viaticum* is an adaptation of the popular medical handbook of Abu Jaʿfar Ahmad ibn Ibrāhīm ibn abī Khālid al-Jazzār (d. 979), *Kitāb Zād al-musāfir wa-qūt al-ḥāḍir* (*Provisions for the Traveler and the Nourishment of the Settled*).[18] Ibn al-Jazzār, a student of the physician and philosopher Isḥāq ibn Sulaymān al-Isrā'īlī (Isaac Judaeus, ca. 855–955), himself the pupil of Isḥāq ibn ʿImran, practiced medicine in the North African city of Qayrawan, the medieval capital of Tunisia. All three physicians considerably influenced the development of medieval medicine in the West through Constantine's Latin translations.

The treatise is divided into seven books with the diseases themselves arranged from head to toe (*a capite ad calcem*). ʿ*Ishk*, or passionate love, is the subject of the twentieth chapter of the first book, immediately preceded by insomnia, frenzy, and drunkenness, and followed by sneezing, epilepsy, and apoplexy.[19] Since the *Zād al-musāfir* was intended as a small book for traveling in case no doctor were available (some of the earliest Latin manuscripts are the size of a paperback), the presence of a chapter on passionate or excessive love reveals how widespread the notion of love as a serious disease requiring treatment was in Islamic culture (Figure 2.2).[20]

In composing the chapter on ʿ*ishk*, Ibn al-Jazzār drew on sources that include Galen, Zeno, al-Kindi, and Rufus of Ephesus. His use of his teacher Isḥāq ibn ʿImran's treatise on melancholy (another Constantinian translation)[21] underscores the close relationship between love and melancholy in Arabic medical thinking: al-Rāzī, ʿAlī ibn al-ʿAbbās, and Avicenna make the same connection. Nonetheless, Ibn al-Jazzār, like his Byzantine predecessors Oribasius and Paul of Aegina, categorizes love and melancholy as distinct diseases in separate chapters. Though the disease of love never severed its ties from melancholy, its separate treatment in the *Zād al-musāfir* granted the idea of morbid love an autonomy that helps account for its ready adoption in the West.[22]

## ʿIshk

Before analyzing Constantine's chapter on love more closely, it will be useful to note the range of meaning for ʿ*ishk* in medieval Islamic culture. The term was widely understood as an "irresistible desire . . . to obtain possession of a loved object or being . . . It betrays, therefore, in one who experiences it a deficiency, a want, which he must supply at any cost in order to reach perfection."[23] As a motion toward perfection, it admits of hierarchical degrees, and as an aspiration toward beauty it can become a passionate quest for God. "Whatever the differences in opinion about its content, ʿ*ishk* is one of the characteristics of medieval self awareness, obsessed with the quest for the eternal, the transcendent, and the sacred."[24]

A wide variety of sources, including not only poetry and *adab* literature

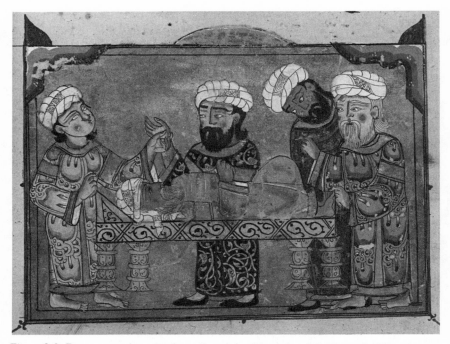

*Figure 2.2.* Doctor treating a patient. From the *Maqāmāt* of al-Ḥarīrī (1122). Vienna, Bildarchiv, Österreichische Nationalbibliothek, Cod. A.F. 9, fol. 64v.

but also theology, jurisprudence, philosophy, and medicine analyzed, debated, extolled and excoriated ʿishk. The scholar Ibn al-Jawzi (d. 1200) declares that ʿishk is "the acute inclination of the soul (*nafs*) towards a form (*sura*) which conforms to its nature (*tabʿ*). If the soul thinks intensely on this form, it imagines the possibility of obtaining it and begins to hope that it may. From this intense thought is born the malady [of love]."[25] The conception of a certain affinity between lovers has its roots in Neoplatonic and Platonic traditions inherited by Islamic culture.[26]

Among Arabic physicians who write on ʿishk, Ibn al-Jazzār gives most prominence to this "doctrine of affinity" when he writes in his chapter on love that "when the soul sees within itself a consimilar form, it goes mad, as it were, in order to fulfill its desire." Like the author of the pseudo-Aristotelian *Problem* 30, then, he fuses a Platonic conception of frenzy with a medical view of madness.[27] This Platonic theme in the chapter on ʿishk offered a point of contact in the West, through Constantine's translation, between medical views of love and those of other disciplines influenced by Platonism, such as philosophy and literature.

If, on the one hand, ʿishk was assimilated to divine love in Islamic culture, on the other it permeated literary depictions of passionate love. "It is a state of spiritual servitude to an idealised female figure, upon which the 'courtly' sentiments of a soul in ebullition . . . crystallize."[28] Since the term *ʿishk* carried significant cultural resonances that strikingly parallel the interplay of mystical madness (*alienatio mentis*), lovesickness, and "courtly" love in the West, to what degree, if any, was their conjunction imported? Or are we dealing instead with parallel manifestations in two cultures equally heirs to the legacy of antiquity? Recently Ioan Couliano has argued that "the phenomenon of courtly love has . . . more in common with Arab medicine and mysticism [than with Catharism]."[29] He points out that idealization of the feminine pervaded Arab mystical poetry and was rooted in the Platonic assumption of a continuum between sensory and intelligential beauty. Couliano locates the genesis of courtly love in this strain of Platonizing mysticism (Sufism) and the concept of *ʿishk*. He argues that it emerged from a shift in the idea of health: "Through this *Umwertung*, the gloomy equilibrium of psychic forces recommended by learned treatises was transformed into a sickness of the intellect [i.e., the medical idea of lovesickness], whereas, on the contrary, the spiritual sickness induced by love ended by being extolled as the real health of body and soul."[30]

Though he argues for the priority of Islam in the development of courtly love, Couliano does not take up the question of whether and how Islam influenced the West on this score. In her re-evaluation of the Arabic, specifically Andalusian, influence on medieval European literary history, María Rosa Menocal makes a strong case that the poetic form called the *muwashshaha* mediated between the two cultures.[31] Originating in Andalusia, this type of poem contained a number of stanzas in classical Arabic and a refrain (*kharja*) in the Mozarabic vernacular. Several passages in the examples she prints show that lovesickness was a standard theme:

> Meu l-habib enfermo de meu amar.
> Que no ha d'estar?
> Non ves a mibe que s'ha do no llegar?

[My beloved is sick for love of me. How can he not be so? Do you not see that he is not allowed near me?]

Oh you, my sickness and my healer, in but a word from you lies the cure of my illness. And yet, because of you, I have melted away to nothing. (93–95)

The Islamic notion of *ʿishk* in all its complexity, then, may have penetrated Europe from two directions: from North Africa (by way of Italy) through

Constantine's medical translations and at about the same time (1050–1150) from Spain in Andalusian poetry. The Spanish route was then later reinforced by Gerard of Cremona's (d. 1187) Toledan translations of other Arabic medical works dealing with the disease of love.[32]

## Viaticum I.20

Constantine translated the *Zād al-musāfir* into Latin with the title *Viaticum peregrinantis*. Since his translation is actually a paraphrase that expands and omits where necessary in order to present Islamic medicine to an uneducated Western audience—those who found the *Pantegni* hard going, as he says in the preface to the *Viaticum*[33]—I will henceforth refer to the Latin version as "Constantine's" *Viaticum* to distinguish it from its Arabic source, the *Zād al-musāfir*.

The chapter on "amor qui et eros dicitur" (love that is also called eros) closely follows the structure of its source, beginning with a definition of love, followed by its causes, symptoms and cures. In reworking Ibn al-Jazzār's chapter, he abridges the definition of love and the catalogue of potential love objects. He also cuts out Arabic names in the attribution of quotations while leaving those of Galen and Rufus.[34] Finally, he omits material at the end of the chapter—an explanation of the type of basil to be used, and an invocation to Allah. One interesting result of Constantine's alterations is the implication that excessive love is directed solely at people. The Arabic and Greek versions indicate that the lovesick patient may desire objects as well as people. Though later Western physicians occasionally use *amor hereos*, as they called it, in reference to horses or other objects—Richard de Bury even uses it of a passion for books—the most common understanding of the disease in the Latin Middle Ages restricted it to sexual passion for a person of the opposite sex.[35]

## Eros and Pleasure

The particular type of love that is also called *eros*,[36] begins Constantine, is. a disease (*morbus*) of the brain involving desire and "affliction of the thoughts." The definition follows Galenic tradition in localizing sensation and passions in the brain rather than in the heart, where Aristotle puts them.[37] Constantine then refers to certain philosophers who claim that *eros* is the word designating the greatest pleasure. Just as fidelity is the ultimate form of affection, so *eros* is the extreme form of pleasure.

The definition of love as a pleasurable disease (*morbus*) suggests the paradoxical inversion of the concept of health found in "courtly" love in medieval Islam and Christian Europe (that is, it is salutary to be sick with love). The parallel makes the definition a locus where we can observe what Couliano calls the "selective will" of the *Viaticum* commentators, by which they read their author through a "hermeneutic filter," an "interpretive grille," which reveals structures and emphases of the appropriating culture.[38] If we accept this hypothesis, the commentaries ought to tell us as much about medieval conceptions of pleasure as they do about love and disease. For Constantine's first surviving commentator, Gerard of Berry (late twelfth century), wealth and leisure—that is, pleasure in daily life—are the prerogatives of the nobility, and it is they who suffer the disease of love. To this localizing of lovesickness in the courts he adds another element generally associated with courtly literature: the coupling of pleasure with intense love for a single individual.[39] For Peter of Spain, as we shall see in detail in chapter six, pleasure is a function of the psychophysiology of gender, and gender affects whether and how intensely one suffers from lovesickness. Viewed as a form of extreme pleasure, morbid love thus evoked cultural assumptions about pleasure in the body politic and in the intimate recesses of the gendered body. These in turn became avenues (among others) for the passage of lovesickness into particular locales of cultural topography—the literature of "noble love" and scientific discourse on sexual pleasure.

## Causes

Erotic love can arise from the body's need to expel excess humor, for which Rufus (says Constantine) recommends intercourse as the best remedy. Erotic love can also arise from the perception of a beautiful form, when the soul goes mad with desire to fulfill its pleasures. Although this Neoplatonic strain is underplayed by *Viaticum* commentators, Gerard of Berry does briefly gloss it as the cause of true love. Mind and body interact closely in this disease: the balance between somatic and psychological causes is also paralleled in symptomatology and therapy. Compared with his symptomatology and therapy, however, Constantine's etiology is the least satisfactory part of the chapter and the section that was to be most amplified by commentators, as will be detailed in the following chapters.

As Constantine presents it, it is difficult to decide whether *amor eros* is more akin to Neoplatonic striving for beauty or to an attack of sexual need. The chapter as a whole embodies the Galenic premise that "man's behavior depends on his somatic constitution and disposition."[40] This medical materialism implies a kind of moral determinism, a consequence that Galen himself was not fully prepared to draw. He maintained that free will was not thereby infringed; dietetic medicine, study, and philosophy could ameliorate the effects of one's bodily composition, allowing moral behavior to overcome the dictates of somatic temperament.

Constantine takes no overt stand on the issue. The allusions to Galen and their application to untreated lovesickness, however, imply a deterministic view, one that also surfaces in his conception of etiology. The adventitious sight of a beautiful object and the presence of excessive or corrupt humors involve chance and the material composition of the body; free will or domination of matter through one's philosophical attitude are passed over in silence. The ambiguity of the *Viaticum's* causality enabled lovesickness to be idealized in poetry, to be compared with mystical love, and to be condemned as cupidity.

## Symptoms; Melancholy

The symptoms of lovesickness, in contrast, proved far less problematic. Those that can be traced back to Greek and Roman literature through the intermediaries of Arabic and Byzantine medical works include the alteration of appearance (sunken eyes, jaundiced color) and of behavior (insomnia, anorexia, depressed thoughts [*profundatio cogitationum*]).[41] The consequences of untreated lovesickness are even more dire. As Galen says, "the power of the soul follows the complexion of the body"; furthermore, "the body follows the soul in its action, and the soul accompanies the body in its suffering." This dynamic interaction of body and mind increases the lover's bodily suffering while the disturbed balance of his physical complexion further unbalances him psychologically. He may lapse into a melancholy passion.

Whereas the *Viaticum* considers love a forerunner of melancholy, in another Constantinian translation, the *Pantegni theorica*, love is a type of melancholy.[42] And in Constantine's translation of Isḥaq ibn 'Imran's treatise on melancholy, those who lose a beloved, scholars who suddenly lose their books, those who are exceedingly religious, indeed, anyone who suffers from excessive thought, which is "labor of the soul" according to Hippocrates, may fall prey to melancholy. The symptoms of lovesickness correspond to those listed in *De melancholia*, and in fact the *Viaticum's* chapter on love parallels *De melancholia* in a number of places.[43] The kinship between love and melancholy in the Constantinian corpus reinforced the notion that love could become a disease; it provided an authoritative medical background for the figure of the "melancholy lover" in European literature; and it suggests that the psychodynamics of melancholy may illuminate the genesis of lovesickness, a point to be taken up in the last chapter.

## *Cures*

The longest section of the chapter, embellished with frequent quotations from medical authorities, deals with therapy. In keeping with the dual causality, the cures—intercourse, wine, baths, conversation, music, and poetry—are directed at both body and mind. Therapeutic intercourse, a cure that ancient medicine particularly recommended for melancholy and mania, was a therapy whose aim was to restore proper humoral balance. It was considered one of the six "non-naturals" (air, food and drink, waking and sleeping, motion and quiet, evacuation and repletion, and the emotions), whose regulation was essential to health (Figure 2.3). Constantine's *De coitu*, for example, sets forth the circumstances in which intercourse is healthful or harmful and describes how it best may be accomplished. Not only does coitus expel superfluous humors, but in addition, according to the widely-quoted Rufus of Ephesus, it also chases out fixed ideas, which is particularly valuable for the melancholic. Among its benefits he also reckons that of "dissolving love."[44]

Therapeutic intercourse seems to have posed no ethical dilemma to most of the doctors who wrote on lovesickness, most likely because it fit lay European sexual morality: men's sexual activity outside marriage, especially with prostitutes, seems not to have been viewed very seriously, since it posed no threat to "household order or the purity of the lineage."[45] The easy availability of prostitutes, at least in the larger urban centers where academic physicians, medical students, and their well-to-do patients congregated, suggests that there would have been little practical difficulty in carrying out this particular cure.[46] Though Constantine and his commentators never address the topic explicitly, it seems clear that "honest" women were excluded from the enjoyment of this therapeutic practice.

Other physical cures, drinking wine and bathing, were also calculated to restore the proper balance of humors. At the same time, they helped the patient regain a more cheerful disposition by counteracting his tendency to isolation and depression. Of all the cures, wine elicits the most fulsome praise. Three ancient authorities in turn endorse its powerful benefits. According to Rufus, it is a strong medicine for the timid, the sad, and lovers. Galen reckons the first winemaker among the wisest men, and Zeno describes its ability to leach discontent from the soul. The benefits of wine are at their best, says Constantine, if the drinking is among friends who are outstanding in beauty, knowledge or morals.[47] The physical and moral excellence of the lover's drinking companions redirects his fixation toward more worthy objects. If this relaxing but not somniferous conversation can take place in gardens, so much the better. It will be most pleasant if they

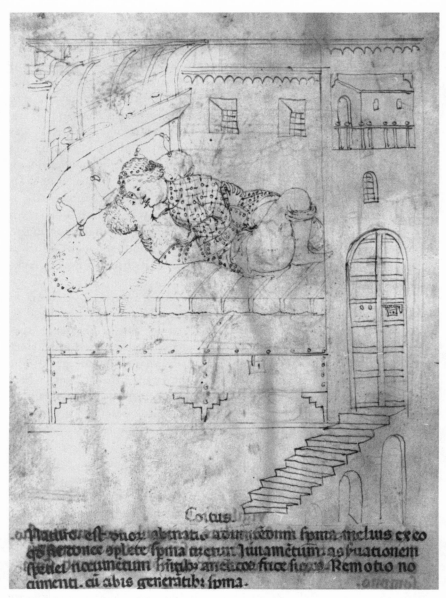

*Figure 2.3.* Coitus, one of the "non-naturals" upon whose regulation health depends, is illustrated in the health handbook *Tacuinum sanitatis*. Bibliothèque générale, Université de Liège, MS 1041, fol. 69v.

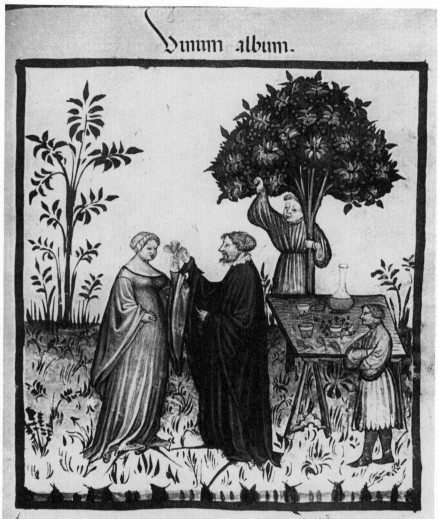

*Figure 2.4.* Drinking wine with a good-looking companion in a fruit-bearing garden. Vienna, Bildarchiv, Österreichische Nationalbibliothek, Cod. ser. nov. 2644, fol. 86r.

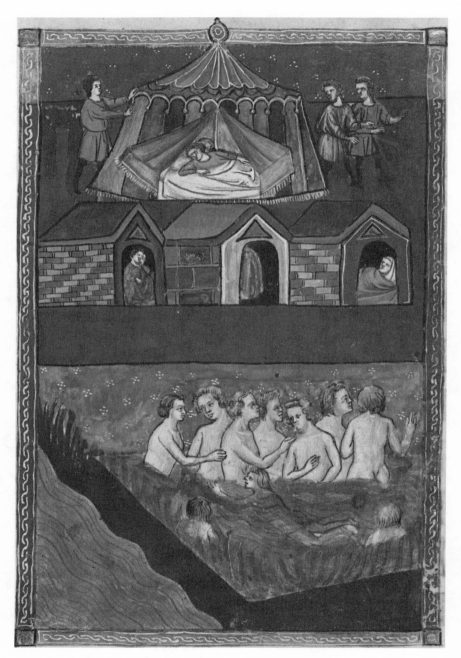

*Figure 2.5.* Bathing was often a social activity in the Middle Ages, offering distraction from preoccupation as well as physical therapy. Bath of Iuncara, from Pietro da Eboli's *De balneis Puteolanis.* New York, The Pierpont Morgan Library, G 74, fol. 6.

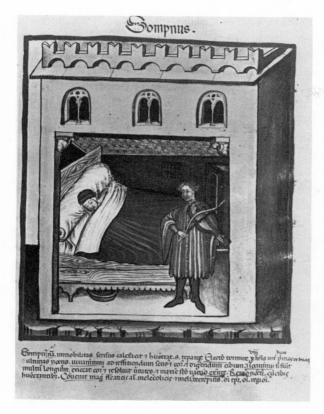

Ṡompnꝰ.

Ꝼompnꝰiũ. immobilitas fenſuſ caleฟacit �7 huฟecʊꞇ.ง. ꞇepaꞇꝛꞇ Ꝯꞇecꞇꝺ ꞇꞅꞇmꞇꞃ.p̃ꞃ̃iꞃ tū̃ Ꞇิꞇnꜳꞡꞻ cꞇbuꜳꞡ
ultⱳꞇ iꞃ̃ꞇꞇꞇꞃ.uꞇꞇꞇꞇꞇꞇꞇꞇ ꜳꞡ ꞇꞻꞇꞇꞇꞇꞇꞇꞇꞇꞇꞇꞇ feꞃꞻ ꞇ ꞇ ꞇ ꞇ ꞇ oiꝺꞡꞇꞃꞇꞇꞡꞇ cꞇbuꜳꞡ ᶴꞇcꞇꞇꞃiꞡꞇꞻ ꞇ ฟㅇ̃uⱳꞇ
mulꞇฟ ꞇꞇꞇꞡꞇꞇꞇ. ꞇꞃꞇฟꜳꞇ ꞇꞡꞇꞇ 7 ꞇฟfoluⱳꞇ ꞇฟꞇꞇꞇꞇꞇ.ᓇ ꞇꞇꞇฟꞇꞡ ㅇꞻꞇ uⱳꞡꞇuꞇ ꞇꞇꞇฟꞇꞇꞇꞇ ᶴꞡꞇ̃ꞇꞇꞇꞡꞇ̃ꞇ. ꞡꞇฟ ꞇฟbꞇꞻ
ฟuꞇꞇꞇꞇꞇꞇꞇꞇบꞻ. Ꝯꞇꞇ̃uⱳꞇ̃uⱳꞇ ꞇꞇꜳꞡ ฟꞇꜳꞇꜳꞇꜳฟꞇ.ꜳꞇ.ꞇꞇꞇฟꞇ̃ฟꞇฟꞇ ꞇꞇꞇฟꞇꞇꞇꞇꞇꞇฟꞇꞇꞇฟ̃.ㅇꞇ ꞇꞇꞇ.ㅇꞇ.ꞇꞡꞇㅇꞇ.

*Figure 2.6.* According to the *Tacuinum sanitatis,* sleep is a suitable cure for, among others, the melancholic. The power of music to soothe is also implied in the illustration. Vienna, Bildarchiv, Österreichische Nationalbibliothek, Cod. ser. nov. 2644, fol. 100r.

are bright, sweet-smelling, and fruit-bearing (Figure 2.4). If this is not possible, the rooms where the people are to sit should be strewn with salutary herbs like roses ("good for inflamed brains" according to the *Tacuinum sanitatis*), myrtle, willow, and basil.

Bathing, like wine drinking, was supposed to alter the humoral balance as well as to restore equanimity. Constantine recommends that bathing follow sleep, and that the water and air be bright and temperate. Some patients are so heartened when they enter the baths, he notes, that they begin to sing. Since bathing in the Middle Ages was a social activity (Figure 2.5),[48] Constantine cautions that the patient should be shielded from repugnant people while bathing, and reinforces the point with a brief anecdote. Philosophers once asked someone why a horrible man is worse than any burden (*pondus*). He replied that while other weights are borne by body and soul together, a horrible man is a burden to the soul alone.

Music too is a therapy with both physical and psychological benefits.

Some philosophers even claim a kind of synergy for music and wine: sound, they say, is like spirit, and wine like the body, each of which aids the other. Both ancient and medieval medicine prescribed music for its therapeutic effects.[49] Constantine quotes "Orpheus" to reveal music's power to alter moods. Though emperors invite him to perform for their pleasure, he in turn takes pleasure in them because he can change their souls as he pleases—from anger to mildness, from sadness to joy, from avarice to generosity, from fear to boldness (Figure 2.6).

"Recitation of verses" was also supposed to alleviate the patient's obsession with a particular woman.[50] As Avicenna recognized, sometimes this strategy only served to reinforce the lover's preoccupation, especially when the songs were about unsuccessful love. Constantine, in contrast, though giving the cure only the briefest mention, introduces no doubts as to its efficacy. This particular cure provided a fertile point of convergence between the medical tradition of lovesickness and literary representations of passionate love. From the twelfth century onwards, fictional characters or lyric personae claim to compose or sing in order to relieve love-sorrow, and in the hands of Dante, Boccaccio, and Chaucer, the lovesick poet or poetic lover was variously reinterpreted according to medical ideas about lovesickness.

## Johannes Afflacius and the "Liber de heros morbo"

The study of Constantine's chapter on love and the Western understanding of lovesickness has been both enriched and complicated by the discovery of a "second edition" of Ibn al-Jazzār's chapter on ʿishk. As I have argued elsewhere, its author may have been Constantine's pupil Johannes Afflacius, who used both the Arabic version and the *Viaticum* to produce a smoother, less ambiguous text which circulated under the manuscript rubric *Liber de heros morbo*.[51] That the *Viaticum's* chapter on lovesickness enjoyed a second edition as an independent treatise suggests that European readers were sufficiently interested in this new technical discourse on passionate love to justify the effort of retranslation.

·   Appended to the text is the explicit: "Finit liber heroice passionis" (here ends the book of the disease heros); throughout, forms of the word *heroicus* replace Constantine's *eriosis* and *eriosos* as designations of the patients. In the context of the *Liber de heros morbo, heroicus* means "those who suffer from the disease *heros*"—a new and unique meaning. The previously attested semantic range of *heroicus* includes the obvious "belonging to a hero" as well as a peculiar medieval sense "belonging to a lord or nobleman," documented as early as the sixth century. Just as Constantine introduced the neologism *eriosis*, so Johannes (or whoever was the author of the *Liber*) reforged *heroicus* as a technical medical term for passionate lovers. Whether *heros* was adopted from a *Viaticum* manuscript or whether it was intended as a deliberate contrast to *eros* finds no easy answer in the evidence at hand. Whatever its origin, does the translation of ʿishk as *heros* testify to a nascent concept of love as a "noble passion"? One change made in the Latin definition of ʿishk suggests that some of the usual meanings of *heros* consciously or unconsciously shaped the explanation. Whereas Constantine says that just as loyalty is the most extreme form of affection, so eros is the most intense form of pleasure, the *Liber* alters the terms of the contrast. Instead of distinguishing between the *qualities* of love (affection, pleasure), it does so between the *objects* of love: "Just as fidelity is immoderate love for a lord, so heros is immoderate love for those to be possessed (sexually)." By comparing intense sexual love to loyalty to a lord, the *Liber de heros morbo* collocates passion and service as early as 1100 in a way that was to become conventional in certain twelfth-century literary traditions. Though there is "a long and large difference," as Chaucer's Merchant would say, between *heros morbus* and the erotic suffering of stylized love service in later medieval literature, the *Liber heroice passionis* is nonetheless a harbinger of the cultural transvaluations of both *amor* and *passio* in the twelfth and thirteenth centuries, when idealized love-suffering gradually shifted from cultural fantasy to social reality.[52]

## *The* Viaticum*'s Popularity and Influence*

With its flourishing scriptorium and its proximity to the medical school at Salerno, Montecassino was well-placed for the diffusion of Constantine's translations. Although the degree of Constantine's immediate impact on Salernitan medicine has been controversial, recent scholarship has affirmed his early influence on Salernitan writers.[53] Johannes Afflacius may have been instrumental in introducing his mentor's works to the Salernitans.[54] Constantine's other student, Atto, who was chaplain to empress Agnes, also helped the diffusion of his master's works by either paraphrasing them in Latin or translating them into the vernacular. Though none of these versions appears to have survived (unless the *Liber de heros morbo* is the joint work of Johannes and Atto), they suggest an immediate interest in the newly available medical learning on the part of lay readers as well as physicians.

Through imperial courtiers like Atto and through Montecassino's wide-ranging ties in Europe the new Constantinian corpus spread relatively quickly throughout the West. His works are found as early as the 1130s in

Chartres, 1161 in Hildesheim, and appear in twelfth-century library catalogues in St. Amand and Durham.[55] In the first half of the thirteenth century Richard de Fournival listed the *liber passionarius quem Viaticum vocat* in his library catalogue, and in the fourteenth Simon Bredon, a physician and Fellow of Merton College (d. 1372), bequeathed a glossed copy to Roger Aswardby, asking him to return it to the owner; if the owner could not be found, he was to give it to any physician who lacked it, which suggests that many doctors were expected to own a copy.[56] The German physician Amplonius Ratinck (d. ca. 1434), whose library is now at Erfurt, owned five glossed copies of the *Viaticum*.[57] Private owners of the work are well attested in England, where they have been traced through donations to libraries.[58]

With the rise of more formal medical education at the medieval universities, the *Viaticum* entered the standard medical curriculum. Alexander Neckham's list of textbooks shows that the *Viaticum* was read at Paris by the end of the twelfth century, and in the statutes of 1270–74, the bachelor of medicine was required to hear it in order to be licensed.[59] Though documentary evidence is not as abundant for the medical school at Oxford as it is for Paris, Oxford seems to have followed Parisian practice; thus it is likely that the *Viaticum* was read there as well.[60] Constantine's work may have been known to an even wider audience than the candidates for medical degrees, since many students at Oxford studied medicine without receiving a degree in it.[61] The statutes for the medical school at Cambridge date from the late fourteenth century (a fire in 1381 wiped out earlier records) and were based on those at Oxford. Since the *Viaticum* was among the required texts there, we may infer its use at Oxford as well.[62]

Though legend attributes the foundation of the medical school at Montpellier to a student of Constantine the African, the *Viaticum* seems not to have been intensively studied there in the middle of the thirteenth century. By the early fourteenth century, however, Montpellier physicians quoted it in their own works.[63]

*Concordantiae*, which were general medical dictionaries arranged alphabetically, attest to the particular importance of the *Viaticum*'s chapter on love. Entries were usually brief and referred the reader to the standard authorities on the subject.[64] Jean de St. Amand ( Johannes de Sancto Amando), a professor of medicine at Paris in the late thirteenth century (d. before 1312), drew up a concordance, or as Sarton calls it, "a dictionary of internal pathology," based primarily on the works of Galen and Avicenna.[65] The *Viaticum* is occasionally cited and appears in the entry for *amor hereos*. The reader of this entry in Jean's concordance, after learning of Galen's famous diagnosis of lovesickness by alterations of the pulse, is referred to Constantine and Avicenna: "De ista materia habes I° (primo) viatici et III° (tertio)

Avicennae" (Concerning this material see the first book of the *Viaticum* and the third book of Avicenna).[66] Jean's concordance was revised by Pierre de St. Flour (Petrus de Sancto Floro), who received his degree as bachelor of medicine at Paris in 1349.[67] Under the entry *amor hereos* Pierre lists al-Rāzī, Averroes and Constantine as authorities, and he also quotes Avicenna's definition of *ilisci* (ʿishk) from the *Canon*. These concordances testify that Constantine and Avicenna were considered the standard authorities on the subject of lovesickness in the thirteenth and fourteenth centuries. The final form of medical writing that allows us to judge the importance and influence of the *Viaticum* in the Middle Ages, glosses and commentaries, is the subject of the following chapters.

The *Viaticum's* division of the causes of passionate love into physical and psychological paralleled the growing dualism of twelfth-century habits of mind, with their tendency to see reality in terms of matter and spirit, outer surface and inner reality. As a disease caused by humoral imbalance, *amor eros* reminded the medievals of their materiality, their subjection to environmental forces and to time. Perhaps medicine even gave them license to enjoy that materiality a bit, by prescribing actual pleasures—women, wine, and baths—to replace the anticipated pleasure of union with the beloved.

The historical record has left no details on patients treated by practitioners who consulted the *Viaticum*. Using recent investigations of the implications of literacy, we can, however, sketch the probable effect of the *Viaticum* and the *Liber de heros morbo* on medieval society. Among the consequences of the spread of literacy, Stock argues, are the formation of "new rituals of everyday life."[68] In the eleventh and twelfth centuries, new texts and changed methods of interpreting old ones introduced new values that in turn reshaped social behavior. This was likely to happen with medicine, which is by its very nature a pragmatic social interchange among healer, patient, and family.[69] New ideas from Arabic medicine—ʿishk and *amor eros*—had the potential for transforming the social practices associated with love. While it is true, as I have argued in the first chapter, that Biblical and classical literary conceptions of lovesickness, as well as folk ideas about love madness, aided the reception of Arabic medical ideas, the new medicine gave the West a different sort of model of erotic action and passion.

As medical texts, they had scientific authority and were viewed as empirical descriptions of reality, that is, of the social reality of humans in health, disease, and states in between. They *had* to be seen as empirical descriptions if medicine was to have any practical effect—and we need to recall that the *Viaticum* was above all else intended as a practical handbook.

The love that was the subject of the physician's concerns was neither literary fable nor spiritual allegory, but a psychosomatic disorder requiring treatment. The disease of love, as we may gather from the commentaries on Constantine and Avicenna, from medical texts and vernacular literature, gradually rooted itself in medieval mentalities, shaping both intellect and affect. By the late Middle Ages, lovesickness had become an effective ploy in the amorous intrigues of the nobility.[70] The medical texts also confirmed the "reality" of the disease in a second way, by granting the physician the authority to intervene in the patient's emotional life. His power to diagnose a certain pattern of behavior as love turned disease and to prescribe cures for it also gave him the power to reshape perceptions of love. In other words, medicine offered a new interpretive model for explaining certain symptoms of appearance and behavior.

The shift from oral to scribal culture enabled people to pattern their lives on texts to a new degree; as Stock claims, interpretive models influenced experience. With the diffusion of *Viaticum* manuscripts and their assimilation into intellectual life, Constantine's description of intense, debilitating love was available for conscious or unconscious imitation. It potentially generated both a particular experience of love and the means for reflecting upon or classifying that experience. Finally, the description of love as illness lent a powerful and ongoing presumption of reality to the evolving love conventions of the literature emanating from courts and urban centers of medieval Europe. The growing body of medical discourse on love made it possible for the literary representations of erotic passion to be interpreted mimetically or realistically, as reflections of real life. The cultural authority of medicine may have in part enabled the poetic fantasies of the troubadours to become the social realities of the late Middle Ages and early modernity.

## §§ 3 §§

# "NOBLE" LOVE
## Gerard of Berry's
## *Glosses on the Viaticum*

Ecstatic love is taken in another way, for love that alienates the mind . . . which indeed is called among physicians *amor ereos*. For *amor ereos* is a great desire with excessive concupiscence and affliction of the thoughts. *Ereos* are said to be noble men who, because of softness and pleasures of life are subject to this sort of passion.

Hugh of St. Cher[1]

In the century after Constantine had renewed the vigor of European medicine, the discipline itself and its relations to medieval culture underwent profound transformations. The Constantinian translations awakened medicine's philosophical aspirations, which were strengthened by encounter with the new translations of Aristotle and Arabic science issuing from Spain. Institutionally, medicine became associated with the newly-formed universities, where it entered into dialogue with other disciplines, particularly in the arts faculty. Increasingly professionalized and secularized, medicine in the late twelfth and early thirteenth centuries began to achieve recognition both as an intellectual discipline and as a socially important profession.[2]

Between Constantine and Gerard of Berry, who wrote the earliest surviving commentary on the *Viaticum*, also lies the first flourishing of vernacular courtly literature, in which the European nobility fashioned its dream of romantic love. Lyric poems, lais, and romances depicted the passions of "noble hearts." Drawing upon Ovid and perhaps the *Viaticum* and/or the *Liber de heros morbo*, vernacular poets explored the process of falling in love and noted its tell-tale signs.[3] By the end of the century love in imaginative literature had become so conventionalized that Andreas Capellanus (d. after 1191) could codify and spoof the rules for loving in *De amore* (ca. 1181–86), a treatise with which Gerard's chapter on love shows a number of similarities.[4]

Gerard's commentary on *amor (h)eros*, marked by the Aristotelianism of Salerno and the Arabism of Montpellier, reveals the complex crosscurrents of medical, literary, and religious languages on the subject of passionate love around 1200. The importance of his contribution to technical medical discourse on love can be gauged by the large number of surviving manuscripts of his *Glosses on the Viaticum* and by the frequency with which he was quoted by other medical writers on lovesickness. Amplonius Ratinck, a fifteenth-century physician and bibliophile, collected no fewer than five copies of Gerard of Berry's commentary on the *Viaticum*.[5] The medical community of the thirteenth and fourteenth centuries shared Amplonius' high appraisal of Gerard's work: at least seventy-five manuscripts of the *Glosule super Viaticum* (*Glosses on the Viaticum*) have survived into the twentieth century. His work was so influential because, as we shall see, he gave physicians a language for analyzing the pathology of love, for tying emotional states to material conditions in the body.[6]

Calling himself "Magister Gerardus Bituricensis, professione phisicus," Gerard says in the prologue that he compiled his commentary at the request of his Parisian colleagues in order to remedy the excessive brevity of the *Viaticum's* discussions of causes, signs, and cures, and to supplement what was ignored by his predecessors.[7] He also says that he will omit *experimenta*, that is, empirical formulations that cannot be theorized, from Salerno and Montpellier, except for a few that have been well-tested by experience. We may infer, then, that he taught medicine, and that his commentary, like the others in this volume, grew out of classroom instruction (Figure 3.1).

Gerard's work may be provisionally placed in the last decades of the twelfth century. At the latest it must have been composed by 1236, the date of the earliest manuscript, a date also supported by Hugh of St. Cher's quotation of Gerard on *amor hereos* around 1235.[8] However, another citation of Gerard points to an earlier date. The Salernitan master Bernardus Provincialis explicitly attributes to Gerard a discussion of monstrous afterbirths called "brother of the Lombards" in a commentary on the *Tables of Salernus*.[9] De Renzi argues that Bernard's commentary should be dated around 1150–60, based on his failure to quote Salernitan authors from the second half of the century.[10] The one citation that would cast doubt on the date, he says, is of Gerard on the *Viaticum*. De Renzi's solution was to see in a certain Gerard, nobleman and physician, whose activities are attested near Salerno in 1184, the author of the commentary on the *Viaticum*.[11] There are problems with this solution. First, Gerard explicitly says that he wrote at the instigation of his Parisian colleagues. Given the relatively backward state of Parisian medicine before Gilles de Corbeil's (ca. 1140–ca. 1224) arrival

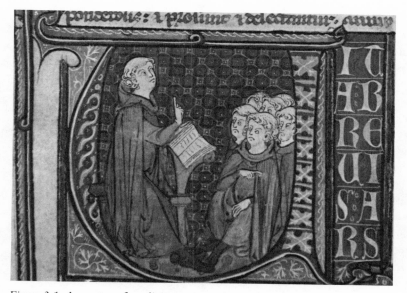

*Figure 3.1.* A master of medicine apparently teaches to the back of the room while a disgruntled student points to the text "Life is short" (the opening words of the first Hippocratic Aphorism). Vienna, Bildarchiv, Österreichische Nationalbibliothek, Cod. 2315, fol. 1r.

around 1194, it is difficult to imagine that Gerard wrote the commentary in Paris before 1160 and then moved to the preeminent medical center of Europe, Salerno, to continue his activities.[12] Second, Gerard uses Avicenna's *Liber de anima* and *Canon medicinae*. The *Canon* was translated before 1187 (the death of Gerard of Cremona), the *De anima* between 1152 and 1166.[13] A date as early as 1150–60 therefore seems unlikely for either Bernardus Provincialis or Gerard.

Several other discussions of *arpia* or *frater lombardorum* do however suggest a general date of 1180–1200 for Gerard's activity, as well as corroborate his Salernitan and Parisian connections. The anonymous Salernitan commentator of about mid-century and the Salernitan master Bartholomaeus, active in the third quarter of the twelfth century, both mention the unusual condition.[14] It also appears in a *Prose Salernitan Question* attributed to "master Alan," who may be identical with Alain de Lille (d. 1203), in a manuscript that originated in Paris in the late twelfth century; Gilles de Corbeil also mentions it.[15] Gerard thus seems to have borrowed from and contributed to this tradition, which would place his activity in roughly the last quarter of the twelfth century.

Although Gerard drew together his glosses on *amor hereos* in Paris in the age of Philip Augustus (1165–1223), the case of the *frater lombardorum* suggests a Salernitan background or strong Salernitan connections. As we have seen, the Salernitan author Bernardus Provincialis was familiar with Gerard's commentary not long after it was written, which suggests close ties to that center. Gerard's treatise also shows affinities with the works of Maurus (d. 1214) and Urso (d. 1225), Salernitan authors of the late twelfth century, and indeed, the commentary form itself is in line with the commentary tradition of twelfth-century Salerno.[16] Furthermore, his choice of the *Viaticum* as an authoritative text on which to comment again suggests connections with Salerno rather than with Montpellier, since the *Viaticum* had little impact at the latter school before the middle of the thirteenth century.[17]

Yet Gerard's relatively early use of Avicenna points to the influence of Montpellier, first of the medical centers to come to terms with the Toledan translations.[18] It is possible that Gerard's refusal to discuss the *experimenta* of Salerno and Montpellier is a response to his Parisian colleagues' expectations that he bring them up to date on the practices of those leading medical centers of the time based on his experiences there. Travel among medical schools was not uncommon: Gilles de Corbeil (ca. 1140–1224), for example, in whose Parisian medical circle Gerard may have been active, studied at Salerno, stayed briefly in Montpellier, and then settled in Paris.[19] However, in the absence of any direct evidence for Gerard's peregrinations among the medical schools, one can say at the minimum that the major currents of late-twelfth-century medicine (Salernitan Aristotelianism and the Arabism of Montpellier) are evident in his commentary, and that he is one of the earliest witnesses in Paris for the reception of Avicenna's psychology and medicine.

## Scientific Interests

Gerard's prologue reveals that the *Viaticum* was important enough to be worth glossing, but at the same time was felt to be inadequate in some respects. Though the work is clear in many places, he says, "if anyone wishes to scrutinize it carefully, he will find many difficulties in the causes, signs and cures of the diseases." Gerard remedies this deficiency by adding what he considers necessary from Avicenna, al-Rāzī, Alexander, and others.[20]

The prologue is worth a brief analysis because it provides an overall context for the specific content of Gerard's chapter on *amor hereos*. It amounts to a defense of medicine as a science—that is, a discipline whose subject is capable of being known through its causes. It is divided into three parts: a general exposition of why a physician must know elements and causes; an explanation of the work's origin; and an *accessus* to Constantine's text.[21]

The argument of the first part runs as follows. Every element and the human body as composed of elements share materiality and thus the capacity for mutual changing and being changed. The human body does not escape these motions and changes, not only because of its diverse material composition, but also because it suffers passions (*passiones*) by reason of which the medical "artifex" considers the human body as subject. Therefore the artifex must know and consider each element and bodies generated from elements so that the causes of the subject and its passions may be plainly evident.[22] Indeed, in every art the causes of the subject and of passions are interlinked; the physician recognizes that they are necessarily generically the same, since they are principles of knowing and of being. As Avicenna says, a thing is truly known when it is known of what it consists and from what it receives perfection in being.

Gerard is concerned, then, to place the microcosm of the human body within the macrocosm of elemental change. In so doing he can establish the claim of medicine to scientific status, since it can proceed through knowledge of causes, reduced, in this approach, to their material and efficient aspects. The human body is subject to illness and is the physician's subject insofar as it is material and resolvable into elements, analytically and actually.

Not every aspect of elemental causality is relevant to the different forms of medicine. The natural philosopher (*phisicus naturalis*) considers the "four radical causes" in themselves without comparison to other things. Theoretical medicine considers the elements in comparison with the human body and the balanced temperament. Practical medicine considers elements in comparison with particular conditions, like place, time, complexion, age, and sex. Practical medicine in turn may be general or particular—what to do in particular circumstances—and this is the heading under which Gerard places the *Viaticum*.

In light of the prologue, then, the chapter on *amor hereos* can be seen as Gerard's effort to establish a truly scientific, that is, natural philosophic, discourse on morbid love, one that offers a knowledge of causes. To construct his account, he draws upon two works of Avicenna (d. 1087), the *Canon medicine* and the *Liber de anima*. From the former he borrows the definition and some symptoms and cures for lovesickness (ʿishk). The latter work gives Gerard the means, through faculty psychology, to relate mental and emotional conditions to physical states, that is, to specify their material basis.

The essay on *amor heros*, as Gerard terms it, is bipartite: a definition, causal analysis, and discussion of symptoms and cures are followed by a series of glosses on specific words of Constantine's text.[23] Though brief, the glosses are of particular interest, since their emphases on the master text as well as their content reveal the interpreter's "selective will."[24] While Gerard's essay on love develops within the bounds of Galenic medical materialism and Avicennan faculty psychology, his glosses on particular phrases of Constantine's text suggest a broader intellectual and literary understanding of love. They are a particularly revealing "hermeneutic filter" through which a medical view of love situated itself in a broader cultural context.

## Causality

Paraphrasing Avicenna's definition of love in the *Canon*, Gerard describes it as a melancholic worry. It is similar to melancholy because the entire mental attention and thought, aided by desire, is fixed on the beauty of a form. Gerard then explains why this type of love is melancholic and how the fixation occurs, giving both material and dynamic aspects of the process.

Gerard begins by noting the difficulty of causal analysis, but continues anyway to explain that the disease of love is caused by a misfunctioning of the estimative faculty. This term derives from faculty psychology, which localizes mental functions such as perceiving, judging, and remembering in specific parts of the brain. The condition of the brain's substance in turn affects the function of the mental faculties or "inward wits." The classification of the mental faculties was by no means uniform; it varied from author to author and sometimes within the work of a single author.

According to Avicenna, on whose account of mental faculties in *Liber de anima* Gerard draws,[25] the estimative faculty is the one that makes "instinctive" judgments about what is to be pursued or avoided: when the lamb flees from the wolf, it does so at the prompting of the *virtus estimativa*. In lovesickness the estimative faculty misfunctions because it is misled by an excessively pleasing sense perception, so strong that it eclipses other sense impressions that might contradict it. Hence the estimation judges a form to be better, more noble, and more desirable than all others: it has "overestimated" the object. Because the estimative faculty is working too hard, innate heat and *spiritus* rush to the middle cerebral ventricle where the faculty resides, leaving the first ventricle, the site of the imaginative faculty, too cold and dry—melancholic, in fact (Figure 3.2). This produces a "bad complexion" or balance of humors that in turn affects the imaginative faculty's operation: the image adheres abnormally strongly on the "screen," so to speak, of the first ventricle; as Gerard puts it, the imaginative faculty becomes fixated on the image.

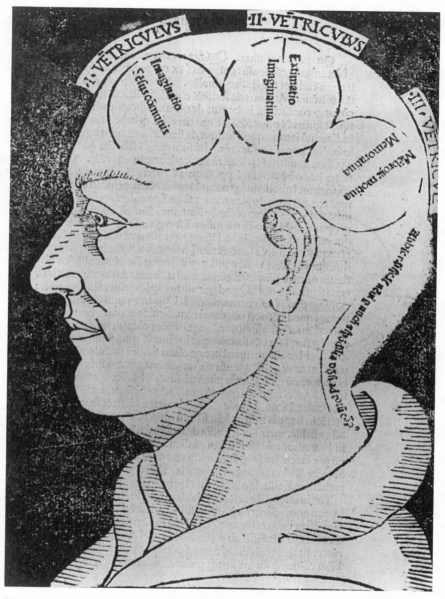

*Figure 3.2.* A diagram of the three cerebral ventricles and the mental faculties located within them. The first ventricle contains common sense and imagination, the second the imaginative and estimative faculties, the third the faculties of memory and bodily motion. Albertus Magnus, *Philosophia pauperum, sive Philosophia naturalis,* 1490. Bethesda, Maryland, History of Medicine Division, National Library of Medicine.

When he localizes the imaginative faculty in the first ventricle of the brain, Gerard departs from Avicenna's account of the mental faculties. Moreover, Avicenna places little emphasis on the *spiritus*, a key feature of Gerard's attempt "to fuse psychology, physiology, and physical causation."[26] Both imagination and *spiritus* are, however, central to Salernitan teachings on the psychophysiology of desire. Urso of Calabria, a contemporary of Gerard's whose works were much read in Paris, wrote extensively in his *Glosses on Aphorisms* about the interactions of body and soul, and on the psychological and physiological processes of desire. Very similar to Urso's teaching is one of the *Prose Salernitan Questions* (before 1200) attributed to Alain de Lille ("Master Alan"). The parallels between Gerard's account and the Salernitan question are striking, particularly on the roles of *spiritus* and imagination in generating lovesickness. In answer to the question "Why do we strive for the forbidden?" Master Alan explains:

> The soul has three cells destined for its operations, the first of which is the fantastic, in which occurs imagination, which is called the appetite of the soul, which is hot and dry. *Spiritus* are so to speak instruments of the soul by which it works. Appetite thus is aroused by nature through heat and dryness, and if the desired thing is denied, heat and dryness do not cease; rather they increase more and the consumption of humors is greater, and the humors rarefy further; once rarefied, they are moved more, and, moved, they excite the appetitive faculty, and thus appetite grows greater and greater. Whence the appetite must be satisfied or the destruction of the subject follows. . . . Because of excessive pleasure the *spiritus* are moved more, and frequently, and immoderately, and [so is] the imagination, whence its cell grows hotter and dries out and the *spiritus* rarefies more. Once rarefied they are moved more, whence follows greater imagination, and it replicates the desired thing more. Thus we see lovers sometimes become mad (*maniacos*) because of excessive thought and imagination.[27]

Master Alan outlines a psychophysiology of desire in which the *spiritus* mediate the dynamic, destructive interchanges of mind and body. Gerard may well have blended Salernitan theories of imaginative desire such as those of Alan or Urso with Avicenna's faculty psychology in order to explain the causes of *amor heros*.[28]

Unlike Master Alan, however, Gerard describes the interplay of mental faculties responsible for the lover's affliction in hierarchical metaphors. Closely following Avicenna's *De anima*, he retains the language of male governance that the "prince of physicians" uses to describe the functioning of the mental faculties. After receiving a powerfully pleasing sense impression, the estimative faculty, the *noblest* of the perceptual faculties, *orders* the imaginative faculty to fix its gaze on the mental image of the beloved. The imaginative faculty in turn *orders* the concupiscible faculty to desire that person alone. The concupiscible *obeys* the imaginative, which *obeys* the estimative, at whose *rule* (*imperium*) the other faculties *are inclined toward* the desired person, even though she may not be desirable in reality.[29] The inner world of perception and desire is thus structured like the outer system of hierarchical rule: those at the top rule and give orders, those below bow and obey. The pathological moment thus subverts the "noble" faculty of estimation from below.

Finally, the glosses to individual phrases of the *Viaticum* reinforce the foregoing etiological analysis. In explaining Constantine's dual causality (the need to expel excess humor and the sight of beauty), Gerard remarks that the humoral cause is not the cause of "true love" (*amorem verum*); rather, the sight of beauty that sends a soul mad "touches the cause of true love." Thus, while he accepts an ultimately Platonic notion of love as generated by the sight of beauty, he nonetheless materializes it by reducing it analytically in the foregoing essay to its material and mechanical components.

In addition, six of the glosses focus on statements in the *Viaticum* that suggest the close relation of body and soul. Gerard emphasizes their reciprocal effects: the soul is moved to its actions according to the various natural and accidental complexions of the body, yet the soul's passions in turn can affect the body. For example, Gerard says that Constantine compares sound to spirit (*sonitum esse quasi spiritum*) because the soul intensely delights in music; that joy is transferred to the body, because the soul is greatly "befriended" (*amicatur*) by the body. Hence Constantine teaches remedies for both body and soul.

The technicalities of faculty psychology and humoral theory can easily obscure the implications of Gerard's analysis of the causes of love for the notion of subjectivity in the Middle Ages. If it is true that the subject is constituted by "a distinct inner space with a law of its own," as Bloch says, then Gerard's chapter on love, together with the Salernitan and Avicennan texts on which it rests, may be seen as an important contribution to medieval subjectivity.[30] The medical writers trace out the interior space that defines man both as the subject of medicine and as a desiring subject who suffers the *accidentia* of that desire. Faculty psychology and the mixing of elements provide the "laws" that regulate the interior space and its exterior manifestations. Earlier than the thirteenth-century allegorical poems to which Bloch refers, writers like Gerard, Urso, and Master Alan offer "full-blown dynamic model[s] of the mind."[31] Evidence that medicine did provide such a model, and that its utility was quickly perceived, lies ready to hand in the adoption of the medical language of love for the innermost world of mystical experience by William of Auvergne, William of Auxerre, Hugh of St. Cher and others.[32]

## Love and Nobility

In general Gerard prefers to offer knowledge based on causes rather than the form of cognition represented by Isidore's etymologies, which conflate "the qualities of things and their origin," and which assume the natural unity of linguistic signs and their referents.[33] Nonetheless, the Parisian physician's explanation of the name *amor heros* betrays the persistence of the etymologizing habit of mind Isidore bequeathed to the Middle Ages. The "confusion" of *eros, heros* (hero), and *herus* (lord) invoked to explain the transformation of *eros* to *hereos* in fact reveals that etymology was a useful prop for a medical theory whose causal explanations did not extend to social factors.[34]

The manuscript of the *Viaticum* upon which Gerard based his glosses contained the reading: "love that is called *heros*." The Parisian master glosses: "Heroes are said to be noble men who, because of their wealth and the softness of their lives, suffer the more from this disease." Did Gerard know the *Liber de heros morbo*, which, as I have argued elsewhere, linked love and nobility as early as the early twelfth century?[35] In view of the currently limited manuscript evidence for the *Liber*, such a claim would be difficult to maintain. Gerard's explanation may simply reflect the fact that "noble" was available as a meaning of *heros* as much in the late twelfth

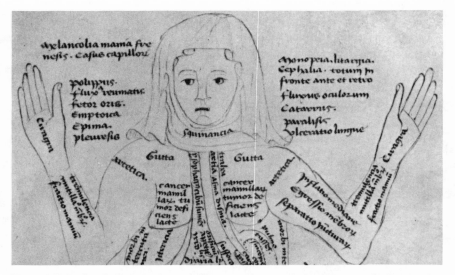

*Figure 3.3.* Melancholia, mania, and phrenesis, but not lovesickness, which was thought to be a disease of noble men, are listed among the diseases of the head on this "disease woman." Paris, Bibliothèque Nationale, MS lat. 11229, fol. 31r.

century as when the *Liber* was composed. The *Liber* and Gerard's chapter would then be parallel manifestations of the same cultural need to attribute an extreme form of passionate love to the nobility.

For Gerard that linkage is firmly based in medical considerations. In keeping with his materialist bent, he argues that the material conditions of wealth and leisure, typical of the nobility, predispose an individual to lovesickness. As Constantine's *De coitu* indicates, "a leisured heart (*cor ociosum*) and daily joy increase libido."[36] Given that Gerard associates lovesickness and melancholy, *De melancholia* may offer another relevant gloss on Gerard's attribution of love to the nobility. It teaches that a great deal of sweetness, rest, and sleep allow digestive products to collect, which can in time turn into black bile and cause melancholy.[37] Because the noble way of life ran the double danger of generating excessive libido and melancholy, it is easy to see how the medical profession could label love an occupational hazard of the nobility. It became another mark of precedence, like wealth and leisure themselves.

Gerard may likewise have found support for the nobility's melancholic love in the pseudo-Aristotelian *Problem* on melancholy. As translated into Latin by the Parisian master David of Dinant (before 1210), the problem asks why all those principally concerned with philosophy, civic affairs, poetry, or other arts appear to have been melancholic and to have suffered from diseases of black bile. Among the heroes (*de heroibus*) Hercules was one such victim of melancholy. Many of those who suffer from melancholy are also libidinous, because sexual desire arises from the fumosity or smokiness of black bile.[38] The conjunction of black bile and libido in men of accomplishment, who in the Middle Ages would have ordinarily belonged to the nobility, would have lent further scientific weight to Gerard's designation of lovesickness as "heroic love."

As a deferral, albeit unwilling, of instinctual satisfactions that wealth and leisure can command, *amor heros* distinguished the noble from the base. It does not appear, for example, among the common ailments described in the *Thesaurus pauperum* (*Treasury of the poor*), a handbook for those too poor to afford the elite care of a university-trained physician.[39] Nor is it found among the diseases of the head in the schematic guide to common diseases and their bodily localizations in Figure 3.3. The absence of love from this and similar diagrams suggests the restricted epidemiology of *amor heros*.

## Lovesickness and Noble Love: Gerard and Andreas Capellanus

In its association with the nobility, *amor heros* begins to resemble the conventionalizing and aestheticizing of erotic life known variously to modern scholars as "noble love," "courtly love," "fin'amors," and so on. Andreas Capellanus, who may have been a contemporary of Gerard's in Paris, defines love as follows: "Love is a certain suffering (*passio*) born within, proceeding from the sight and immoderate cogitation on a form of the opposite sex, on account of which one desires above all things to enjoy the embraces of another and by mutual wish to fulfill all the precepts of love in the embrace of the other" (1.1.1).[40] Though rhetorically more elaborate and lacking reference to melancholy, his definition resembles Gerard's: "This disease (*passio*) . . . is very similar to melancholy, because the entire attention and thought, aided by desire, is fixed on the beauty of some form or figure." Like the physician, Andreas too recognizes imagination's role in passionate love. "The true lover is engaged without interruption by the continual imagination of his beloved" (2.8.48). Imaginative preoccupation in fact defines the type of love that Andreas spoofs.

The two works also share an interest in the nobility's relation to passionate love. In keeping with his interest in the effect of class difference on erotic behavior, which structures the dialogues of the first book, Andreas insists that love not only makes an ugly woman beautiful, but also makes a low-born one noble in the sight of the lover (1.6.181), a claim that is reminiscent of Gerard's description of the lover's "overestimation" of the beloved as more noble than she is in reality. Andreas also contends that nobility derived from moral excellence is the best reason for loving (1.6.13–15). Granted that Andreas' definition of nobility is ethical and Gerard's socioeconomic, the two nonetheless localize passionate love in an elite, be it moral or social.

Despite their commonalities, the two works diverge in key respects. In the first place, "love" in each work has a different ancestry and network of affiliations. I have elsewhere argued that Salernitan theories of imagination and desire, rather than the discussions of lovesickness by Constantine and Avicenna, underlie Andreas' account of passionate love; Gerard's lacks the theological heavy artillery Andreas brings to bear in Book 3.[41] Moreover, as Karnein has shown, Andreas appropriates medicine in order to unmask courtly pretensions, to lay bare the libido masquerading as refined love.[42] The thrust of *De amore* is anti-courtly, and the blunt realities of medicine are meant to drive the point home. Gerard, in contrast, has no such polemical agenda, though the concerns of his masculine, scholastic milieu permeate his exposition of Constantine's chapter.

## Signa Amoris

As love assumed new importance in twelfth-century culture, both vernacular and Latin, so too did the signs that betray—or pretend to betray—erotic passion.[43] The symptoms of love, *signa amoris*, reveal particularly well the confluence of medical, literary, and religious discourses on love in the first part of the thirteenth century. In Marie de France's lai *Guigemar* (ca. third quarter of the twelfth century) the hero, whom love had "pierced to the quick," "spent a sleepless night, sighing in anguish. In his mind he constantly recalled her speech, her appearance, her sparkling eyes and beautiful mouth: the pain she caused reached deep into his heart. . . . A little comfort would have gone some way towards assuaging the suffering which had drained his face of colour." The lady, in turn, rose before daybreak "bewailing the fact that she had spent the night awake. Love, which was torturing her, was the cause. The maiden, who was with her, could see from her appearance that she was in love with the knight who was lodging in her chamber for his cure."[44] The *Art d'amours* advised readers to fake the symptoms of love in order to be successful with the ladies: "It is worth much to be pale and discolored, for it seems that it is from the pangs of love, and then the women feel pity because of it."[45] Richard de Fournival (d. 1260) likewise claimed that a lady could identify a true lover by his appearance: "When he is before you humble, pensive, full of sighs and has a piteous and loving look, and it seems when he looks at you as though he will cry while laughing, know that it is one of the most beautiful and true proofs that one can find in one's friend, whether he loves from the heart or not."[46]

Gerard divides the symptoms of love into those arising from the soul and those from the body, and joins to Constantine's list a number of signs from Avicenna's chapter on ʿishk in the *Canon*.[47] He also makes a modest effort to relate symptoms to causes, but it is not until Arnald of Villanova's *Liber de amore heroico* (before mid-1280s) that a comprehensive physiological mechanism for explaining the symptoms emerges.[48] Several bodily symptoms arise from overheated *spiritus*. The eyes are hollowed because they "follow the spirits racing to the place of the estimative faculty." The dryness of the eyes, absence of tears, and general drying of the body may similarly be attributed to a consumption of moisture by the overheated *spiritus*. Interestingly, the only one of Constantine's remedies that Gerard chooses to gloss is wine; wine is recommended because it humidifies the body, rectifying its excessive dryness. This group of symptoms literalizes the common literary figure of "burning love," which is signalled by the flames on Amor's clothing in Figure 5.2.

A second group of symptoms indicates that passionate lovers lack emotional control. Avicenna mentions their emotional lability—they easily swing between crying and laughing (compare Richard de Fournival's "plourer en riant"). Gerard borrows Avicenna's observation that the lover will cry when he hears love songs, and especially if they are about rejection or separation. Though this symptom originally described a feature of lovesickness in Islamic culture, Gerard's decision to incorporate it into his commentary on the *Viaticum* suggests that he considered its inclusion warranted by the plights of contemporary Europeans in love.[49] The prologue to Gottfried von Strassburg's (d. ca. 1210) *Tristan* similarly alludes to the same deep emotional identification with amorous tales:

> All are agreed that when a man of leisure is overwhelmed by love's torment, leisure redoubles that torment and if leisure be added to languor, languor will mount and mount. And so it is a good thing that one who harbours love's pain and sorrow in his heart should seek distraction with all his mind—then his spirit will find solace and release. . . . Now we hear too much of one opinion, with which I all but agree, that the more a lovesick soul has to do with love-tales the more it will despond. . . . The noble lover loves love tales.[50]

Gerard will specify distraction as one of the cures for love, but fails to say whether love tales are an efficacious diversion.

The final symptom that calls for explanation is found neither in the *Viaticum* nor in the *Canon* and may represent Gerard's addition to the tradition. Preoccupied with depressed thoughts and worries, Gerard observes, the lover scarcely understands when other people speak; but if the topic is love (or the beloved), he is suddenly moved. This recalls Origen's symptomology of *amor languens* (the lover can think and speak of nothing else but the beloved) and Andreas Capellanus' description of an impassioned lover:

> If someone broaches a topic with him, he does not listen closely to his words, and normally fails fully to understand any entreaty unless the other makes reference to his love, in which case the talk could continue for a month without the lover's forgetting a scrap of the whole conversation.[51]

The symptom also recalls an item appearing in various lists of the signs, rules, or precepts for love, namely that the lover or friend gladly listens to talk of the beloved.[52] Whether Gerard drew from such collections or from his own experience, the symptom reveals in any event that love abstracts the lover from language and from the social discourse of masculine society (recall that Gerard defines erotic lovers as noble men).[53] The lover's helplessness and inarticulateness seem those of an infant, *in-fans*, the one who cannot speak. The fifteenth-century physician Jacques Despars characterizes the lover's loss of language as infantile-seeming behavior in his commentary on Avicenna. The *spiritus* and breathing of the patient are uneven or interrupted, he explains, on account of the violent rapture of the mind in the beloved object, just like that of an infant or boy crying with heaving sobs.[54] Gerard's addition of the symptom, then, obliquely indicates that *amor heros* is incompatible with the conventions of masculine adult social behavior.

This latent contradiction becomes apparent if we step back for a minute to review the entire complex of symptoms that signals morbid love. The symptoms of the disease, as outlined by Constantine and Avicenna, and as synthesized by Gerard and other medieval physicians, essentially feminize the male lover. Beyond the passivity inherent in being a patient, with the helplessness and vulnerability that it implies, the symptoms connote traits customarily associated with the feminine in medieval culture. Emotional lability, excessive or inappropriate laughing or crying, fasting, misregulation of speech, that is, inappropriate speech or silence—all these symptoms of lovesickness are corporeal signs associated with the feminine.[55] Isidore of Seville, as we have seen, calls excessive love *femineus amor,* "womanly love." "There is no order or decency in their gestures," says Jacques Despars. "They ramble in speech, are completely fickle, variable, and unstable" (*totus inconstans, varius et mobilis*)—classic misogynist descriptions of the feminine. "Every woman is by nature fickle," says Andreas Capellanus, and Boccaccio reiterates: "Giovane donna è sempre mobile." Such lovers are difficult to cure, claims Despars, because their minds are little exercised in "virile virtues."[56] Through the *signa amoris* and the disease of love the lover's body and behavior are thus metaphorically assimilated to the unattained object of his desire, yet in the male lover this "feminine" state signifies pathology.[57]

The mistrust of passionate love implicit in medical semeiology surfaces elsewhere in Gerard's chapter. According to Constantine, "Just as loyalty is the ultimate form of affection, so eros is a certain extreme form of pleasure." Gerard selects *loyalty* as a key word and glosses it as follows: "Whoever intimately cherishes another reveals all his secrets to that person, and conceals what has been revealed to him." I presume that Gerard wishes to discriminate between the behavior of loyal friends and erotic lovers. Yet that contrast becomes muddled, because in this gloss the rhetorics of vernacular literature and of clerical didacticism intermingle. In vernacular lyric the poet/lover and lady have a mutual obligation to hide their love from others and to reveal their hearts to each other (*celar-retener*).[58] Yet secrecy is also one of the key elements in friendship according to numerous schemes of the "signs of love" (*signa amoris*). In the French translation of the *Twelve signs of true love,* "The first sign of true love is a loyal heart, which can conceal nothing from his friend."[59]

The tradition of the "signs of love" still awaits a thorough investigation; Karnein has traced a number of its strands in connection with the *praecepta* and *regulae amoris* in Andreas' treatise.[60] According to Karnein, Andreas transposes signs derived from a learned tradition of friendship based on Cicero's *De amicitia* into literary rules for love. Andreas assumes that the audience perceives both the distinction between spiritual and erotic friendship and the ironic transfer that he accomplishes. Yet Karnein has also shown that the distinction was lost when the interpretive paradigm for *De amore* shifted and the rules were henceforth read as straightforward precepts for noble love.

Though as technical prose Gerard's text is less ambiguous and therefore less open to major interpretive shifts than Andreas', his chapter nevertheless blurs rather than clarifies discursive boundaries. One would expect the *signa amoris* to permit better and finer discrimination among the types of love, and yet the reception history of Gerard's gloss shows that the opposite result occurred.

The chapter entitled "De scissione cordis per amorem" ("On the cutting of the heart through love") in Hugh of St. Cher's chapter of *De doctrina cordis* (*On the Doctrine of the Heart*, ca. 1235) borrows Gerard's symptoms of lovesickness, point for point, to describe the signs of ecstatic love, "commonly called loving par amours (*amare per amores*)."[61] Ecstatic love may be taken *in bono* or in another way, as a mental alienation that the physicians call *amor ereos*. Although the latter type of love is greatly reprehensible, Hugh nonetheless declares: "Let us prove one love by the other." As Lee Patterson has noted, Hugh conflates and confuses the rhetorics of earthly and spiritual loves by using the same *verba* to describe dissimilar *res*; Gerard's symptoms of love enable him to do so.[62] Hugh's work was immensely popular, surviving in over 180 manuscripts, and was translated into Middle English. His incorporation of Gerard's *signa* not only sanctioned the authority of the medical view, but helped to create contrary conditions for its reception. The *signa* could point to morbid love, or to reprehensible love, or they could signal spiritual love; *amor heros* could be viewed as a disease, as lust, or as true love. Like the allegorizations of love-languor in the Song of Songs, this ambiguity enabled the symptoms of illness to become signs of love's positive value. As Richard of Fournival explains in the *Consaus d'amours*: "Nevertheless, I have often recognized the great value and the great sweetness of love when I ceased to drink and eat, to sleep and rest from the distress of loving well. The hope of my desire comforted me such that it seemed to me that it cost me nothing; rather it pleased me so much that it seemed to me there was no other paradise than to love *par amours*."[63]

## Cures

Gerard adds a number of passages from Avicenna to Constantine's list of cures. By far the most significant of these involve therapeutic intercourse. Avicenna considers it the best cure for lovesickness, though it must be exercised according to "law and faith," a proviso not in the *Viaticum*. What did this stipulation mean? Marriage, first of all, as in Figure 3.4. The illus-

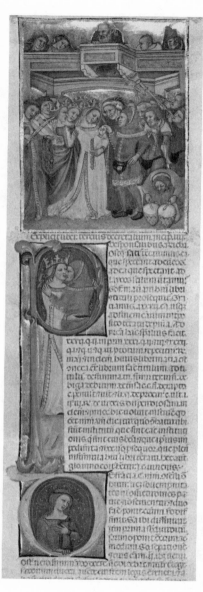

*Figure 3.4.* Detail from manuscript of Pope Gregory IX's *Decretals,* illustrated by Niccolò da Bologna: The Marriage, The Kiss of the Bride, and The Bride Abandoned. Washington, D.C., The National Gallery of Art, Rosenwald Collection, B-22, 225.

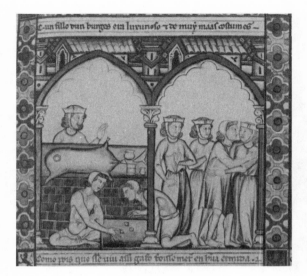

*Figure 3.5.* Tavern scene with wine, women, and dice. *Cantigas de Santa María,* of Alfonso X, the Wise. Escorial, Bibl. MS T.I.1, Cant. XCIII. Photograph granted and authorized by the Patrimonio Nacional, Madrid.

tration perhaps suggests what could happen in "therapeutic" marriages. But there were also plenty of opportunities for sexual activity outside of marriage, at least for men.[64] In particular Gerard recommends (again following Avicenna) consorting with and embracing girls, multiple intercourse with them, and switching to new ones (Figure 3.5). Jacques Despars, an expositor of Avicenna, clarifies the relation of this cure to law and faith. "Insani amantes" can make love with those whom the law permits: prostitutes, public women, and slaves ("meretricibus aut publicis feminis aut de servis emptis quas sclauas vocamus") but not virgins, religious women, married women, or close relatives. In terms that smack of a connoisseur's appraisal, he specifies that the "bought women" ought to be slim, beautiful, clean, "full of juice" ("succi plenas"), and animated ("corde vivido").[65]

As with Constantine, we are once again confronted with the problem of the West's receptivity to the system of sexual morality underlying Islamic medicine. At a time when the Church was attempting with some success to regulate sexuality outside marriage and to enforce clerical celibacy, Gerard and the other physicians who write about lovesickness appear to stage a rearguard attack on "official" sexual morality. In view of this and other aspects of medieval medical teaching on sexuality, Jacquart and Thomasset have questioned Foucault's assumption that medicine is a "normalizing discourse," a force of regulation and repression. They advance the hypothesis that medieval medical discourse on *amor hereos* and sexuality opened a space of freedom in which a Western *ars erotica* could develop untrammeled by theological repression.[66] The physicians who dealt with lovesickness, how-

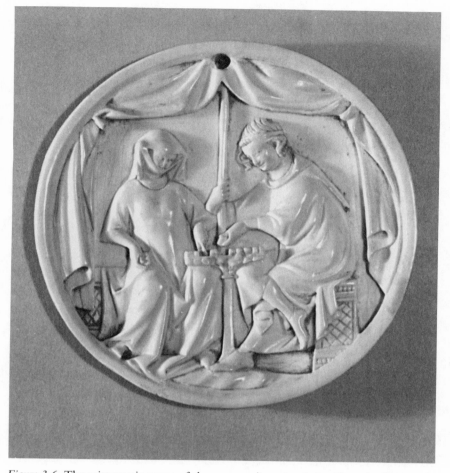

*Figure 3.6.* The aristocratic game of chess was a diversion in itself, or doubly so if the opponent were a lovely lady. Ivory mirror back, France, 1320–40. The Cleveland Museum of Art, Purchase from the J. H. Wade Fund, CMA 40.1200.

ever, may have found it easier to theorize about sex therapy than to implement it. That, at least, is the implication of Boccaccio's story of the young physician, who, after diagnosing the noble Giachetto's love for the servant Giannetta, placed responsibility for the execution of the cure in the hands of Giachetto's mother (*Decameron*, II.8). Like Hippocrates who dared not advocate the obvious but incestuous remedy for Perdica's malady, Boccaccio's doctor (though not Giachetto's mother!) shrinks from arranging a therapy condemned by the Church.

Though Jacques Despars' vivid description of therapeutic lovemaking may well substantiate Jacquart and Thomasset's claim, in Gerard's case the *ars erotica* amounts to little more than rewarmed Ovid.[67] For the rest, Gerard's cures follow the lines laid down by his two authorities. Sleep, humectation (to counter the heat and dryness generated by the disease), good nourishment and baths are to be prescribed.[68] The patients should be occupied in various ways so that they will be distracted from thoughts of the beloved. Hunting and games (Figure 3.6) are helpful, as are the counsels of old women. Gerard somewhat abbreviates Avicenna's recommendation that an old woman disparage the beloved, speaking of her "stinking dispositions." This aversive therapy, whose roots can be traced back to Lucretius and Ovid, easily became a lightning rod for clerical misogyny, of which Bernard de Gordon's version of the cure is perhaps the most famous example.[69]

## The Price of Subjectivity

Throughout this chapter I have been concerned to illustrate how Gerard's chapter on love contributed to and benefited from contemporary discussions in medicine and broader developments in literate culture. Though in general the physicians tell us much about the material causes of lovesickness, they are rather more reticent about the particular social and psychological conditions that lead to morbid love. Gerard's attribution of lovesickness to the nobility and his description of its causality are therefore important clues to the place of the disease in medieval culture.

In the late twelfth and early thirteenth centuries the most important non-medical representation of "noble love" appeared in courtly literature. Though there was no rigid system of "courtly love" as such, a number of conventions appear frequently enough in literary texts to be taken as general symptoms. Two are relevant here: the idealization of the beloved woman, and the lover's service to her. The lover becomes as it were subject to the lady as to a feudal lord (Figure 3.7). As Bloch puts it: "Courtliness is, in many ways, synonymous with the psychologizing of social reality—the conversion of a set of reciprocal social relations, sensed as external and objective, into moral values."[70] It is precisely this attribution of moral value to an erotic relation constituted in the guise of a feudal relationship to which Andreas Capellanus objects. Though the extent to which literary conventions of love were played out in twelfth-century aristocratic society is still obscure, we needn't go far for evidence to suggest that by the early thirteenth century erotic behavior in literate circles was influenced by literary conventions. The Old French translators of Ovid's *Art of Love* gloss the text in a naively realistic way. For them love service is real and necessary:

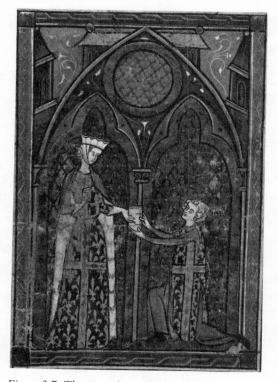

*Figure 3.7.* The poet, in a posture of submission, offers his work to his lady. From the *Roman de poire,* a poem in Ovidian style. Paris, Bibliothèque Nationale, MS fr. 2186, fol. 10v.

The author says, and it is true, that one who wants to begin his love affair well must pretend that he is prepared to do every service, every wish and every private duty that he can for his lady. Because of this the youth say in their songs that they want to show their loves that they are prepared in word and deed. They sing this in their little song: "To serve my lady / I have given my heart and myself." [71]

Richard de Fournival counsels that the lover should address his lady in such words of submission as these: "Je sui votre sers, et apparelliés a faire vos commandemans. . . . si vous pri, dame, pour Diu, que vous me retenés pour vostre ami et pour vostre serf, ou autrement la grans valours de vous et haute amours qui s'est en moi herbergie m'ont mis a le mort!" [72]

If courtliness psychologized social relations by transforming them into moral ones, courtly values in turn influenced social relations—at a price. As the Ovidian passage above makes clear, in some circles lovers had to *pretend* to serve their ladies in order to have a chance of success. Richard de Fournival warns against dissemblers who assume the posture of service without meaning it from the heart.[73] And even his own stance in this regard is not above suspicion, since he claims at the end of the work to have been skeptical of love in his youth: "I held love of so little worth that it seemed nothing to me; it seemed to me a very illusion and a foolishness of those lovers I heard complain that they were dying of love."[74]

Erotic subjectivity as defined by literary conventions that contravened the realities of gender roles and power relations bore the price, as I shall argue in the last chapter, either of duplicity or of the mental alienation of lovesickness (Figure 3.8).[75] In Gerard's analysis of love, we can see that the patient's "overestimation" of the beloved woman corresponds to the idealization of the beloved in literature. The patient considers her better, more noble, and more desirable than other women, even though this may not objectively be the case.[76] The overestimation of her desirability immobilizes the lover's mental faculties in meditation on her mental image. Although the woman's overestimated nobility and superiority mirror at a psychological level the lover's own social elevation, the metaphorical language of Gerard's causal analysis reveals that her ennoblement threatens the inner hierarchy of self-rule. Gerard's chapter thus reveals a kind of fault line where the clerical intellectual culture of the universities intersects vernacular literature. Set against the idealization of the beloved object, which is a narcissistic mirroring of the noble lover in the ennobled love object, a process familiar in courtly literature, there is a loss of inner control and governance in the noble subject, a degradation of the mental faculties expressed in the infantilization or feminization of the lover's body and behavior.

Gerard's aim is to bring Constantine's chapter on love up to date in light of recently available medical and psychological texts; it is not to critique "courtly love." Nonetheless, if we read the metaphoric language of his causal analysis and the signs of love in light of later medical texts, a profound ambivalence toward idealized passionate love, "noble love," emerges. The lover's mind is subjected to the imaginary dominion of a woman who seems more noble than she is; the psychological and physiological degradation that follow threaten to result in the "destruction of the subject," as the question of Master Alan puts it. Gerard's chapter refracts these cultural stresses concerning erotic love. In chapter one I argued that the high medieval celebration of Christ's Passion endowed human *passio* with new value and meaning. Within this general revaluation of suffering, assigning lovesickness to the nobility tended to elevate the disease further, to mark love-suffering as itself noble, refined, a testimony to the sensitivity of "noble

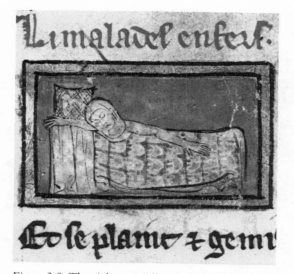

*Figure 3.8.* The sick man ("li malades enfers") shown bed-ridden after he has been wounded by the arrow of desirous thought. "He must uncover the wound to cure the malady, or otherwise he cannot be healed" (Bernier de Chartres, *La vraie médecine d'amour*). Vienna, Bildarchiv, Österreichische Nationalbibliothek, Cod. 2609, fol. 1v.

hearts." "When we are deeply in love," says Gottfried, "however great the pain, our heart does not flinch. The more a lover's passion burns in its furnace of desire, the more ardently will he love. This sorrow is so full of joy, this ill is so inspiriting that, having once been heartened by it, no noble heart will forgo it!"[77] And Chaucer's Troilus claims to prove the nobility of his love through his ability to suffer from it.[78]

On the other hand, the same fusion of the courtly and the morbid implies that there was a price to be paid for subjection to eros. It disrupted the lover's place in the order of things, and threatened him with psychological and/or social abasement. We need to recognize how profoundly disturbing the "feminization" of love in the late twelfth century was to intellectuals and clerics, university men whose sense of self was rooted in ontological, intellectual, social, and legal superiority to women.[79] Traces of that disturbance are inscribed in the scientific discourse on love in Gerard of Berry's glosses and in the works of later physicians.

# WHAT PART OF THE BODY
# DOES LOVE AFFLICT?
## Giles' *Gloss on the Viaticum*

From Gerard's essay and glosses we move to a different form of textual exegesis with the briefest of the *Viaticum* commentaries on love, attributed to Giles (Egidius) and preserved in a single manuscript. Whereas Gerard, in addition to clarifying the letter of the text, essentially rewrote Constantine's chapter in light of Avicenna, Giles instead disputes two short questions about lovesickness. Since he covers diseases of the head contained in the first book of the *Viaticum* selectively, the two questions on *amor*, brief as they are, indicate that the nature and cure of morbid love were intellectually compelling problems that warranted dialectical inquiry.

It is not easy to determine the particular historical audience for which Giles undertook that investigation, since his identity is uncertain. A heading on the first folio of the unique late thirteenth- or early fourteenth-century manuscript records the author's name; there are no other explicit clues to his biography or milieu.[1] Nonetheless, of all the thirteenth-century men named Egidius with attested interests in medicine or natural philosophy, it seems likeliest that the author of the *Viaticum* commentary was Aegidius Portugalensis, also known as Giles of Santarem (d. 1265), a Dominican friar and physician in Paris in the 1220s. Though it is of course possible that Egidius is someone who has been lost from the historical record, the case for Giles of Santarem is worth making, since it provides a context for understanding the questions on love.

Giles was born around 1184 in Vaocela, Portugal into a family of local nobility.[2] He was first educated in Coimbra, where he studied philosophy and also medicine, in which he rapidly excelled. Because the King saw in him a future royal physician, he supported his studies and granted him a number of benefices. In order to advance his studies, Giles set out for Paris. Legend has it that, fired by ambition for worldly glory and reputation, he was persuaded en route by the devil to detour to Toledo so that he might learn necromantic arts. He supposedly made a pact with the devil, signed with his own blood, and then spent seven years in apprenticeship as a sorcerer. He set forth for Paris once again, where his magic arts as well as his own skill won him great acclaim as a healer. But a horrifying vision convinced him to renounce magic, burn his books of magic, and return home.[3]

We are on firmer historical ground with the records of his entry into the Dominican order around 1220 in Portugal. Once admitted to the order, he returned to Paris once again, this time to study theology. There he was a close friend of Humbert of Romans, who entered the order in Paris in 1224 and persuaded his own teacher and friend, Hugh of St. Cher, to do so as well.[4] The novices Giles and Humbert served together in the Dominican infirmary. During this period of his life it also appears that Giles taught medicine. Though no formal records of the medical faculty survive from this period, a fifteenth-century manuscript of Giles' remedies for various ailments contains a brief biographical notice which claims that the Dominican Giles of Portugal, master in arts and medicine, compiled the work: "Questa opera e trattato fu compilato perlo Venerabile religioso Maestro Gilio diportugallo dellordine disancto domenico. Il quale . . . fu maestro in artj et in medicina et compilo lodicto tractato. Et apresso che fu nellordine fu grande Theologho et uisse nellordine .XL. annj."[5] Giles' designation as master of medicine implies that he taught the subject. Since the *Viaticum*, as Gerard's commentary shows, was a standard text in Paris in the early thirteenth century, Giles would very likely have had the opportunity to lecture on it.

Sometime before 1233 Giles left Paris for Spain; it may have been in the general exodus of masters and students of 1229 that resulted from violent conflicts between town and gown.[6] From 1233 to 1245 Giles was prior of the Dominican province of Spain. He lived in the convent of Santarem (Scalabitano) until his death in 1265, and was canonized in 1748.

Apart from the *Viaticum* commentary in question, two of Giles' medical works have survived. One is the previously-mentioned collection of remedies, the other a translation from Arabic of al-Rāzī's *De secretis in medicina* into which was incorporated John Mesue's *Book of Medical Aphorisms.*[7] The manuscripts indicate that the translation was accomplished at Santarem, probably in the last period of Giles' life.

Can the *Gloss on the Viaticum* be attributed to Giles? His biography, as we have seen, certainly admits it as a reasonable possibility, and other indications support it as well. Giles' questions appear to have more in common with earlier thirteenth-century problem literature such as the *Prose Salernitan Questions* than with medical and natural philosophical works of the later part of the century. For example, although Giles' questions on lovesickness resemble those of Peter of Spain's *Questions on the Viaticum*, Version A, and although Giles' questions on other topics in the *Viaticum* parallel some of Peter's, Giles' commentary is nevertheless much shorter than Peter's, having both fewer questions and shorter argumentation within each question. The similarities may result from Giles' use of Peter's questions (or very similar ones); however, were this the case, we might expect rather more of Peter's arguments to appear.[8] His commentary thus seems to precede Peter's, and to stem from earlier in his career (i.e., Paris) rather than later (i.e., Santarem).

Textual citations also help to situate the commentary. The most useful among them for this purpose are quotations from Aristotle's *De animalibus*.[9] The *Gloss* had, therefore, to be composed after around 1210–17.[10] It would thus fit well into Giles' Parisian period in the 1220s. Because his citations of *De animalibus* are among the earliest, one might be tempted to place him after Peter of Spain, whose medical and natural philosophical works are generally taken as the first significant engagement with that Aristotelian text. However, the legend of Giles' "Toledo episode" may hide a kernel of truth about his career that explains his relatively early use of *De animalibus*.

During the time when Giles is supposed to have studied magical arts in Toledo (before ca. 1220), that city was home to Michael Scot, who translated *De animalibus* into Latin. For half a century or more it had sheltered the scholars whose scientific translations from Arabic had transformed European learning. As J. Ferreiro Alemparte has recently shown, the city's reputation as a place where necromancers had their own "school" is a polemical inversion of its scientific preeminence. Many of the authors who report stories of Toledan necromancy and necromancers are religious who, at bottom, denigrate any purely scientific knowledge.[11]

Behind the story of Giles' necromantic apprenticeship in Toledo, then, may lie the reality of a scholarly sojourn. His youthful interest in medicine may have drawn him to the city whence issued so many recent medical translations from Arabic. As we know, he himself in later life translated one of al-Rāzī's medical treatises into Latin.[12] Youthful study of Arabic scientific texts in Toledo may thus have earned him a reputation as a necromancer among religious writers mistrustful of worldly accomplishments. In Toledo he may have learned of or even known Michael Scot, who at that very time was translating Aristotle's *De animalibus*. Such contact would help to explain Giles' relatively early use of this Aristotelian work.[13]

Giles' commentary on the *Viaticum*, though called a gloss in the manuscript heading, takes the form of disputed questions. As a method of conveying information, the question had a long history in natural philosophy, reaching back to such collections from antiquity as the pseudo-Aristotelian

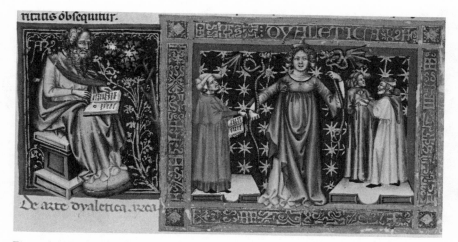

*Figure 4.1.* In this emblem of "Aristotelian dialectic art," Aristotle himself is seated on the left. In the scene on the right, Dialectic holds two opposed winged serpents. To her right two scholars are engaged in a disputation, while on her left a master makes a point about a text. Cassiodorus, *Institutiones*. Paris, Bibliothèque Nationale, MS lat. 8500, fol. 33r, detail.

*Problems.* The Salernitan questions of the twelfth and thirteenth centuries taught medical and natural philosophical ideas independently of an authoritative text. However, beginning in the twelfth century questions were used to explicate texts in the schools, and in the early thirteenth they were regularly used in university lectures on standard texts. Differing opinions on a controversial passage obliged the master to resolve the problem through the application of dialectic (Figure 4.1). This type of *quaestio* thus involves four elements: the text, dissonant opinions on the text's subject, dialectic method, and the master in the process of regular teaching.[14] Disputed questions in medicine, then, had a double pedigree, the older problem literature and the newer form of textual commentary.[15]

Peter of Spain's contribution (ca. 1246 and following) to the development of disputed medical questions has recently been emphasized.[16] If Giles' work truly antedates Peter's, then he must be seen as one of the earliest medical writers we know of to blend Salernitan-type questions with the question-commentaries coming into use in the other faculties.[17] The intellectual climate of Paris, where both forms of question were in vogue, favored the union of the two types of questions in a medical commentary.

The surviving manuscript may not, however, do full justice to Giles' ideas. In many cases our documentation of scholastics' teaching depends on a student's transcription of the lectures (*reportatio*) that may or may not have been edited and polished by the lecturing master. If they were not edited, what survives is what the student heard and was able to jot down, not necessarily what the master said. In addition, both hasty notation and the shared knowledge of an intellectual community, which can be assumed rather than explicitly articulated, contribute to the abbreviated style characteristic of *reportationes* and classroom questions. Often an argument is summarized as "therefore et cetera." The compressions and ellipses of argumentation in the *Gloss on the Viaticum* suggest that it indeed stems from the classroom rather than from the author's study, where he would presumably have had more control over its form.

Disputed questions, as Bernardo Bazàn has noted, were the site where the most pressing intellectual problems of the age were raised and discussed; as such they are an important guide to the period's intellectual interests.[18] Though the section on *amor hereos* in Giles' commentary is quite brief—was it too disturbing a topic for a Dominican novice to dwell on?—it can be profitably read in the context of Parisian learning of the early thirteenth century.

The first question on *amor heros*[19] asks why the *Viaticum* classifies love as a disease of the head when, as an emotion, it would seem rather to be located in the heart. Giles' question can be seen as a response to the challenge posed by Aristotelian physiology and psychology.[20] The location of emotions in the body became controversial after Aristotle's biological and psychological works began to circulate in the West in the late twelfth and early thirteenth centuries. Medical writers traditionally maintained that the brain was the seat of sensation and emotion, but Aristotle claimed that joy and sadness, hope and fear, hate and love, and so on all originated in the heart. Giles' contemporary, the Aristotelian David of Dinant, set forth Aristotelian teaching on the affections in his noteboooks (*Quaternuli*) containing excerpts, paraphrases, and interpretations of Aristotle's writings.[21] His notebooks conveniently summarize some of the Aristotelian biological and psychological notions that the Galenic-Arabic medicine of the early thirteenth century had to grapple with.

In David's account of the Stagyrite's teaching, no affect in the soul can take place without a "suffering" or "being affected" of the heart (*cordis passione*). But it then remains debatable whether the affect in the soul occurs because of the heart's being affected, or whether the heart's being affected results from the affect in the soul. Because illness or even death can result from excessive love or other emotion, David argues that although the *passio* of the heart and the *affectus* may be simultaneous, the heart's *passio* is the cause of the soul's affect. He defines the heart's *passio* physiologically, as a change in the systole and diastole. So, for example, in love the dilation of the heart is faster, its constriction slower, and slower is the dilation of the arterial pulse, which feels "deep" or perhaps "depressed" (*profundus*).[22]

Rather than tackling the physiological issues of the first question directly, Giles instead constructs his argument around the semantic ambiguity of *passio*. Whereas, following Constantine's usage, he initially terms love a *morbus* afflicting the brain, in subsequent steps of reasoning on locating love in the heart he calls it a *passio*. On the one hand, *morbus* and *passio* were synonymous medical terms for "disease"; on the other, *passio* also had a broader range of meaning that included various senses of "undergoing" or "being affected." This broader sense of the word allows him to argue that hate and love are *passiones* of the heart, and that therefore lovesickness is an affliction of the heart.

This apparent bit of scholastic logic-chopping in fact rearticulates, in medieval terms, problems raised in antiquity about the passions of the soul: can a "passion" affect the soul in the same way that a "passion" (*morbus*) affects the body? What is the dividing line between somatic disease and illness of the soul?[23] And where on that axis is the disease of love located? Giles' conclusion sides with the physicians' traditional views on love's bodily location: love is not actually a disease except by virtue of its consequences, and these affect the brain. Like Gerard of Berry, then, only in indirect fashion, Giles uses the subject of *amor heros* to probe the psychosomatic unity of the human subject.

If Giles is identical with the Dominican novice infirmarian, then professional tensions may have motivated, whether consciously or not, his engagement with this particular question. As we have seen, lovesickness and its cures highlighted certain tensions between those who cured bodies and those who cared for souls. Some bodily cures, like therapeutic intercourse, endangered the soul's health. We can readily see why a question on lovesickness whose terms implicated profound questions on the relations of body and soul would attract a mind like Giles', scientific by training and religious by commitment. Such a question delineates the site of potential conflict between medical and pastoral care, but in its abstraction and formulaic style, it also distances itself from the overt professional interests of either discipline. By so doing, the disputed question enables the conflict to be mediated, if not resolved, through intellectual inquiry.

An interest in the puzzling relation between body and soul subtends the remainder of Giles' commentary on *amor heros*, a question on the efficacy of wine in curing love (Figure 4.2). Of all Constantine's therapies, why is this one singled out for special attention? Therapeutic intercourse, for example, was more obviously controversial, especially for a Dominican novice in an age of sexual reform. Perhaps it was a topic too hot to handle. Perhaps,

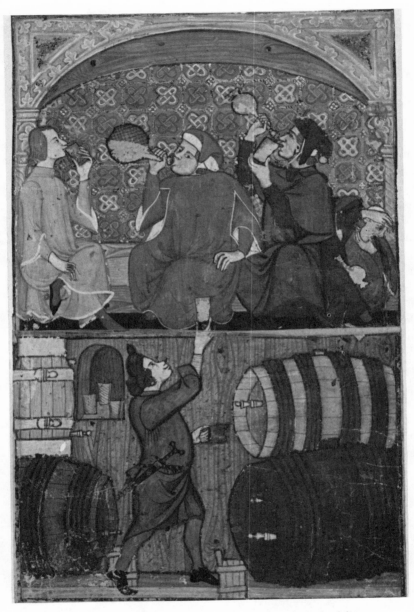

*Figure 4.2.* Is wine a suitable cure for love? From the relatively delicate enjoyment on the left to the excess depicted on the right, various stages of inebriation are shown in this scene from a public house. British Library, MS Additional 27695, fol. 14.

since the topic preceding *amor heros* in the commentary is drunkenness, the pedagogical desire to give thematic continuity to adjacent chapters dictated Giles' choice. Finally, practical and theoretical considerations may have impelled the question.

From a medical point of view, wine is a tricky spirit. Not only does it affect both body and mind, but it has opposite effects at different dosages. It will make a silent man initially loquacious, but in greater quantity he will become contentious. Beyond that wine will make him mad (*amentem*), and finally it will render him senseless and motionless.[24]

For medieval physicians, the nature of wine's action in producing these varied effects was enigmatic. If curative effects were supposed to derive from the nature of medicinal substances, why was it, for example, that the hot and dry nature of wine produced "cold" diseases like apoplexy and paralysis?[25] As Giles argues in the chapter on stupor, every agent acts by means of its own complexion (that is, its substantial composition) and brings about an effect similar to itself. Because wine is an agent in the human body by virtue of its heat and dryness it should cause similar effects.[26] As Giles poses the problem for lovesickness, wine's beneficial effects on the disease are questionable because the lover's malady is accompanied by depressed thoughts and by excessively heated *spiritus*, as we saw in Gerard of Berry's explanation. Though Constantine recommends wine as a cure for love, other authorities disagree. Isaac (Judaeus) says that it sharpens and deepens thinking, but this is counterproductive in lovers already given to depressed thoughts. And in the *Remedies for Love* Ovid says that wine should not be given to lovers.[27] Giles concludes that wine deepens the minds of the "wise," that is, those who are of sound mind, and quotes a Goliardic jingle to make his point: "Cum bene sum potus, circa versibus influo totus; cum sim ieiunus, sim de peioribus unus" (When I'm well soused, in poetry I'm doused; when I'm athirst, I'm one of the worst). Lovers' minds are not sluggish, however, but depressed instead (*non est profundata in bono sed in malum*). Since wine washes away "bad thoughts" (*cogitationes malas*), it gladdens the soul and thus is a suitable cure for "heriosis" when drunk in moderation. It is hard to resist the conclusion that beyond the dialectic play of authorities, the realities of practical treatment influenced Giles' choice of question and its elaboration.

Giles' questions on the classification and cure of lovesickness emphasize the challenge the disease posed to medical theory and to medical practice by probing the subtle links between matter and spirit. In this respect they evince an interest in the lover's malady similar to Gerard's more comprehensive effort to clarify the corporeal dynamics of desire, and one that also anticipates Peter of Spain's elaborate sequence of questions on the psycho-physiology of love. Given his selective coverage of the diseases of the head contained in the first book of the *Viaticum*, the two questions on *amor*, brief as they are, testify to the importance of lovesickness as a locus for exploring various dimensions of man's psychosomatic unity.

# PETER OF SPAIN
## Questions on the Viaticum

In quella parte     dove sta memora
prende suo stato . . .

. . . . . .     . . . . . .

L'essere è quando     lo voler è tanto
c'oltra misura     di natura     torna;
poi non s'adorna     di riposo mai.
Move, cangiando     color, riso in pianto,
e la figura     con la paura     storna.
Poco soggiorna.     Ancor di lui vedrai
che 'n gente di valor,     lo più, si trova.

Guido Cavalcanti, "Donna me prega"[1]

Guido Cavalcanti's (d. 1300) philosophical poem on love, "Donna me prega," owes much to the medical tradition of lovesickness. The Florentine physician Dino del Garbo (d. 1327) explicated the poem at length; his commentary is preserved in a manuscript written by Boccaccio. Dino quotes Avicenna and "Aly Abbas," and alludes to "medical authors" to elucidate Cavalcanti's stanzas on the lover's appearance, behavior, and the deadly threat that unsatisfied love poses.[2] One such author may well have been Peter of Spain (d. 1277), a Portuguese logician, philosopher, and doctor who taught medicine in Siena from 1246 to 1250. His series of questions on *amor hereos* in the *Questions on the Viaticum*, composed in Siena and extant in two versions, represents one type of poetic raw material that Guido Cavalcanti, whom Boccaccio calls "most excellent natural philosopher" (*Decameron* 6.9) and whom Dante names as his "first friend" (*Vita nuova* 3), wrought into his difficult, beautiful poem on love.[3] The only contemporary pope whom Dante placed in paradise (he was elected John XXI in 1276), Peter of Spain wrote the most philosophically ambitious of the surviving *Viaticum* commentaries. Like Cavalcanti and Dino del Garbo, Peter read deeply in Aristotle, whose influence is evident throughout his work. Peter's questions on love range over a wide variety of topics, from the workings of faculty psychology and the physiology of appetite to the age of patients, why there is pleasure in intercourse, and the role of gender in lovesickness. While not all of Peter's questions on lovesickness are original—several appear to derive from Giles of Santarem and the loose body of scientific problems known as the *Salernitan Questions*—his way of handling them opened new ground that later physicians worked more thoroughly.[4]

Remembered by a chronicler of the lives of the popes as "most accomplished in the art of healing," Peter is best known to medical history for the *Thesaurus pauperum*, a medical textbook popular for its brevity and practical nature.[5] His career, however, was that of a medieval polymath: not only was he one of the most important physicians of the thirteenth century, but as a logician, psychologist, philosopher and theologian he also has a fair claim to be one of the principal scholastics of the era.[6] His life is relatively well attested. Born, according to his most recent biographer, in Lisbon, Portugal sometime before 1205, Peter attended Lisbon's cathedral school as a boy. In the 1220s he then moved on to Paris to study logic, physics, metaphysics and theology.[7] His era in Paris was that of Alexander of Hales, William of Auxerre, and William of Auvergne rather than that of Albert the Great and Thomas Aquinas, as earlier biographers supposed.[8] Peter may conceivably have studied medicine under his fellow countryman Giles of Santarem (Aegidius Portugalensis), who taught medicine in Paris in the 1220s and whose questions on the *Viaticum* are similar to Peter's.

It is thought that in 1229, when there was a general exodus of masters and students from the city owing to disputes with city authorities, Peter left Paris for the north of Spain. There he most likely taught logic and composed the *Summule logicales* in the early 1230s. This widely-used textbook of logic was instrumental "in developing a dialectical method of interpreting Aristotelian science."[9]

In 1246 Peter reappears as a master of medicine at the newly-organized medical faculty at Siena, where he remained until around 1250. He then returned to Portugal and held a number of ecclesiastical offices, eventually becoming *magisterscholarum* at the cathedral school of Lisbon from 1263 until 1272. During this time, he visited the Papal Court in Viterbo and Orvieto several times.

Peter composed most of his surviving medical and psychological works, which provide a fruitful context for his ideas on lovesickness, in the period 1246–72. Many of his medical treatises are versions of lectures on the texts he taught at Siena: Johannitius' *Isagoge,* Galen's *Tegni,* Isaac's (Isḥāq al-Isrā'īlī) *De dietis universalibus et particularibus* and *De urinis,* and Constantine's *Viaticum.*[10] In addition to commentaries on standard medical works, he also compiled the earliest surviving Western commentaries on Aristotle's *De anima* and *De animalibus,* the latter forming the basis for Albert the Great's own *Quaestiones super de animalibus.*[11] Peter did not limit himself to commentaries, however; he also wrote a textbook of psychology, *Scientia libri de anima,* "das umfassendenste Lehrbuch der Psychologie aus der Zeit der Hochscholastik."[12] Its doctrines on the mental faculties illuminate, as we shall see, several questions on lovesickness.

In 1272 Pope Gregory X summoned Peter to Viterbo to become court physician. At the papal court he probably met other leading scientists, including the perspectivists Witelo and John Peckham, who were drawn to the flourishing court school.[13] In 1276 he became Pope, taking the name Johannes XXI. He died May 12, 1277, fatally injured by the collapse of the ceiling in his newly-built study in the papal palace.

## *The Two Versions of the Questions*

A number of Peter's commentaries, including the *Questions on the Viaticum,* survive in multiple versions.[14] They most likely record the changes in his teaching over a span of years. The two versions of the *Questions on the Viaticum* allow us to trace changes in Peter's thinking on love over a period of five or more years (assuming that relative chronology can be established). In both versions he continues Gerard of Berry's assimilation of Avicenna's psychology into medical doctrines on lovesickness. Aristotle, however, also provides *loci* or starting places for arguments in the questions on *amor hereos.* Peter's fusion of Avicenna and Aristotle anticipates, and may even have helped to shape, the later Montpellier synthesis of classical and Arabic natural philosophy.

Because many of his arguments focus on the physiological bases of love psychology, Peter's ideas on morbid love assume a decidedly somatic bias, one that is more evident in what I call the B version than in the A. The A version is further distinguished from the B in that it quotes Gerard of Berry's commentary on the *Viaticum* almost verbatim (lines 33–46; not in B), and contains two questions that appear to derive from Giles. If we assume that Peter developed greater intellectual independence as he gained experience teaching medicine, then perhaps the A version is indeed the earlier.[15]

Since it is sometimes difficult to penetrate the thickets of Peter's procedure, Table 1 gives an overview of the two versions. The form of Peter's commentary, like that of Giles, is that of disputed questions, a method of

## Table 1
### Outlines of Versions A and B

---

*Version A*

---

Of which psychological faculty is love a disease, the imaginative faculty, the cogitative faculty, the estimative faculty, or the fantasy? Solution: Love is a disease of the estimative faculty because it is damaged first and primarily.

Of which part of the body is love a disease, the heart, the testicles, or the brain? Solution: One must distinguish between love as a *passio* of the heart, which is not a disease, and love that is accompanied by the symptoms of melancholy, which is a disease of the brain.

In which humoral complexion does it occur the most, in the melancholic, or in hot complexions (choleric and sanguine)? Solution: Since sexual stimulation is the major cause of *amor hereos*, it occurs most frequently in hot complexions.

In which sex does it occur most frequently? Solution: Lovesickness occurs more frequently in women because they are less hopeful than men and are more easily sexually stimulated. However, it is more tenacious and difficult to cure in men.

In which age does it occur most often, in youths (*iuvenibus*) or in boys (*pueris*)? Solution: In youths, especially at the end of adolescence when they desire intercourse the most.

Is traveling abroad useful in curing lovesickness? Yes, because one sees beautiful (hence distracting) sights. No, because one's suspicion and fear of losing the beloved increase. Solution: Traveling is beneficial because one is distracted by the scenery and consequently will forget the beloved.

Are ugly women to be brought before the patient? Yes, because they are contrary to the woman he thinks beautiful, and cures are effected by contraries. No, according to Avicenna. Solution: No, because contraries illuminate each other and thus his beloved will seem more beautiful by contrast.

Are beautiful women to be brought before him? No, because like added to like causes the disease to grow worse. Yes, according to Avicenna. Solution: Yes, because the patient will be distracted by more beautiful forms from his previous preoccupation.

Is drunkenness a useful cure? No, because it is sexually stimulating. Yes, according to Isaac. Solution: It is useful when it completely hinders the inner wits, so as to cause oblivion, but not useful when it merely impairs these mental functions.

Questions on certain texts. 1. al-Rāzī says that fasting is beneficial but Avicenna says that temperate food is useful. 2. Avicenna (*actor*) says that the beloved should be scorned; on the contrary, this will only make the lover remember her. Solutions: Fasting reduces the seminal matter which arouses sexual desire, while good food produces subtle and laudable humors that do not lead to erections and aid in combating weakness and wasting. Even though scorn causes the lover to bring his beloved to mind, nonetheless it withdraws his mind from its obsession with her.

---

Lecture: Definitions, causes, symptoms, cures

Incidental Questions: Of what part of the body is love a disease, the testicles or the brain? Solution: the brain.

Why does a cold complexion increase appetite in the stomach and diminish it in the testicles, while heat does the contrary?

Why does appetite in the stomach cause the *villi* to become rigid through cold while appetite for coitus causes the member to become rigid through heat?

Why is appetite in the stomach aroused through cold, but appetite in the womb aroused through heat, since both stomach and womb desire to be filled?

Of which psychological faculty is love a disease, the imagination or the estimative faculty? Solution: the estimative faculty.

Whom does this disease befall the most, those of melancholic complexion or youths (who are not of melancholic disposition like the aged)? Solution: Love is called a melancholic worry not on account of its humoral material, but because of symptoms similar to melancholy. [Therefore the young are more subject to it.]

In which sex does the desire for coitus occur more and in which sex is the pleasure greater? Solution: Love is more intense in men but women enjoy intercourse more.

Why is there so much pleasure in intercourse? 1. The sensible and nervous disposition of the genitals. 2. Each faculty delights in its own operation. 3. The motion of moisture through the genitals induces a certain itching and pleasurable movement. 4. The rubbing of members against each other. 5. Some assign a final cause, the fetus, lest generation cease.

Which sex enjoys coitus more? Solution: Men enjoy it more, but women have a twofold pleasure, in emission and in reception.

Do the eyes suffer more in love? Yes, since they are close to the brain and are of a watery and fluid substance. No: Constantine says that all parts of the body except the eyes are attenuated. Solution: The eyes appear larger when the rest of the face grows thin from insomnia and wasting.

Is intoxication a useful cure in this disease? Yes, say Ovid and al-Rāzī. No, because it disturbs the mind's operations. Solution: Two things are useful in the cure—restoring proper judgment, for which intoxication is not useful, and relieving preoccupation and anxiety, which Ovid recommends.

Are baths useful? No, because like good food they stimulate desire. Yes, say al-Rāzī and Serapion. Solution: Baths and good food are useful because they relieve melancholic worry.

Is it useful for patients to see ugly shapes? Yes: cures are achieved by contraries. No, says Constantine. Solution: No, because the sight of an ugly woman will cause the patient to become even more ardent about the woman who seems more beautiful to him.

teaching based on an authoritative text in which the master voiced, evaluated, and resolved opposing views on various passages.[16] The full structure of disputed questions (arguments, counterarguments, solution, response to arguments) is, however, more fully apparent in Peter's commentary, whose questions are both longer and more numerous than Giles'.

Common to both versions of Peter's work are questions about the psychological and bodily "place" of the disease, categories of patients, the role of gender in susceptibility to lovesickness, and whether wine and ugly women are useful cures for morbid love. Five questions are unique to the B version, though some of them are paralleled elsewhere in Peter's medical works. They explore the physiological and psychological bases of sexual desire as it affects the genesis and severity of *amor hereos*.

## Version B: The Introductory Lecture

One manuscript of the B version (Vatican pal. lat. 1166) contains the only copy of the Portuguese master's summary exposition of *amor hereos*, titled *Lectura super Viaticum*. Opinions on lovesickness from the authorities (Avicenna, al-Rāzī, *Pantegni*) are arranged in the usual order of definition, causes, symptoms and cures. Although the *lectura* offers no developments in medical thinking about *amor hereos*, it does anticipate some of the topics addressed in the debated questions. It provides a convenient epitome of what might, in the absence of similar surviving works, be called "standard" scholastic doctrine on lovesickness ca. 1250.

Peter opens his lecture by summarizing various definitions of lovesickness. To Avicenna's definition of *ilisci* as a "melancholic worry," he joins that of the *Pantegni* and a versified definition of love sometimes found in the margins of *Viaticum* manuscripts.[17] The poem, which defines love as the sickness (*mentis insania*) of a mind moving among phantoms, bringing more sorrow than joy, is found in Old French and Middle English as well as Latin sources. According to a recent study, the poem, extant in several forms, developed from twelfth-century religious and philosophical literature.[18] As we saw above with Gerard of Berry's commentary, clerical mistrust of love filtered into medical teaching on lovesickness; in Peter's commentary it did so through this poem. Bernard de Gordon, the most misogynistic of writers on lovesickness, incorporated the versified definition, now commonplace in the generations after Peter of Spain, into his own exposition of *amor hereos* in the *Practica dicta Lilium medicinae*.[19]

Peter's etymology of *amor hereos* is curious and more difficult to explain than many. He derives *hereos* from *heremis* and explains: "that is, from nobility who are most accustomed to contracting this disease." The explanation recalls that of Gerard of Berry, but the term itself is a mystery, since *heremis* ordinarily means "hermits." It may be a ghost word resulting from a copyist's error (especially since elsewhere in the *Questions* morbid love is called *amor hereos*), or it may bear a significance dimly reflected in Domenico da Ragusa's (fl. 1394–1427) distinction between *hermete* (?), a type of melancholy caused by the sight of beautiful forms, and *amor* which is called *herios*.[20] Whatever the word means, Peter reaffirms the connection between lovesickness and the nobility, and reinforces it by explaining that the material cause of the disease is an excess of seed produced in those who live in leisure, quiet, and bodily pleasure.

When Gerard of Berry lectured on the *Viaticum* in Paris a generation before Peter assumed his position at Siena, he noted that the causality of lovesickness was a difficult topic. By the middle of the thirteenth century, however, increased study of the Aristotelian corpus led to an interest in and ease with more complex causal analysis. As a result, the sections on causes in medical treatises expanded significantly. A little more than a generation after Peter of Spain's treatises were written, William of Corvi compiled a catalogue of causes of *amor hereos* that begins with the *causa primitiva*, moves through *cause extrinsece, causa antecedens, causa antecedens humoralis*, and ends with the *causa coniuncta*.[21] Peter's list of causes here is far more modest, limited to the material cause of excess seed, and to three psychological roots of the disease: the desired object, the desire itself, and frequent thoughts about the object. He then lists four factors necessary for intercourse: a hot complexion, imagination, "an elevating windiness," and an abundance of seed. The presence of conditions for intercourse in the section on causes exemplifies the underlying premise, we might call it, of the B version: that *amor hereos* can be understood as the result of the physiological processes of appetite.

Though Peter passes over the symptoms of lovesickness quickly, without any notable addition, he does mention the pulse test from Avicenna's chapter on *ilisci*. He follows Gerard of Berry once more (and anticipates Arnald of Villanova) in declaring that the prognosis is poor for lovesick patients who fail to satisfy their desires. The body will generate black bile (*cholera nigra*), the brain will grow too cold, and as a result, the patients will suffer from melancholy. Peter thus reaffirms Constantine's view that unless treated, *amor hereos* will lapse into melancholy or mania; in the last sentence of the lecture he stresses that "this disease generates the matter and disposition for melancholy unless it is cured."

Peter turns to Avicenna and al-Rāzī for his discussion of cures. "Avicenna says that the better cure is to lie with the beloved" (B 46–47). Al-Rāzī recommends wise counsel and stories, freshwater baths, travel, listening to songs, and drinking wine. He also says that melancholic humor should be purged with the appropriate medicine. At this point in his presentation there follow the disputed questions on love that are contained in the other manuscripts of the B version. My discussion is organized by the sequence of topics common to both versions. Because Peter's questions on gender and lovesickness deserve more detailed commentary than is possible in this summary, they have been reserved for separate treatment in the next chapter.

## The Psychology of Love

### VERSION A

The *Viaticum* posits a dual causality for the disease of love. Against the psychological cause of love—sight of a beautiful form—it balances a somatic one, the body's need to expel excess humoral matter. As we have seen, Gerard of Berry's causal explanation outlines how the inner senses or mental faculties are derailed by the perception of an excessively pleasing form. Peter tackles the problem of causality by inquiring about the precise mental and physical sites of morbid love, devoting a question in each version to the mental faculty and part of the body affected by lovesickness. Though he acknowledges in the second question of the A version that the psychological cause of *amor hereos* is more important than the physical cause, nonetheless, by investigating causality through love's place in the body, Peter lessens the Platonism evident in Constantine's and Gerard's chapters on love. Correspondingly, he augments the sense of material determinism associated with the disease.[22]

The first question of version A seeks to determine which of the internal senses or inner wits is primarily damaged by *amor hereos*, for which there are four possibilities. To Gerard's analysis of the roles of the estimative and imaginative faculties, Peter adds consideration of the *virtus cogitativa* and the *fantasia* (Figure 5.1). Since one faculty (*virtus*) could exercise several different functions, each of which had its own name, the terminology of the inner senses and their functions can be confusing.[23] Fortunately for our understanding of the debated question, Peter himself composed what is in effect a handbook of psychology (*Scientia libri de anima*), in which he catalogues the mental faculties and explains their functions.

Peter's first argument simply claims that since lovesickness damages the imaginative faculty, it is therefore a disease of that faculty. The imaginative faculty, located in the first cell of the brain, receives the forms of sensible objects (through sense perceptions) and transfers them to "higher" mental faculties for further processing.[24]

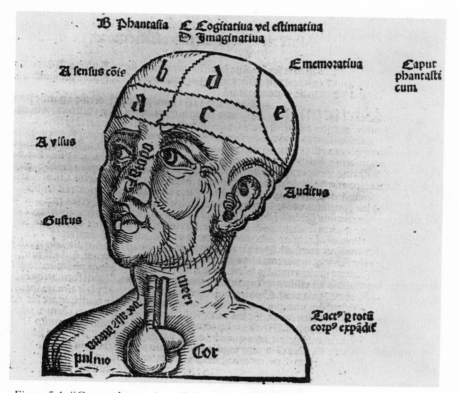

Figure 5.1. "Caput phantasticum" showing the internal senses and their locations. This diagram separates *phatnasia* (B) from the imaginative faculty (D), and shows the cogitative and the estimative faculties in (C). Matthias Qualle, *Parvuli . . . philosophie naturalis cum comentariis* (Hagenau, 1513). Bethesda, Maryland, History of Medicine Division, National Library of Medicine.

One of the higher faculties to which the imagination transmits images is the estimative faculty, whose definition Peter, like Gerard of Berry, derives from Avicenna: it is that power by which we judge non-sensible "intentions" of sensible forms—whether something is to be pursued or avoided (the sheep's estimative faculty judges it is time for flight when it perceives the "intentions" of a wolf). Since the lovesick patient errs in his judgment about the desirability of pursuing the beloved, so runs the next argument, his estimative faculty must be damaged by the disease.

Peter next argues that when Constantine speaks of the lover's "assiduous thoughts," he refers to the workings of the cogitative power as it reflects on the image of the beloved woman. In the *Scientia libri de anima* Peter explains that the cogitative faculty is the *fantasia* or "fantastic faculty" (*virtus fantastica*) when acting under the direction of the intellect in considering and reflecting upon sensible forms.[25] The *virtus fantastica* is situated in the middle cell of the brain and works on images after they have been received by the common senses and imagination.

Last of all, Peter proposes the *fantasia* as that faculty which is primarily damaged by lovesickness. Its task, according to the *Scientia*, is to "judge, distinguish, compose and divide" sensible forms in the absence of the objects themselves. By so doing, it produces a judgment concerning the object. It can be led astray either by not heeding the evidence of the senses, or by refusing the rule of the intellect. Peter focuses on the comparative function of the *fantasia* in the question on lovesickness. *Amor hereos*, he declares, is a suffering (*passio*) of that faculty whose task is to compare one object with another. Since the lover judges one woman to be more beautiful than all others, or one object to be better than others, the *fantasia* must be the affected faculty.

The plethora of inner wits as possible victims of "sensible damage" from lovesickness may seem a particularly fine bit of scholastic hairsplitting. Because the solution to the question is borrowed almost wholesale from Gerard's discussion of misestimation and because in the replies to the arguments the roles of the *fantasia* and cogitative faculty are never really discussed, Peter may have advanced the four faculties more from a desire for thoroughness than from a concern to pinpoint the exact psychological process by which love overwhelms the mind and body. But to dismiss the arguments without further consideration would be to miss an important aspect of Peter's approach to *amor hereos*. Even where he adopts the opinions of previous authorities, whether *moderni* or *antiqui*, he does so critically, enriching the field of intellectual play with additional possibilities in order better to test the truth of their statements. In this instance, as psychology had become more complex through the assimilation of Aristotelian and Avicennan psychologies, Peter lays out a fuller continuum of those mental functions involved in perceiving and responding to a desirable form. Gerard may have been correct in his assessment of the psychological damage involved in *amor hereos*, but Peter tests that view against a fuller understanding of psychological functioning.

## VERSION B

In the B version of the *Questions*, lovesickness potentially affects only two mental faculties, the imaginative and the estimative. As a result of this reduction in scope, the underlying causal issue stands out more sharply: is the image itself or the overappreciation of the image more important in the etiology of lovesickness?

Peter first proposes the imaginative faculty as the locus of disorder.

*Amor hereos* impairs both its function (*operatio*) and its organic substance. On the other hand, the estimative faculty, which apprehends "non-sensible forms" that entail pleasure or pain, may be the damaged faculty. Because love is generated by judgments about intangibles like good and evil, rather than about sensible qualities like heat or odor, the disease of love, so Peter argues, must damage the faculty responsible for such judgments, which is the estimative. Moreover, love is a disease of the faculty that "operates as it apprehends," that is, that composes and divides images as part of its function. Since lovesickness involves the comparison of one woman to others, as we have seen from Gerard of Berry's analysis, and since comparison and evaluation belong to the estimation, love must be a disease of that faculty.

Peter concludes, as in the A version, that the *virtus estimativa* is the place of disturbance in lovesickness; the lover's malady is rooted in faulty judgment rather than faulty perception. Whereas the A version reconciles the arguments for the imagination and the estimative faculty by distinguishing between immediate and mediated damage caused by lovesickness, the B version offers a somewhat different distinction. Peter draws a temporal division in the operation of the internal senses affected by *amor hereos*. Love is a *passio* of the imagination in its initial motions, but in its completed form (*complementum*) is a disease of the estimative faculty.

Peter's focus on perception and the initiating role of the imagination anticipates the later thirteenth-century interest in the stages of visual perception in lovesickness that was stimulated by contemporary interest in optics.[26] Furthermore, his distinction between initial and completed stages of the disease proved fruitful for later analyses of *amor hereos*. Gerard of Solo, one of the leading masters at Montpellier in the middle third of the fourteenth century, took as the theme of his disputation on lovesickness (*Determinatio de amore hereos*) Peter's question on which part of the body love is a *passio*. The most interesting intellectual problem of the *Determinatio*—when does love leave the realm of health (*latitudo sanitatis*) and become morbid?—develops from Peter's temporal distinction between initial and completed phases of lovesickness.[27] Both Peter and Gerard thus investigate time and, as we shall see in Peter's case, matter as ways of discriminating *amor* that is called *hereos* from other types of *amor*.

## *The Locus of Love: Heart, Brain, or Testicles?*

### VERSION A

The opening words of Constantine's chapter on love define it as a disease of the brain, yet he gives the body's need to unburden itself of excess humors a causal status equivalent to the sight of a beautiful form. Where then, Peter asks in the second question, is lovesickness actually located in the body? His dialectic efforts to localize love somatically paradoxically reveal a broader view of love psychology.

At the same time that it exemplifies the intimate connections between physiology and psychology, the second question also serves as a model of dialectic method. As the editor of Peter's philosophical works has pointed out, Peter exemplifies the doctrines of his textbook on logic, the *Summule logicales*, in his philosophical teachings.[28] The same can be said of his medical pedagogy. If we read the chapter on lovesickness in light of the *Summule logicales*, we find illustrations of *equivocatio*, arguments from contraries (ll. 55–58), from genus (59–62), from similarity (74–77), and from definition (77–82).[29] Furthermore, recognition of the semantic ambiguity of *amor* (*equivocatio*) unlocks the sometimes cryptic arguments of this question.

The first argument that Peter advances, that opposites are predicated of the same subject, derives from Aristotle's *Categories*. To take Aristotle's examples: disease and health require as their subject the body of an animal; white and black require as their subject a body without further qualification; and justice and injustice have as their subject the human soul. In an argument that corresponds closely to Giles of Santarem's first question, Peter contends that since the heart is the seat of emotion, and since hate lodges in the heart, so too will love. The crux of the argument, of course, is the silent substitution of "love" for "lovesickness."[30]

The next argument for placing love in the heart defines it as one of the "accidents of the soul" or emotions, themselves one class of the "non-naturals" (*res non naturales*)—air, rest and movement, food and drink, sleep and vigils, excretion and repletion—that affect health and disease.[31] In the psychology Peter sets forth in the *Scientia libri de anima*, the brain and the heart interact closely in the development of emotions, or "passions (accidents) of the soul." The power that governs the diversification of the emotions according to the type of stimulus is the *virtus affectiva* (affective faculty), whose seat is the heart. Since, however, the genesis of emotion depends on perception and the workings of the imaginative and estimative faculties, and since emotion in turn disturbs perception and judgment, the *virtus affectiva* in its workings is closer to the brain (*proximius est cerebrum*).[32] The emotions then "return" to their source, the heart, which is also the origin of motion, from which point the appetitive faculty (*virtus appetitiva*) can direct pursuit or avoidance. Although brain and heart interact dynamically, Peter focuses for the sake of this argument on the role of the heart in the generation of emotions.

The counterargument, in which the testicles are proposed as the site of lovesickness, is a study in equivocation. Capitalizing once again on the am-

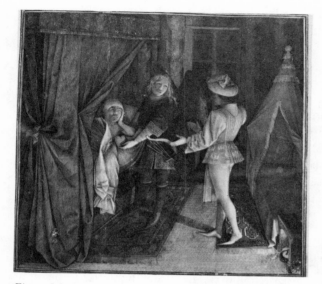

*Figure 5.2.* Amor removes the heart from a dreaming
King René and hands it to Desire. King René d'Anjou,
*Le cueur d'amours espris* (1457). Vienna, Bildarchiv,
Österreichische Nationalbibliothek, Cod. 2597, fol. 2r.

biguity of *amor* and also playing on the meaning of *actus*, Peter defines it as
the sexual act and calls it a *passio* of the testicles. But what exactly does
*passio* mean in this context? Not "disease" (*morbus*), certainly, but rather the
philosophical sense of "being affected, suffering, undergoing." Yet in the
conclusion to the question *passio* shifts to mean *morbus*—because the act of
love involves the testicles it is a *morbus* that afflicts them.

The next argument, which links diseases and their humoral substances,
"materializes" the origin of lovesickness. Since the offending substance in
lovesickness is excess seed, *amor hereos* must be a disease of the testicles.
Moreover, since the cure, as he rather crudely puts it, involves the application of "plasters or women to the testicles," the disease must be located in
this organ. The instrumental use of women makes it clear that the patients
are assumed to be male, and that *testiculi*, which can refer to the organs of
either sex (gonads), are here assumed to be the male sex organs. Whereas
women may receive special consideration as possible sufferers of lovesickness, as we shall see in the next chapter, most of the questions presume that
men are the patients.

Finally, the last two arguments locate *amor hereos* in the brain, "the principle member, noble . . . the foundation of the whole body and the seat of
the soul," as Peter calls it in his treatise on preserving health.[33] Because the

classic medical authorities on love, Avicenna and Constantine, place the disease in the brain, and because *amor hereos* is defined as a melancholic worry accompanied by depressive thoughts, and a disease similar to melancholy, lovesickness must be located in the brain, where these originate.

Peter distinguishes between two types of love in his resolution of the debate: One is located in the heart, but is not morbid; the other is located in the brain, and is a true *morbus*. Aristotle is right, but so is Avicenna: it all depends on what you mean by *amor*. "Cardiac love" may be a passionate emotion, but "cerebral love" can become a disease (Figure 5.2). To the arguments about testicular localization he responds that coitus is not a *morbus*, but rather the failure of the estimative faculty is, and that the application of women or plasters to the testicles cures the symptoms but not the disease *per se*.

## VERSION B

Though the corresponding question in the B version duplicates some of the arguments of A, it also contains new material. The possible locations of love are reduced from three (brain, heart, testicles) to two (testicles and brain). This reduction not only sharpens the dichotomy between mind and body, but also strengthens the bond between corporeality and sexuality. Without the mediation of the heart, man's upper and lower halves seem to polarize. If we step back to consider this intricate debate from some distance, it begins to resemble one of the dialogues in Andreas Capellanus' *De amore*, in which a man and a woman from the higher nobility converse together. The lady sets her suitor a problem: Which is a lover to prefer, the solaces of the upper half of the body, or of the lower? Their ensuing debate introduces analogies between appetites for food and sex, alludes to the interplay of mind and body in sexual desire, and considers whether sexuality is the efficient and final cause of love.[34] The central issue of the controversy (as of *De amore* as a whole) is clear: what is the relationship between sexual desire and love? This, too, is the problem in Peter of Spain's questions on the *Viaticum*, articulated in the language of scholastic medicine rather than in that of courtly badinage.

To return, then, to Peter's debate: The first argument, which posits that love is a disease of the testicles, echoes the A version's contention that a disease belongs to that part of the body which it affects. Since love *per se* involves the testicles, lovesickness is located there. As in the A version, here too the reasoning depends on the unacknowledged ambiguity of *amor*, which means both "love" (sexual act) and lovesickness.

The second reason for locating *amor hereos* in the testicles leads Peter to consider the nature of appetite. Appetite, he claims, is dual: it is both general or "universal," originating in the brain, and particular, located in a specific part of the body. Since love entails an "appetite" or desire for an object, this desire must be located in a particular part of the body, and the testicles are the obvious spot.

The third reason, which echoes an argument of the A version, advances this line of reasoning a step further. Since action and potential belong to the same subject, in this case the testicles, inability (*impotentia* or lack of intercourse) with respect to this action must be attributed to the testicles as well. The disease resulting from this lack is nothing other than *amor hereos* caused by superfluities located in the testicles.

The first counterargument for the cerebral localization of love is two-pronged: since love involves thoughts and cares, and these stem from the brain, love is a disease of the brain; and since it is a melancholic worry, it is of the brain.

The second argument is unique to the B version. If love were really located in the testicles, then eunuchs and those not able to have intercourse would not suffer from it. But since "we see" (*videmus*) that they are in fact liable to lovesickness, it cannot be a disease of the testicles, but rather must originate in the brain.

Like that of the A version, the solution distinguishes between two aspects of love. Love as a disordering and depression of the thought is a disease of the brain. Sexual desire, however, also plays a role in *amor hereos* and itself has two aspects. One is mental (*animalis,* from *anima*), based on the image of the desired object in the mind, and thus is located in the brain. The other aspect of sexual desire, arising from the body's natural functioning, is in turn twofold. One type is "fluctuating," so called from its dependence on the varying amounts of heat resulting from digestion, in which the liver plays an important role. The other type is "fixed," linked to the innate heat that is "rooted in seminal moisture" in all parts of the body, as Peter explains in his questions on *De animalibus.*[35] He apparently means that since the testicles conserve more seminal moisture than other parts of the body, they generate more *naturalis stimulatio coitus* than other members. Thus lovesickness is a disease of both the brain, and, through these elaborate bifurcations, of the testicles as well. Like his *auctoritas* Constantine, then, Peter emphasizes the part man's psychosomatic unity plays in the development of lovesickness, but unlike Constantine, he pursues the precise routes by which mind and body collaborate in the lover's decline.

Such dialectic acrobatics may have tested the extent to which the play of logic usefully enhanced medical discussion. While the final conclusion of the first question reaffirms Constantine's statement that love is a disease of the brain, in general the terms of such discussions may have opened medical discourse to philosophical development, as is apparent in Gerard of Solo's *Determinatio de amore hereos*.[36]

In the B version three subquestions on the relation of heat and cold to appetite in the stomach and the sexual organs amplify the main question. Their appearance in a chapter on *amor hereos* sets the erotic malady in a larger context of appetite and its physiological manifestations. Although Aristotle (*De anima* 414b) could have provided the general inspiration for the collocation of these topics, the more specific rationale for these particular questions appear in a commentary by the Salernitan master Maurus. In his commentary on the *Isagoge* of Johannitius, a general introduction to Galenic medicine, he locates desire (*desiderium*) in the stomach, the penis, and the womb.[37] The *Prose Salernitan Questions*, which incorporated Maurus' statement and which Peter knew well, offered a ready source for comparing and contrasting these appetites.

These questions appear again later in Peter's *Questions on the Viaticum* in the chapters on sexual disorders, as well as in the section on mammalian procreation in Peter's commentary on Aristotle, the *Questiones super de animalibus*.[38] The recurrence of the same set of questions in three different contexts marks Peter's interest in how heat and cold determine the mechanics of appetite. His focus on the mechanics of appetite (heat and cold) lend his exposition a more emphatic materialism than those of other authors in this volume.

## The Patients

In both versions the attempt to classify likely groups of sufferers according to humoral complexion, age, and sex unifies the next set of questions. These questions, a favorite means of inquiry in Peter's commentary on the *Viaticum*, greatly broaden Gerard's restricted epidemiology. In contrast to Gerard's socioeconomic explanation of lovesickness as a disease affecting the nobility, Peter's analysis in Version A concentrates on bodily composition arising from the balance of humors, that is, on material causality.

In the first of the questions on the sufferers of lovesickness, Peter argues that imagining the delights of intercourse provokes adolescent males, of an age most suited for love, to suffer *amor hereos* (Figure 5.3). In general, however, the most important underlying cause of the disease is what we would call a high metabolism—in medieval terms, a hot complexion—that generates what Peter calls sexually stimulating heat. Since of the four humoral complexions two were considered hot, namely the choleric and the sanguine, and two cold, namely the melancholic and phlegmatic (Figure 5.4),

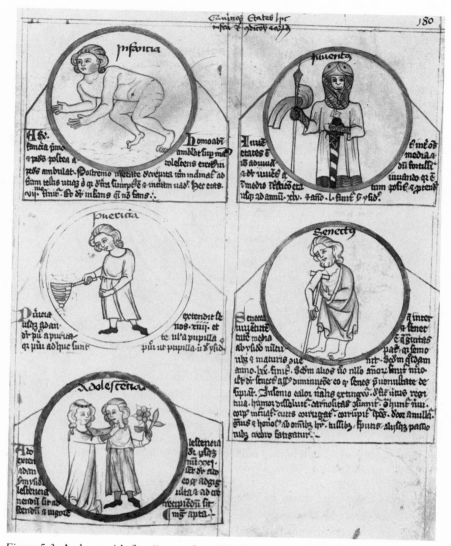

*Figure 5.3.* A chart with five "ages of man": infancy (to 7), childhood (to 14), adolescence (to 21), "youth" (adulthood, to 45), and old age. Adolescence is the age for love and for reproducing (*ad gignendum sit adulta*). Munich, Bayerische Staatsbibliothek, MS lat. 19414, fol. 180r.

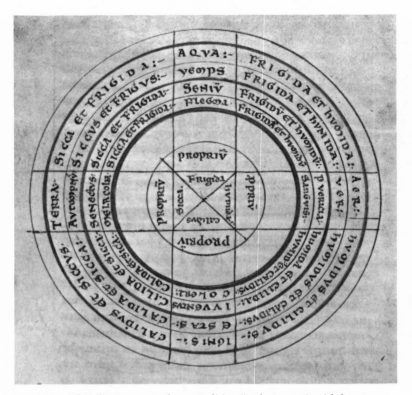

*Figure 5.4.* This diagram correlates qualities (in the center) with humors, ages of life, seasons, and elements. Reading clockwise from the top: Fire, summer, youth, and choler are hot and dry; earth, autumn, maturity, and melancholy are dry and cold; water, winter, old age, and phlegm are cold and moist; air, spring, childhood, and blood are moist and hot. Paris, Bibliothèque Nationale, MS lat. 11130, fol. 48r.

Peter concludes that those of sanguine or choleric complexion are more likely to contract lovesickness.

In the B version Peter treats the roles of age and complexion in *amor hereos* in a single question on melancholy. Throughout the Middle Ages *amor hereos* stood in an ambiguous relation to melancholy. According to the *Viaticum, amor* leads to a *passio melancholica* if the thoughts are not relieved, and this causal role of love in melancholy appears again in the *Prose Salernitan Questions,* a body of literature that Peter of Spain drew upon and reworked throughout his medical career. As Salernitan lore had it, a certain girl who awaited her lover in vain contracted mania, caused by the melancholic humor that her worried thought had generated.[39]

Avicenna calls love a "melancholic worry," intimating a close connection between the two but failing to specify its nature.[40] To confuse the picture further, Constantine's *De melancholia* discusses both humoral and psychological causes for melancholia and mentions lovers as subject to the disease.

Peter concludes that *amor hereos* is a "melancholic" disease only insofar as the symptoms are similar to melancholy; he does not argue for a common humoral origin. Consequently, his analysis stops short of positing a "type" of melancholy lover, whose bodily constitution and temperament predisposes him to lovesickness. In this, he and Arnald of Villanova, who considers melancholy a possible complication of lovesickness, agree.[41]

Fourteenth-century medical writers, on the other hand, tend to assert a closer connection between *amor hereos* and melancholy, classifying the former as a subspecies of the latter. Gerard of Solo (in his commentary on the ninth book of al-Rāzī's *Ad almansorem*), John of Gaddesden, John of Tornamira, and the fifteenth-century author Jacques Despars all designate *amor hereos* as a melancholic disease.[42] By the seventeenth century Burton was able to identify the two in his tome on "Love Melancholy." This shift, if it indeed occurred and is not merely a reflection of the limitations of surviving evidence, may have resulted from more intensive study of Avicenna, who associates love and melancholy, and from the growing popularity of temperamental "types" used to explain behavior (Chaucer's Reeve, for example, is a "sclendre colerik man").

## Symptoms

Whereas the A version lacks any discussion of signs and symptoms, one question of the B version concerns the effect of *amor hereos* on the eyes. Although Constantine had said that all of the body except the eyes wastes away, Peter argues that because of the eyes' aqueous substance, which is, as he puts it, "passible and fluxible," they must suffer from the effects of lovesickness as well. In his book on preserving health, he notes that crying, fasting, and excessive wakefulness all take their toll on the eyes.[43] Since these symptoms accompany lovesickness, it stands to reason that the eyes should be affected. In addition, the eyes, of all the bodily members, have the closest connection with the brain, and must therefore suffer when the brain does, as happens in lovesickness. The solution focuses on Constantine's statement that the eyes of a lovesick patient appear larger: this may, Peter says, either be due to the fact that the face has thinned so much that the eyes seem proportionately larger, or because insomnia causes vapors to distend the eyes, making them in fact larger.

The singling out of this particular symptom for special treatment invites commentary. The question may have offered a chance to integrate Aristotelian physiology with the traditional symptoms of *amor hereos* derived from Arabic medical treatises. When compared to Arnald of Villanova's more completely integrated physiological conception of symptoms in the *Tractatus de amore heroico*, however, Peter's isolated question seems a hesitant step toward harmonizing symptoms with causes.

But perhaps we owe its presence in his lecture to less technical motives. If, as I have suggested, symptoms of illness correspond to cultural values, other considerations may motivate Peter's interest in ocular symptoms.[44] The eyes, which Peter describes as "windows of the soul" admitting light in the manner of stained glass, allow the image of the beloved woman to enter the imagination, where, according to the B version, lovesickness begins.[45] On this point medical theory and literary practice agree. One of the staple conventions of vernacular love literature in Peter's time is the entry of love through the eyes. The Lover in the *Romance of the Rose* is pierced through the eye with the arrow of Beauty, which lodges in his heart (Figure 5.5). The affliction of the eyes, whose radiant and fluxible substance interposed between the outer world containing the beloved and the inner world filled with appetitive desire, is possibly the most fitting symbol of the disease and its causes. The eyes, moreover, betray the patient in a manner unlike the other symptoms. The changes in the pulse require the expert divination of the physician; the obsession with the beloved's image can only be revealed by the patient himself. The hollow eyes, in contrast, enable the knowledgeable to "read" from afar the sign of the patient's secret disease.

## Cures: Travel, Women, and Wine

"The best, readiest, surest way, and which all approve," says Robert Burton of the cures for love melancholy, "is *loci mutatio*, to send them several ways, that they may neither hear of, see, nor have an opportunity to send to one another again."[46] However, travel is not among the cures Constantine suggests, nor does it appear in Avicenna's chapter on *ilisci*. Al-Rāzī does nevertheless recommend it, and in the later thirteenth century it was standard therapy (cf. Bona Fortuna's prescription in the next chapter). The principle underlying the treatment is the familiar (and Ovidian) "out of sight, out of mind." In the A version Peter formulates the principle a little differently, stressing the positive value of the distraction provided by scenery, whose novelty attracts the patient's attention and causes him to forget his erotic obsession.

The cure had its dangers: William of Saliceto, writing in 1250, describes another type of *amor hereos* besides that for a woman—love for a distant

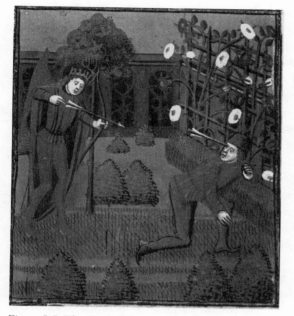

*Figure 5.5.* The God of Love strikes the Lover's eye
with the arrow of beauty. Scene from the *Roman de
la Rose.* Philadelphia Museum of Art, Philip S.
Collens Collection ('45-65-3), fol. 14r, detail. Photo-
graphed by Joan Broderick, 1985.

homeland. Patients languish for their countries and the only cure is to
return.[47]

The next controverted topic, whether ugly or beautiful women should
be led before the patient, is common to both versions and probes apparent
contradictions in Avicenna's therapy. On the one hand, the Arabic physician
advises that horrible old women should disparage the beloved in the patient's presence, but on the other that he should distract himself (as Constantine recommends) with other young women. The pedagogical strategy
of Peter's questions, harking back to that of the second question, seems
designed to provoke reflection on the nature of contraries and similars. He
quotes Galen's principle that cures are effected by contraries: *omnis cura per
contrarium.* This was generally understood to refer to elements and qualities:
hot is cured by cold, moist by dry, and so on. By proposing to apply therapeutic principles generally associated with altering the body to psychological cures, Peter forces his students to think more deeply about the
differences between somatic and psychological cures. Moreover, the question confronts them with the real therapeutic issue: how can the physician

transform the patient's desire to a less damaging form? Does he merely substitute another object, or does he transform desire into loathing? In keeping with the Ovidian dictum that "a new love drives out the old," Peter concludes in both versions that another beautiful woman should be substituted for the unattainable object of the patient's desire. Diversion, in his view, is more successful than conversion.

The last two questions of the series address somatic cures for love: wine and food. While Constantine tempers his praise of wine with a caution against inebriation, another authority on lovesickness, al-Rāzī, recommends a thorough sousing (*ebrietas plurima assidue*).[48] Characteristically, our author chooses to inquire into the contrasting effects of inebriation on the body and the mind. Alcohol generates excesses in the body that tend to stimulate sexual desire, thus thwarting a basic therapeutic principle of *amor hereos* (see lines 117–30), namely reducing sexual stimulation. Nonetheless, the loss of memory that follows diligent drinking lessens the lover's preoccupation.

Peter harmonizes the conflicting authorities by arguing that there two types of drunkenness, just as there are two types of love, and two meanings of *maior*. One type completely befuddles the internal senses, and thus aids the cure of lovesickness since the patient forgets the beloved object. The other type merely perturbs the inner wits, exacerbating the disturbance that causes lovesickness in the first place: this kind of drunkenness, says Peter, is useless as a cure.

In the B version, Peter again counters the authorities' prescription of potation with an argument that drinking will only make lovesickness worse. Whereas in the A version drunkenness is objectionable because it is both sexually stimulating and mentally befuddling, the B version raises only the latter objection. Peter concludes that inebriation is of no help in restoring the mind to an ordered love, which is one way to cure lovesickness; however, the disease can also be cured by thorough intoxication, which frees the mind from cares and worry.

The authorities (al-Rāzī and Avicenna) disagree not only about drunkenness, but also about whether fasting or a moderate diet is to be recommended for the lovesick. According to the A version, two aspects of nutrition need to be considered. Fasting may help to eliminate superfluities that would otherwise augment sexual desire, but the leanness and wasting induced by *amor hereos* have to be countered by "temperate" food, that is, by food that generates beneficial humors rather than potentially harmful superfluities.

The last question of the A version inquires why, given that oblivion is an important part of the cure, the beloved should be scorned when this will only cause the lover to think about her more. Peter admits that she will indeed be brought to mind during this process, but declares that the vilification will in fact detach the patient's mind from its preoccupation with her.

To this array of therapies the B version adds only one new question, on the usefulness of baths. As though he were all too familiar with the bathhouses-cum-brothels that dotted the medieval urban landscape, Peter suggests that baths are counterproductive as a cure because they only increase the desire for intercourse. On the other hand, eminent medical authorities hold that baths are indeed effective. Peter sides with the authorities and explains that baths, which are among the *genus deliciarum* (type of pleasures), and nourishing food distract the mind from melancholy.[49]

## *Influence*

Peter's contemporary fame and long years of teaching insured that his ideas on *amor hereos* found their way into the works of later medical writers. The surviving manuscripts indicate that within a generation or two of his stint in Siena, readers were demanding copies of his commentary on the *Viaticum*. Several of the manuscripts were written at Montpellier in the early fourteenth century, a sign that Peter's ideas interested medical students or teachers there. Nor was his work ignored in the later part of the century. The German physician Amplonius Ratinck acquired copies of both the A and the B versions of the *Questions on the Viaticum*. Moreover, Peter's work enjoyed more than local interest; it circulated outside the medical centers of the Continent, reaching England in the fourteenth century.[50]

Nonetheless, it is at Montpellier that we can trace the deepest engagement with Peter's teaching on lovesickness. The work of one Montpellier physician clearly shows familiarity with the exposition of lovesickness in the *Questions on the Viaticum*. Gerard of Solo is best known to students of *amor hereos* for his commentary on the ninth book of al-Rāzī's *Liber ad almansorem*, in which he discusses lovesickness as a third type of melancholy, called *amorereos* in the Renaissance edition of his *Opera*.[51] His *Determinatio de amore hereos*, however, though it duplicates some of the material contained in the commentary on al-Rāzī's ninth book, offers more thorough treatment and different emphases than the commentary.[52] Most importantly in this context, the *Determinatio* at points resembles Peter of Spain's series of questions on love closely enough that direct influence seems likely.

Like Peter of Spain, Gerard analyzes love as a phenomenon of appetite, and examines its distribution in various classes of people, its relative intensity in men and women, and the sources of sexual pleasure. Like his predecessor, he is, moreover, thoroughly Aristotelian, drawing upon *De anima* and the *Nichomachean Ethics* for the psychology of friendship and love, and the distinctions among action, habit, and passion. Gerard's manner of using philosophical and natural philosophical arguments shows that *amor hereos* had become a topic through which medicine could parade its claims to being a "philosophy of the body." The intellectual ancestry of this philosophical somaticism is rooted, as far as the evidence allows us to judge, in Peter of Spain's inquiry into the lover's malady.

It is harder to pinpoint Peter's contribution to the ideas of other Montpellier masters who wrote about *amor hereos* in the later thirteenth and early fourteenth centuries, since their treatises are not in the form of disputed questions, as is Gerard's *Determinatio*. Bernard of Gordon's chapter on love in the *Practica dicta lilium medicinae* (1305) shows few signs of engagement with Peter's ideas except in the "Clarificatio."[53] There he discusses controversial issues—how much wine? does *amor hereos* afflict the brain or testicles? does it strike men or women more often?—that Peter also raises. Bernard concludes with several lines of verse in which he defines love as *insania mentis*. The same versified definition of love appears in the *lectura* that opens the B version of Peter's commentary.[54] Whether his influence on Bernard was direct or mediated is difficult to tell; in any event, Bernard's chapter suggests that the issues Peter articulated passed into scholastic medical writing on lovesickness by around 1300.

More problematic is the relation of Peter's discussion of *amor hereos* to Arnald of Villanova's *Tractatus de amore heroico* composed before the mid-1280s, and possibly a dozen years earlier. Arnald studied medicine at Montpellier in the 1260s, when the *Viaticum* appears not to have been part of the curriculum.[55] His treatise on heroic love diverges considerably from later treatments of the subject by the Montpellier masters Bernard of Gordon and Gerard of Solo, some of whose concerns, as we have seen, are similar to Peter's. Nonetheless, the two Iberians' discussions of lovesickness share a number of topics.

At the most general level, Arnald, like Peter, integrates medicine and natural philosophy, a feature more evident in the B version of Peter's commentary than in the A. Both address the issue of whether love really is a *morbus*: Peter distinguishes between two types of love, one of which is a *morbus*, while Arnald declares that, properly speaking, love is not a *morbus* but an *accidens*.[56] He also notes that the mind's fixation on the pleasing object is due to the pleasure of intercourse, as does Peter in the B version (ll. 195–247). Both consider whether hope or lack of it has a role in the disease's origins.[57] Though they arrive at opposite conclusions, it may be significant that they raise the same question. As far as therapy goes, Arnald's statement that the *proper* cure (*forma rectae curationis*) for this disease is by contraries, and thus the pleasure associated with the beloved should be turned into revulsion by showing or narrating her odious traits, may be a response to Peter's conclusion that beautiful rather than ugly women should be brought before the patient to distract him.

All this does not add up to proof of Arnald's knowledge of Peter's work, although if Peter were an alumnus of Montpellier, such contact might have been possible. Nor should the differences between the two be underemphasized. Arnald gives a coherent mechanistic explanation of the disease that integrates etiology with semeiology, whereas Peter's treatment is fragmented by the question form and, apart from the *lectura* in the B version (ll. 1–53), does not offer a systematic presentation. Comparison does, however, reveal that ca. 1245–85 a common set of questions and approaches to *amor hereos* emerged in scholastic medicine, and that Peter of Spain's *Questions on the Viaticum* shaped the problematic at an early stage.

Peter of Spain continued the process, begun by Gerard of Berry, of synthesizing Constantine's chapter on lovesickness with more recently translated medical and philosophical texts. To Gerard's incorporation of Avicennan psychology into the *Viaticum's* chapter on love Peter added a variety of physiological considerations: on the nature of appetite in itself; on the contrasts between appetites for food and sex; on the effects of heat and cold on these appetites; and on the relation of sexual appetite to lovesickness. These were important themes in his general medical teaching; they indicate that he approached lovesickness from a broad perspective, viewing it as a specific case of general processes of desire and appetite.

To his teaching on lovesickness he brought his characteristic habits as a thinker: logical rigor, psychological acuity, psychosomatic interests, and philosophical vision. The A and B versions of his exposition of Constantine allow us to see developments in the theory of lovesickness being forged, as it were, in the classroom. Like that of Aquinas, to whom he is often compared, Peter's procedure is both analytic and synthetic. Through his various distinctions and semantic clarifications he resolves the questions into their separate aspects. Lovesickness becomes a specific process in specific organs and faculties. At the same time, the premises drawn from Aristotle's biological works place lovesickness in a wider framework of mammalian activity. At the level of both specific detail and general procedure, we can see in his teaching a gravitation toward a problem expressed otherwise in thirteenth-century philosophy as the interrelation of particulars and universals. Given that *amor* is general and ambiguous, what can be said of the specific variety discussed by the medical authorities Constantine and Avicenna? If it does not yield a scholastic *Summa amoris*, the Portuguese physician's dialectical play nonetheless preserves some of the excitement that must have filled the lecture halls where the young master of medicine and his even younger students matched Arabic medicine against Aristotelian philosophy, pitted authority against authority, and boldly tried to measure the quantity and quality of pleasure.

# THE MEASURE OF PLEASURE
## Peter of Spain on Men, Women, and Lovesickness

Men do not know how to feign their feelings of love, but women do it well. Just as the fire which is covered by cinders is the most ardent and the most dangerous and lasts longer than the one which is uncovered, so the love of women is stronger than that of men. Jupiter and Juno argued about who was the warmer, man or woman . . . To get an answer to their questions, they went to a wise man named Tiresias. He said that women were more ardent than men.

*Art d'amours*[1]

In one of the last stories told in the *Decameron* (X.7), Lisa, an apothecary's daughter, fell in love with King Peter of Aragon. But her lowly condition prevented her from fulfilling her passion, and as her love increased, so did her melancholy until "being unable to endure it any longer, the beautiful Lisa fell ill and began to waste visibly away from one day to the next, like snow in the rays of the sun."[2] Despite this and similar instances of women's love melancholy in medieval literature, modern historians of medicine working from printed medical sources of the Middle Ages have termed lovesickness an "echte Männerkrankheit."[3] Their assessment rests on the opinions of such medical writers as Gerard of Berry and Bernard of Gordon, both of whom claim that *amor hereos* afflicts noble men.[4]

Peter of Spain's *Questions on the Viaticum* invite us to reconsider how medieval medical writers understood the relation of gender to lovesickness. In elucidating the *Viaticum's* chapter on love, Peter inquires which sex suffers more from lovesickness. His answer, in keeping with his somaticism, links susceptibility to lovesickness with the psychophysiology of sexual pleasure. Assuming that the degree of pleasure affects one's likelihood of falling ill with love, Peter applies terms of qualitative and quantitative measurement to sexual experience, adumbrating what John Murdoch has called "a veritable furor to measure" in the later Middle Ages.[5] This analysis spurred other medical writers and natural philosophers to develop further the contrasts of intensive and extensive sexual pleasures and to rethink in turn the relationship between gender and lovesickness.

## Lovesickness and Gender

In literary accounts of love, the torments of lovesickness spare neither sex. Many of the famous patients whose minds were alienated by love are men—one thinks of the young Dante, Boccaccio's Giachetto, Arcite, and Troilus—yet their female counterparts clearly exist as well: Boccaccio's Lisa and Lisabetta, for example, and Christine de Pisan's faithful women in *The Book of the City of Ladies*.[6] Vernacular poems more nearly contemporary with Peter of Spain also offer powerful examples of women stricken by the *aegritudo amoris*.

Ovidian lore from the *Ars amatoria* and *Remedia amoris*, which incorporate ancient medical ideas on love as illness, contributed to the stock of cultural themes about women in love (Figure 6.1). *L'art d'amours* notes that love is a "pure art" that "women and young men of ease" know by nature.[7] In the anonymous twelfth-century adaptation of the *Aeneid*, the *Roman d'Eneas*, heroines like Dido or Lavinia, who were afflicted with the madness of love and all its symptoms, express their torments in the language of love as illness derived from the *Ars* and the *Remedia*.[8] The psychology of thwarted and abandoned women evident in the *Heroides* also influenced literary representations of women in love. Chrétien de Troyes in turn endowed his heroines with the signs of the amatory malady derived from Ovid. Fénice in *Cligés*, for example, complains that she is *dolcement malade* (l. 3044) and her nurse Thessala explains that she is suffering the *max d'amors* (l. 3073).[9]

The Ovidian language of lovesickness found in secular texts partly overlaps that of divine languor in the Song of Songs, which enjoyed a resurgence of commentary in the twelfth century and contributed a richly ambiguous vocabulary of love to medieval spirituality.[10] The female speaker's refrain, *quia amore langueo* (2.5, 5.8), characterizes spiritual love as a type of earthly lovesickness (Figure 1.3). The equivocal meaning of the phrase allowed many vernacular lyrics to borrow the vocabulary of spiritual languor in order to describe a very secular "love-longing"; in a number of these lyrics the speakers are women.[11] Other texts that do not claim to be imaginative literature also show that women used the language of the Song to express both the exaltation and the painfulness of their experiences of love. Among the *Epistolae duorum amantium*, one of the woman's letters to her lover confesses: *tui presencia dum careo . . . permota amore tuo langueo* ("while

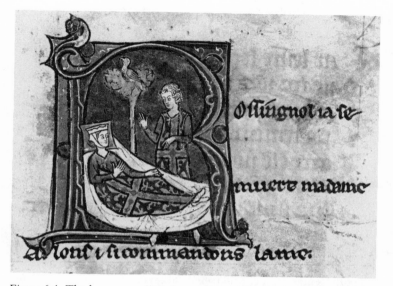

*Figure 6.1.* The lover says: "Nightengale, my lady is dying." From the *Roman de poire.* Paris, Bibliothèque Nationale, MS fr. 2186, fol. 79r.

I lack your presence . . . I languish, frenzied by your love").[12] In the thirteenth century, the biographer of the mystic Julian of Mount Cornillon related that she suffered a divine love-languor that her companions mistook as an earthly illness.[13] Whether directed toward a sacred or a secular object, women's passionate love, figured as illness, was thus a familiar part of thirteenth-century culture.

Natural philosophy, in contrast to love literature, investigated women's sexuality rather than their erotic maladies. Twelfth- and early thirteenth-century natural philosophers, with the notable exception of Hildegard of Bingen, considered women to be more libidinous than men, and to take greater delight in sexual activity.[14] As the encyclopedist Bartholomaeus Anglicus, Peter's contemporary, puts it, women are "hasty in likinge of Venus." Moreover, "the femel desireth more than the male and is more ymoeued to loue in alle kynde of bestes, as Ysidorus seith *libro xi°.*"[15] Constantine the African asserts in the *Pantegni* that women enjoy intercourse more than men do because men receive pleasure only from the expulsion of seed, whereas women enjoy themselves doubly (*dupliciter delectantur*), in expelling their own seed and in receiving that of the male, an idea still current as late as the eighteenth century.[16] Constantine's physiological view about women's double pleasure achieved wide currency in the Salernitan questions.[17] An inquiry of this type, incorporated into the *Art d'amours*, adds a psychological twist to women's sexual desire. In answer to the question about why animals love only during the rutting period but women love all the time, the author says that women have reason and memory "and they remember the pleasure they have had of love and the delight; therefore, they desire it always."[18]

There are, however, some few indications that physicians before Peter of Spain had considered the problem of women's lovesickness. One of the prose Salernitan questions mentions a girl who fell into mania because the lover whom she awaited never showed up. Though it is not explicitly designated as such, the incident might be construed as a case of lovesickness.[19] Bernardus Provincialis, a late twelfth-century physician, states more clearly that *amor hereos* is no respecter of sex in his *Commentarium super tabulas Salerni*. He says that if any youth or girl is afflicted with love for someone unobtainable, he or she, with hands held or tied behind the back, should bend over to drink water into which glowing iron has been plunged. This, he claims, is a "physical and empirical and rational remedy" because it settles the humors aroused by *amore illicito vel hercos* [for *hereos*?].[20]

Bernard's commentary aside, other medical texts before Peter of Spain's *Questions* that describe *amor hereos* both imply and explicitly claim that men are the primary class of patients. Avicenna's suggestion (repeated by Gerard of Berry and others) that the patient purchase and enjoy girls as part of the cure is clearly meant to benefit male patients. Gerard's claim that *amor heros* is a disease of noble men who suffer from it more often because of their wealth and the softness of their lives proved long-lived. The author of the *Art d'amours*, a cleric no doubt, somewhat scornfully described their amatory disposition in terms that recall Gerard's: "When rich young men are at leisure, they want to practice the art of love. They want to amuse themselves, to ride horses, and to be prized and praised for having love and riches with which they are fat and puffed up."[21] In the late thirteenth century Bernard of Gordon repeated Gerard's view that noblemen are most subject to the disease, as did Jacques Despars in the fifteenth.

Gerard's masculinization of the *morbus amoris* is difficult to explain. He implicates social and economic factors—leisure and wealth—in lovesickness, but why he should attribute the disease to men is unclear. The *De amore* of Andreas Capellanus, which, as we have seen, parallels Gerard's gloss in a number of ways, also corroborates the physician's views on this point. Though Andreas concedes the *imperium* of love over both sexes, he addresses the treatise to Walter and the how-to advice exemplified in the dialogues and the chapters on the love of nuns and prostitutes is tailored for men who must possess *nobilitas* and *probitas morum* in order to attain their aspiration of loving *curialiter*. Moroever, Andreas generally reserves the rhetoric of love-as-illness for aristocratic male speakers.[22] Gerard's claim that

noblemen are predisposed to suffer *amor hereos* coincides with literary representations of aristocratic young men as the primary victims of lovesickness
or as the ones likely to experience love as illness, as in, for example, the
*Roman de la Rose*.[23]

This view may have been a commonplace in Parisian academic circles
in the 1220s, when Gerard's gloss had circulated for one or two decades and
when Peter of Spain pursued his studies at the University. As noted in chapter one, William of Auvergne, bishop of Paris (1228–49) and teacher of
theology, offers a bit of evidence for the incidence of morbid love among
the young Parisian clerks. He tells his students: "You ought to remember
some things which you experience continually. You see that love is a certain
*raptus*, just like that which is called *morbus eros*, which is a most violent
and intense illness, in which someone who loves is in such rapture that it
barely permits him to think of anything besides the woman he loves in this
way."[24] The apparent offhandedness of the remark suggests that love as a
medically-defined illness was both common knowledge and common experience, as does its pedagogical strategy of moving from the more familiar
(*morbus eros*) to the less (*raptus*). William attributes *morbus eros* to men explicitly in the phrase "the woman he loves" and implicitly in the reference
to the experiences of the male audience. His contemporary and colleague,
William of Auxerre, agreed that *amor morbus* for some woman drives many
mad, who must then be cured through diet and medication.[25]

Important university thinkers during Peter of Spain's intellectually for-
mative period thus assumed that men were the usual patients of *morbus
amoris*, an idea embodied in some contemporary imaginative literature. Yet
other vernacular poems provided numerous examples of women who suffered *max d'amors*, and some physicians in turn recognized that lovesickness
affects all. Within this complex context, then, Peter of Spain framed his
controversial questions on lovesickness and gender.

## Peter of Spain's Questions

The surviving manuscripts of Peter's *Questions on the Viaticum* contain three
facets of his thinking on lovesickness and gender. The first reflects the influence of Gerard: Peter claims that noblemen suffer more than others from
love. The second and third aspects compare men's and women's susceptibility to lovesickness; the third is distinguished by its use of the language of
measurement to compare sexual pleasure.[26]

Peter strikes out into new territory (as far as the sources permit us to
judge) by raising the problem of women and lovesickness. Though in both
versions he debates whether men or women are more subject to *amor hereos*,

the distinction in the B version between intensity of pleasure in men and quantity of pleasure in women proved more attractive to later writers searching for a vocabulary to compare sexual experience. A discussion of the A version will highlight by contrast the novelty and difficulty of B's argumentation on the measure of pleasure.

## VERSION A

Several questions of the series of ten on *amor hereos* in the A version consider in which complexion, sex, and age this disease occurs most often. The fourth question concerns the relative susceptibility of the sexes. Peter argues that because women are, according to Aristotle in *De animalibus*, "weaker in hope" than men, they are therefore more subject to *amor hereos*.[27] The lean syllogism tells us no more about women's hopelessness, but Aristotle's remark is part of a passage dealing with similarities and contrasts of disposition and habit in male and female animals:

> Woman is more compassionate than man, more easily moved to tears, at the same time is more jealous, more querulous, more apt to scold and to strike. She is, furthermore, more prone to despondency and less hopeful than the man, more void of shame, more false of speech, more deceptive, and of more retentive memory.[28]

Peter investigates women's despondency in his unpublished *Questiones super de animalibus*, the earliest surviving Western commentary on Aristotle's text.[29] In that work Peter asks why women despair more than men, have less confidence, and are more jealous. The answers rest on medical–biological commonplaces and unwittingly reveal something of the psychological stresses that women in medieval society labored under. Starting from the medical commonplace that women are moister than men, Peter argues that because moisture retains an impression less easily than dryness, women lack confidence concerning things promised to them.[30] They are jealous because they realize that they are by nature less perfect than men, and so envy the superior sex, or because they are occupied with children or a business (Figure 6.2). Fearing that others are out to cheat them, women become envious.[31]

This biological–social explanation for women's despondency helps to explain the argument for men's susceptibility to *amor hereos* in the *Viaticum*. Since men have drier brains than women, the image of the desired object is imprinted more deeply in the imagination, and since lovesickness is partly caused by a strong impression upon the imagination, men, with their drier brains, are more likely to contract it.[32] The solution to these opposing arguments denies neither sex the chance to suffer from love. Although *amor hereos* "is more quickly and frequently generated in women because of the

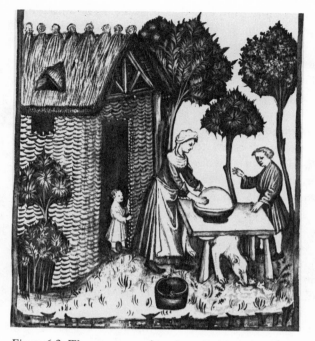

*Figure 6.2.* Woman engaged in cheesemaking and child-care, from the *Tacuinum sanitatis.* Vienna, Bildarchiv, Österreichische Nationalbibliothek, Cod. ser. nov. 2644, fol. 61r.

lack of hope in them and because they are more frequently sexually stimulated," in men the disease is more difficult to cure because "the impression of any desirable form in the brain of a man is deeper and more difficult to eradicate than the impression of a form in the brain of a woman."[33]

As far as epidemiology is concerned, then, female patients seem to predominate numerically (*frequentius*), but men are more profoundly stricken by the disease. Peter thus links predisposition to *amor hereos* to biological dispositions humans have in common with other animals, and—apart from an unelaborated phrase about women's sexual excitability—to different physiologies of the brain in men and women, determined by the basic polarity of dryness and moisture.

## VERSION B

In contrast to the A version, the B version of the commentary focuses on the intensity of sexual pleasure as the key to understanding susceptibility to *amor hereos*. The arguments are at first sight confusing, because Peter seems to claim that each sex suffers more from love than the other. The ambiguity stems from his attempt to reconcile Constantine's pronouncements on women's greater sexual pleasure with other medical and philosophical traditions that grant preeminence in this regard to the male sex. Replying to the question "In which sex is the desire for intercourse greater and in which is pleasure greater?" he argues first that men have a greater *desire* for intercourse because the four factors stimulating sexual desire—imagination of the desired object, an imbalanced complexion, an "elevating windiness" (*ventositas elevans*, the *spiritus* necessary for erection), and an abundance of seed—occur more in men than in women.[34] Women, however, have a greater *pleasure* in intercourse, and where there is a greater pleasure, he argues, there is a greater desire. "Therefore the desire for intercourse is greater, and love is greater and more intense in women than in men." In addition, women fall in love more easily than men and thus desire both sex and love more than men do.[35] The solution to these arguments sounds paradoxical, if not downright contradictory: love is more intense (*intensior*) on the part of men than on the part of women, but pleasure is greater on the part of women.[36] What, then, is the intended distinction between *intensior amor* and *maior delectatio*?

The meaning of the contrast is clearer if we compare a second question on pleasure raised in the same section: Which sex delights more in intercourse? The argumentation reveals that Peter perceives a qualitative difference between the experiences of men and women. For his claim that men's sensations are more intense than women's he gives three pieces of evidence: they have an inherently more intense sense perception, they emit more during intercourse, and are "more consumed" by it. Women, on the other hand, have a double pleasure, but it is not of the same quality as that of men.[37] Despite his failure to specify this qualitative difference, Peter clearly uses contrasting terms, intensity and quantity, to compare pleasure in men and women. The comparison leads to an assessment of sexual pleasure as "separate but unequal": intensity of pleasure in men is "greater" than quantity of pleasure in women. And since in the terms of his analysis, sexual pleasure partially determines lovesickness, he can conclude that men have *intensior amor* but women have *maior delectatio*. The philosophical and physical bases for this duality are apparent if we turn again to his commentary on Aristotle, the *Questions on* De animalibus.

## *Evidence from the Commentary on Aristotle's* De animalibus

In this work Peter raises the same questions on appetite and pleasure as he does in the *Viaticum* commentary, this time, however, in the context of mammalian procreation rather than in that of lovesickness, and poses the problems of sexual appetite and sexual pleasure separately. In determining which sex takes greater pleasure in intercourse, he adduces a principle from Aristotle's *Physics* that grounds the distinction between intensive pleasure in men and quantitative pleasure in women. He cites the famous dictum that (in his words) "matter desires forms just as the ugly the good or the beautiful and the female the male" (*Physics* 192a 22–23).[38] By appealing to the traditional association of women with matter and men with form, he not only rationalizes the superiority of men's pleasure, but reveals the ontological basis for that superiority. Since form is a greater perfection than matter, and since an early theory of intensity held it to be a perfection of a thing's form, men, by nature more perfect and "formal" than women, must experience a greater intensity of pleasure.[39] The association of women with matter suggests a lesser pleasure to the extent that matter is inferior to form, and this is supported by another statement in the commentary. To the question of why there is shame in the act of generation, Peter replies that in this work women hold the place of matter and men the place of form, "in which a man glories; a woman reviles herself in this."[40] Little wonder that, oppressed by the consciousness of serving the place of matter instead of form, the intensity of her pleasure might be less than his.

Further debate on sexual pleasure follows from the Aristotelian premise. The familiar quotation from Constantine on women's double pleasure makes its appearance once again. However, the conclusive argument for greater masculine pleasure hinges, as it does in the *Viaticum* commentary, on a qualitative difference between the sexes. Men are hotter than women (another medical commonplace), and since heat stimulates intercourse, Peter concedes that men take greater pleasure in it. A second qualitative difference distinguishes men and women, yielding greater delight to the masculine sex: male seed is more digested, i.e., refined and perfected, than female seed, hence its emission gives men greater pleasure. In summary, Peter says that "although women take pleasure in a number of ways, a greater pleasure increases more in men than in women."[41] As in the *Viaticum* commentary, he contrasts a numerical superiority of pleasures in women with a qualitative superiority in men. Women's association with matter links their pleasures with quantity rather than quality, suggesting a mensuration of number and extent, the attributes of matter, rather than of intensity, which is reserved for qualitatively superior men.

## Quantification of Qualities

Perhaps prompted by Constantine's remark that "eros is a word designating the greatest pleasure" and by Avicenna's inclusion of unfulfilled desire as a coadjuvant cause in his definition of lovesickness, Peter systematically compares the experiences of men and women in order to obtain a relative measure of which sex experiences greater pleasure during sexual activity. He refines the understanding of the causal mechanisms of lovesickness beyond Constantine's "necessity of expelling superfluous humor" and the "sight of a beautiful form" with the psychological acumen of a three-time commentator on Aristotle's *De anima* and with the physiological concerns of an Aristotelian biologist.[42] Attributable to both his Aristotelianism and his psychological interests is the implicit recognition of *delectatio* as a final cause of *amor hereos* (Figure 6.3). Later writers, among them Arnald of Villanova and Gerard of Solo, explicitly acknowledge the final causality of pleasure among all the other immediate, mediate, and coadjuvant causes of the disease.[43] John of Tornamira expresses the extent to which physicians assimilated the correlation of sexual pleasure with lovesickness when he defines *hereos* as *multum delectabile*, because the lover desires ultimate carnal delight from a woman.[44]

The contrast between intensity and quantity that Peter applies to sexual pleasure is a rather early and not wholly clear attempt to formulate a relative measure of the quality of pleasure. The quantification of other qualities, such as charity or heat, for example, had been discussed in early thirteenth-century philosophy, but a rigorous analysis of the problem of qualitative change or measurement became possible only in the late thirteenth century or early fourteenth century, when the conceptual tools for these problems were fully developed.[45] Michael McVaugh has shown, for example, that although Peter of Spain was aware of the problems involved in quantifying the quality of heat, his analysis was limited by the lack of an adequate terminology.[46] Still, a writer at mid-century who wished to discuss alterations in heat or charity had at least a traditional context and some points of reference for his analysis; one who attempted to assess the relative sensations of pleasure with the language of intension and remission was undertaking something quite new. Peter's analysis does not represent a conceptual breakthrough or a development of the language of intension or of methods of quantification; rather, it extends current terminology to a new subject. In this Peter not only anticipates the "mania to measure" that invades fourteenth-century science and philosophy, but also evidences the close connection between medicine and philosophy in the later Middle Ages.

Peter of Spain's cogitations on the measure of pleasure were immediately imitated and extended by both natural philosophers and physicians, who clarified the terminology of the discussion while maintaining the basic distinction between intensity and quantity or extensivity. The first and clearest reaction to Peter's work on this topic is contained in Albert the

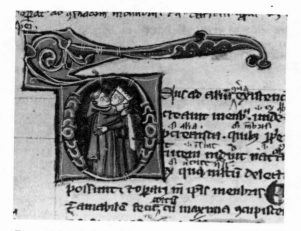

*Figure 6.3.* Cleric and woman embracing in the "D" of *Deus,* the first word of the *Viaticum's* book (6) on sexual disorders. The passage explains that God created sexual pleasure so as to ensure procreation. Cambridge, St. John's College, MS D.24 (99), fol. 146. By permission of the Masters and Fellows of St. John's College.

Great's questions on the *De animalibus* (1258), which are "closely modelled" on Peter of Spain's questions on Aristotle, indicating their importance in the eyes of the greatest thirteenth-century natural philosopher.[47] The changes Albert makes in his discussion of sexuality and pleasure, however, both reaffirm and clarify the philosophical basis of Peter's ideas on measuring the relative intensity of sexual experience. Albert, like Peter, cites the analogy between men and women, form and matter, from the first book of Aristotle's *Physics,* but unlike Peter, goes on to argue explicitly that men's participation in the act is *formalius* (more formal) than that of women, and hence gives greater pleasure.[48] The language used to describe women's delight is rooted in the analogy with matter. In addition to the familiar *delectatio duplicata,* they are said to enjoy themselves *in pluribus modis,* which he terms "extensive" pleasure. He phrases it in another way: "Quantitatively, pleasure is greater in women, but intensively it is greater in men."[49]

Since Albert's and Peter's discussions of pleasure are so similar, it is difficult to sort out indebtedness among later writers who adopt the distinction between extensivity and intensity. In fact, the contrast becomes a commonplace in late thirteenth- and fourteenth-century medical and natural philosophical texts on sexuality, appearing in such diverse places as Pierre de St.-Flour's *Concordancie,* a fourteenth-century medical dictionary, and a mid-fourteenth-century commentary on the *De secretis mulierum*.[50] These later writers sometimes develop the analysis beyond that found in either Peter's or Albert's works. For example, Pietro d'Abano, while repeating the substance of Peter's argumentation about pleasure in his *Conciliator* (1305), adds yet another dimension to the measure of female pleasure, that of time. Their pleasure is extensively greater than men's because, among other things, it lasts longer. Yet like Peter of Spain and Albert the Great, he grants men a greater intensity of pleasure within its shorter duration.[51]

## Influence on the Medical Tradition of Lovesickness

Peter's analysis influenced, it may reasonably be assumed, the more specialized medical tradition of *amor hereos*. The idea that intensity of masculine pleasure is greater, and hence that men are more subject to *amor hereos*, appears in the chapter devoted to lovesickness in Bernard of Gordon's *Practica*. Bernard notes at the end of the chapter that the disease occurs more often in men, because they are hotter than women and hence receive more intense pleasure from intercourse. Women, however, enjoy themselves more extensively because they delight in both their own and male seed.[52]

Gerard of Solo, active at Montpellier around 1330–50, analyzes *amor hereos* in two works, one a commentary on the ninth book of al-Rāzī's *Liber ad regem almansorem*, the other an unpublished *Determinatio de amore hereos*, both indebted to Peter of Spain's commentary on the *Viaticum*.[53] These works reveal that though the level of detail had increased, the difficulties of quantifying pleasure had not been solved completely half a century later. In the *Determinatio* Gerard raises the same question that Peter had: Who is most likely to suffer from lovesickness? His premises are similar as well: those who enjoy intercourse the most, and desire it the most, are most susceptible to *amor hereos*. He organizes his inquiry around the four complexions, suggesting each one in turn as that most likely to contract the disease, and concludes that choleric youths are most likely to suffer from *amor hereos*. In the distinctions he makes concerning the modes of appetite, however, he discusses the differences between men and women. He says that sexual appetite is twofold, extensive and intensive. The former is greater in women because they delight in more ways than men, for they take pleasure in four things in intercourse: reception of male seed, expulsion of their own seed, motion of the womb, and friction of the male member which induces *pruritum et titillationem*.[54] Gerard then considers why there is so much pleasure in intercourse without returning to explain intensive pleasure in men. Peter's and Albert's definition of quantity or extensivity as "many modes" apparently invited subsequent writers further to define or specify what these modes were, leading to the tetrad just listed here and to Pietro d'Abano's triad above.

Gerard's commentary on al-Rāzī contains a fuller explanation of the contrast between the masculine intensity and the female extensivity of pleasure. The context, like that of the *Determinatio*, is an examination of the types of people susceptible to lovesickness. Unlike the *Determinatio*, however, the section opens with the remark that this disease can befall anyone.[55] As Gerard proceeds, he distinguishes appetite for intercourse from appetite for food on the basis of heat and cold, just as Peter of Spain had done in his questions on both the *Viaticum* and the *De animalibus*. Because appetite for intercourse depends on heat, it will be greater in men, since they are hotter than women—the same argument that Peter had used in his commentary on Aristotle's *De animalibus* and that Albertus repeated in his *Questiones*. Thus, Gerard says, "it is apparent that a man takes pleasure more intensely than a woman, because he is hotter, but a woman takes pleasure more extensively because she takes pleasure in more ways than a man."[56] In fact, one of her pleasures is so great, Gerard remarks with an unusual rhetorical inversion, that poor women *as well as* rich ones become whores in order to satisfy the desire it generates.[57]

The impulse to measure sexual desire and pleasure did not wane with the Middle Ages. In our own time, the sophisticated equipment of Masters and Johnson was in part designed to answer some of the same questions that the Portuguese physician had debated so many centuries earlier.[58] But the twentieth century is not the only post-medieval era to apply available technology to the subject of sexual desire and pleasure. In visual and verbal fantasies of the eighteenth century, "lecherometers" or "Female Thermometers" gauged the level of women's desires, replacing the medieval metric of intensity/extensivity with a mechanics of pressure.[59] Women's relatively hidden physiological responses to sexual stimuli elicited mensurations of their desires and pleasures according to conceptual schemas of the age.

## Women and Lovesickness

Peter of Spain's influence on the application of the language of measurement to sexual pleasure proves easier to trace than his contribution to changing ideas about the relation of gender to lovesickness. That he never finally synthesized his arguments on gender and lovesickness into any clear epidemiological statement may in part explain the difficulty of charting the impact of his ideas. We find, for example, that the opinion of Gerard of Berry on the social origins of *amor hereos* and men's susceptibility to it was still voiced in the fifteenth century. Jacques Despars wrote in his commentary on Avicenna's *Canon* that the disease is called *hereos* or *hereosus* "because it befalls noble men and heroic men more [often] than it does simple men of the common people."[60] Nonetheless, a century later women appear in case histories of lovesickness and in the seventeenth century the physician Jacques Ferrand claimed that women were the primary sufferers of "la maladie d'amour."[61] Since Peter of Spain is the first physician in surviving sources to investigate women's lovesickness in comparison to men's, we may reasonably explore the connection between his ideas and similar ones expressed in later medical texts.

To recapitulate briefly the three aspects of his thinking on lovesickness and gender: In the first, he more or less duplicates Gerard of Berry's opinion that aristocratic men are disposed toward the disease. In the second, embodied in the A version, he claims that women suffer from love more frequently than men do, but that men are harder to cure. The third aspect, evident in the B version, is generated from the equivocal senses of *amor* and *maior* in the statement that men have *intensior amor* but women *maior delectatio*. The wide semantic range of *amor* allows him to interpret it as "sexual desire" and thus to narrow the focus of his argument about the incidence of lovesickness to sexuality, while the ambiguity of *maior* enables him to distinguish the intensity of men's pleasure from the quantity of women's. The coexistence of the first and third aspects within a single manuscript of the B version (Vatican, pal. lat. 1166) suggests that Peter responded in an *ad hoc* fashion to the opportunities presented by Constantine's text, without a focused concern to refashion medical thinking on lovesickness and gender.

Even so, his interest in women invites explanation, especially given Gerard's delegation of *amor hereos* to men a generation earlier. Most speculative, but also most tantalizing, is the possibility that Peter introduced women into medical discourse on lovesickness in order to reflect clinical realities. That is, he may have sought to adjust academic theory to account for female patients seen in practice. We know from medical *consilia*, written advice given by physicians in response to individuals' requests, that university-trained doctors did treat women of the well-to-do classes.[62] Literary representations of lovesick women may also have influenced Peter's deliberations on the topic, especially since he knew his Ovid well. It should not be forgotten, however, that dialectical discourse itself can generate its own subjects. Once the question of which sex is more subject to *amor hereos* is raised, women perforce enter the discussion.[63] The method of his inquiry, then, rather than any particular interest in women, may have spawned the debate. Finally, a certain amount of professional ambition may have led the new teacher of medicine to raise the question in the first place in order to outdo Gerard's magisterial claim.

If the causes of Peter's interest in the topic of women and lovesickness cannot be pinned down exactly, his questions nonetheless express a willingness to consider women as patients of *amor hereos* that is found elsewhere among his contemporaries. Sometime after 1230–35, Hugh of St. Cher (pseudo-Gerard of Liège) composed his immensely popular (180 mss., numerous vernacular translations) *De doctrina cordis* for an audience of women religious. The last part of the treatise, *De scissione cordis per amorem*, describes *amor extaticus* in terms of *amor ereos*, "since we test and recognize one love by the other." [64] Although Hugh too repeats the attribution of *amor ereos* to *viri nobiles*, it apparently posed no impediment to the female audience's understanding of themselves as potential subjects of lovesickness. Hugh's fusion of medical and mystical loves for women of the mid-thirteenth century shows that in the mind of at least one of Peter of Spain's contemporaries, medically-defined *amor hereos* supplied a useful way of describing women's experience of love.

The association of women and lovesickness evident here and in Peter of Spain's *Questions* came to be more clearly defined by later physicians. Historians of medicine have noted a tendency among medical writers of the Renaissance not merely to consider women subject to morbid love, but to deem them, as did Jacques Ferrand, the *primary* victims of the malady, or at least particularly susceptible to it. [65] An admittedly metaphoric description of the change might run as follows: In the Middle Ages, a number of academic physicians viewed *amor hereos* as a disease primarily located in the brain rather than in the testicles, and primarily as an affliction of noblemen. Thus *amor hereos* resided at the top of physical, social and sexual hierarchies. As a result, however, of Peter of Spain's attention to the role of sexual physiology in generating lovesickness, the disease gradually shifted "downward" to become, in the estimation of some later writers, an illness of the sexual organs and of women, thus preserving the homology between the corporal and social "place" of the disease (Figure 6.4). [66] In the generation after Peter of Spain, Arnald of Villanova names a *complexio venerea* or *humiditas titillans in organis generationis* as antecedent causes of *amor hereos*; the shift in localization from brain to testes is thus apparent even before the end of the Middle Ages in some writers. [67] Such a gradual "decline" in the localization of *amor hereos* may help to account for its transformation from a "heroic" malady to a "hysteric affliction."

That transformation was never fully completed; noble men continued to be numbered among love's victims in literature and medical writing. The mutual validation of medicine and literature may help explain why the "melancholy lover" persisted even as the "lovesick maiden" entered pathography. [68] *Amor hereos* reverses the hierarchy of perception and reason, sub-

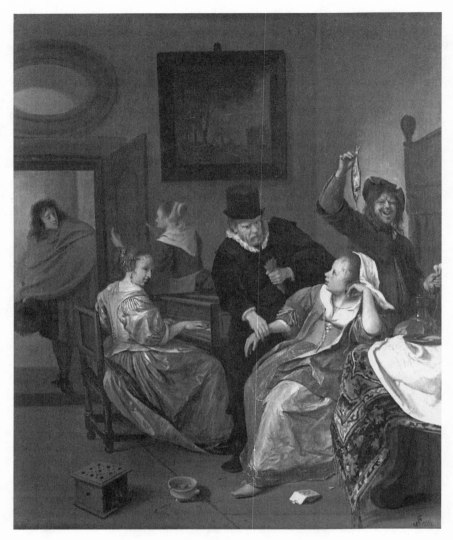

*Figure 6.4.* Women's lovesickness was a stock theme in Dutch genre painting. This burlesque example emphasizes the woman's middle-class status and the sexual implications of the malady. Jan Steen (Dutch, 1626–79), "The Doctor's Visit" (1663–65). Philadelphia Museum of Art, John G. Johnson Collection of Philadelphia (J510).

ordinating judgment to sense perception. As Arnald of Villanova remarks, such an inversion of the proper relation of psychological powers parallels the reversal of the social hierarchy evident in the conventions of *fin'amors*, which subordinates the male lover to his natural and social inferior, the beloved woman.[69] Such a homology betweeen the social and the psychological, between *fin'amors* and *amor hereos*, literature and medicine, would offer a powerful system of analogies difficult for medical ideas alone to displace. In any event, Peter of Spain, the *summus medicorum monarcha*, provides an early and fascinating comparison of the fundamentally similar and yet distinctive sexual pleasures of men and women.

# IS LOVE CURABLE BY HERBS?
## Bona Fortuna's *Treatise on the Viaticum*

*Non est medicabilis amor herbis.*
Love is not curable by herbs.

Ovid, *Remedies for Love*

La sua bellezza ha più vertù che petra,
e 'l colpo suo non può sanar per erba;
ch'io son fuggito per piani e per colli,
per potere scampar da cotal donna.

Dante, *Rime*, 101

In the decades after Peter of Spain debated his questions on the *Viaticum*, some of Europe's leading physicians scrutinized the disease of love, among them William of Saliceto (fl. 1258–75), Arnald of Villanova (ca. 1240–1311), Bernard of Gordon (ca. 1258–1320), William of Corvi (or Brescia, ca. 1250–1326), Dino del Garbo (d. 1327) and Gerard of Solo (fl. 1330–50). Some, like Arnald and Gerard, returned to the topic more than once. Moreover, translations of al-Rāzī's *Liber continens* (1281) and Ibn Jazlah's *Tacuini aegritudinum et morborum* (1280) enriched the store of medical doctrine on love available to Western physicians and other readers.

Bona Fortuna wrote his treatise on the *Viaticum* (*Tractatus super Viaticum*) in this context of active intellectual speculation on the nature and treatment of morbid love. Although in the absence of a firm date for his activity it is difficult to judge the particulars of his indebtedness to his contemporaries, or theirs to him, we can discern in his chapter on *amor hereos* the intellectual currents of the late thirteenth and early fourteenth centuries. But this is not to rob him of his individual contribution to the medical tradition of love; Bona Fortuna has his own distinctive interests and approaches. His therapy for love, for example, with its empirical pharmacy and appeals to experience, seems to embody the attempts of a practitioner to find remedies that work (Figure 7.1). It suggests that medical energies devoted to the problem of love may have been as much practical as speculative around 1300.

Evidence is currently lacking for Bona Fortuna's identity, career, and place of teaching. Codicology and textual evidence suggest that he may have been a Montpellier master who taught a course on the *Viaticum* sometime between 1300 and 1320. The two fourteenth-century manuscripts that contain the *Tractatus* (or *Summa*) on the *Viaticum* list a name, *magister Bona Fortuna*, and codicological evidence dates his activity before the mid-fourteenth century. Although only these two manuscripts survive, their textual difficulties suggest that others now lost once circulated among readers and copyists. Both manuscripts have been carefully read and annotated by a variety of medieval readers; one of them was available in the later fourteenth century at the Sorbonne.[1]

Like the commentaries of Gerard of Berry and Peter of Spain, this treatise reflects the circumstances of medical teaching in a university, but unlike them, it reveals something of Bona Fortuna's presence as a teacher. We are reminded that the *Tractatus* is a series of lectures by such phrases as "I'll say now what I said the other day" or "as I said the other day."[2] Bona Fortuna addresses his students frequently and directly, telling them straightforwardly what they ought and ought not to do as they prepare medicines and treat patients.[3] These crystallized moments of Bona Fortuna's teaching suggest that the text as we have it may be based on a *reportatio* by one of his students.[4] This would account for both the sense of immediacy the text conveys, and also for some of the gaps and omissions common to both manuscripts. Due to the obvious problems of taking lecture notes, even *reportationes* edited by the master are not always fully reliable witnesses for what in fact was said. However, since both manuscripts are by and large intelligible, they may be taken as adequate guides to the master's teaching.

The university milieu offers Bona Fortuna some of his most striking analogies. Parchment and books present themselves as ready objects of comparison. Bona Fortuna instructs his students to note that the skin has three layers, as can be seen in parchment.[5] Elsewhere he explains that *dolor pungitivus* (piercing pain) can be imagined by means of a simile: "For we see that when parchment nears fire, it does not contract equally in all parts, but rather more in one part than in another. Whence also sometimes it is pierced through in one part and not in another. And this type of pain often occurs in pleurisy."[6] The craft of bookmaking also provided material for the prac-

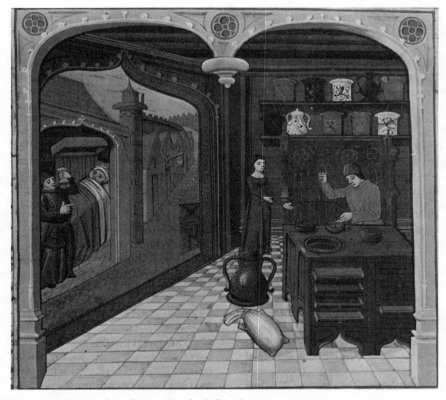

*Figure 7.1.* Practical medicine. On the left a physician inspects a patient's urine. On the right is a scene in an apothecary's shop, where medicines were prepared and sold. Paris, Bibliothèque Nationale, MS fr. 218, fol. 111r.

tical exercise of medicine. Bona Fortuna advises his students to construct casts for broken bones using cloth prepared as in bookmaking.[7] The *Tractatus* thus assumes an audience thoroughly at home with the materials of books and their making, and places itself squarely in a university milieu.

The text contains no clear evidence of its exact place of composition. The likeliest places, however, given its date and the fact that both manuscripts are of French origin, are Paris and Montpellier, between which there was an active commerce of masters and manuscripts.[8]

The evidence for Bona Fortuna's presence at either place is evenly balanced. One manuscript belonged to the Sorbonne, and the text contains references to Paris and to French words.[9] No comparable southern references have come to light. The flimsy weight of statistical probability, however, inclines the scale toward Montpellier. Of medical authors whose university affiliations are known, 10.3% were associated with Montpellier, while only 3% were affiliated with Paris.[10] In fact, many of the physicians writing on *amor hereos* around 1300 were associated with Montpellier. Bona Fortuna's reworking of Constantine's teaching reflects, if not a collegial relationship with the Montpellier masters Arnald of Villanova or Bernard of Gordon, at least a similar approach to the topic of lovesickness. The Paris manuscript of Bona Fortuna's *Tractatus* (Paris, BN lat. 15373) also contains texts by Arnald and Bernard. Since the handwriting in part of the manuscript appears to be southern French, it may have originated at Montpellier—not a guarantee of Bona Fortuna's activity there, of course, but a mark of interest in his work at that medical center.

An ingenious solution to the problem of Bona Fortuna's identity has been offered by Luke Demaitre. Bona Fortuna may be identical with Bernard de Bona Hora, since both names may be translations of the French name "Bonheur."[11] Bernard was a master of medicine at Montpellier whose presence there is documented in 1313 and 1320. Indeed, the chartulary's portrait of the vigorous married cleric who in 1320, along with Jordanus de Turre, did not care to obey either the Chancellor or his deputy and would not do as much for them as for a goose, and who then cursed and beat up another master in medicine, tallies with the forthright personality Bona Fortuna presents in the *Tractatus*.[12] While the *experimenta* bearing Bernard de Bona Hora's name in Montpellier recipe collections do not seem to be duplicated in corresponding sections of Bona Fortuna's commentary on the *Viaticum*, not all Bona Fortuna's *experimenta* would necessarily be preserved in the *Tractatus*.[13] Whether or not Bona Fortuna is Bernard de Bona Hora, either Paris or Montpellier would be a fitting place for his medical teaching.

## The Treatise

The *Tractatus super Viaticum* follows the structure of Constantine's text from first book to last. Bona Fortuna generally divides the exposition of each chapter into definition, causes, signs, and cures, each of which he may in turn subdivide either simply or elaborately. Though the form of his treatment is not syllogistic like that of Peter of Spain, Bona Fortuna's careful *divisio textus* is no less scholastic.[14] Under each heading he quotes and interprets Constantine's words, adding ample material of his own. He cites medical authorities relatively sparingly; none are directly named in the chapter on lovesickness, although it appears that he was familiar with the discussions of Avicenna, al-Rāzī, and Gerard of Berry. Cited authorities are almost exclusively classical and Arabic physicians; references to contemporary writers appear to be lacking. He cites Hippocrates, Galen, and

Avicenna most frequently. Often Bona Fortuna quotes medical authors in order to disagree with them.[15] Even Constantine is not immune from criticism. When Bona Fortuna feels it necessary, he will point out Constantine's errors and advance his own rectifications, sometimes based on his practical experience.[16]

Although the following discussion emphasizes the practical aspects of Bona Fortuna's chapter on lovesickness, since it stands apart from other works in this respect, this does not imply that he is "merely" empirical. In fact, he is quite concerned that his students follow the *via rationis* in their practice of medicine: "one must always proceed rationally."[17] This in turn requires the ability to adjust theory or general recommendations to the individual requirements of the case. The physician's own efforts, his *industria*, bridge the distance between the rules of the art and the individual patient.[18] Bona Fortuna's concern for the harmonious integration of general rules and the varying requirements of the individual patient's circumstances is pointedly expressed in the chapter on *amor hereos*, where he counsels the physician to use his industry to distinguish among universal and particular cures, and to find those most appropriate for his patient. In his concern to adjust theory and practice, and to bridge the gap between universals and particulars, Bona Fortuna agrees with such leading medical thinkers of his time as Bernard of Gordon and Arnald of Villanova.[19]

The *Tractatus* amply documents both the particulars of medical practice and the hazards of late medieval life that physicians were called upon to remedy. The form of such information ranges from lists of *experimenta*—fruits of practice not predictable by theory—to details about patients he has seen recently, to advice about compounding and storing medications. He notes, for example, that one mixture should be boiled for as long as one would cook an egg, or that another paste ought to be shaped into pieces the size of the eucharistic host, or that certain powders will remain potent for up to a year.

He reports several memorable cases. An entire household went bald as a result of mice that had fallen into their stores of oil and had putrefied. In another case, a man was so bitten by lice that he bled in a hundred places. During the treatment of another patient, a *scutella* full of lice was recovered from his body.[20] Anecdotes like these reveal that teacher-practitioners such as Bona Fortuna exercised their callings in both the academic world of scholastic disputation and the "real" world of mice, lice, and other dangers.[21] Among the other medical dangers posed by late medieval life, lovesickness claimed the attention of this practicing physician.

One area of medicine that provides an important context for Bona Fortuna's chapter on *amor hereos* is that of sexual disorders. His teachings on the subject, scattered throughout the *Tractatus*, distinguish medical opinion on sexuality from theological; in this he is joined by other thirteenth-century medical writers. In his discussion of involuntary emission of semen, he notes that one of its causes is the strong *virtus* that accompanies youth or adolescence. One cure, therefore, might be to lessen its strength. Bona Fortuna, however, objects to this method, and parts company from the theologians:

> Then note concerning the cure of this disease. If therefore it is because of excessive seed, and the patient is adolescent or youthful, and other circumstances are suitable, and there is a strong *virtus*, then as far as medical opinion is concerned, whatever theological opinion might be, it is not safe to break such *virtus*. Wherefore note that the generation of seed is one of the good things . . . Whence I, as far as medical opinion goes, would not resist but would do something else.[22]

Our author's freedom from the restraints of theological discourse is perhaps nowhere more evident than in his chapter on the suffocation of the womb. One of the causes of the disease was thought to be retained seed that became corrupted and poisonous, and, consequently, needed to be purged from the body. One means, acceptable in classical medicine and found in the works of Galen and Avicenna, was to arouse the woman to orgasm so that she ejaculated the retained seed. The arousal was often achieved by a woman who manipulated the patient manually. Some scholars have suggested that such practices were problematic in the medieval Christian West. It has been argued that although physicians were familiar with Galen's recommendation, the conventions of decorum obtaining in medical writing prevented them from endorsing it explicitly, assuming that they found it acceptable practice.[23] Bona Fortuna, however, speaks without the least hesitation or circumlocution, recommending masturbation by an *obstetrix* and providing technical directions for it.[24] The manuscripts contain no marginalia expressing surprise or outrage at this therapy, which suggests that the latitude of accepted medical practices was wider than we tend to assume. To judge from the attitudes Bona Fortuna expresses elsewhere in the treatise, his discussion of love unfolds within the liberal bounds of late medieval medical discourse on sexuality.

## *Outline of the Chapter on Lovesickness*

I.  The disease
    A. definition
    B. causes
       1. principal: extrinsic apprehension
       2. adiuvant: beauty; need to expel excess seed

II. Symptoms
    A. those which signal the disease
        1. physical
        2. behavioral
        3. involuntary (pulse, breathing)
    B. those which signify the person provoking the disease
        (the pulse test)
III. Cures
    A. physical
        1. restore the body's composition
        2. restore the balance of humors
    B. psychological
        1. for patients without discretion
        2. for patients with discretion
    C. universal cures
        1. travel
        2. business
        3. litigation
        4. intercourse
IV. Additional helps

## Definition

Unlike Peter of Spain and other writers concerned to localize morbid love in the brain or in other organs, Bona Fortuna skips the controversy by deferring to Constantine's placement of *amor eros* among other diseases of the brain. He does, however, offer his own definition of the illness. Though it is based on Constantine and Avicenna, it more strongly emphasizes the role of the visual image in the generation of the disease. As he notes, the definition includes an understanding of the disease's causality centered in the "extrinsic apprehension" of a form.

The essential role of sight in the birth of love, debated from Plato and Aristotle to Andreas Capellanus, had entered the Western medical tradition of lovesickness in Constantine's *Viaticum*. With the revival of interest in optics in the second half of the thirteenth century, physicians discussed the role visual images played in the disease's causality. Arnald of Villanova, Dino del Garbo, and Gerard de Solo all commented on the *species* or *apprehensum* that the imagination or *phantasia* must store in order for the mind to reflect upon it.[25] Bona Fortuna makes the *species vel passio*—a likeness of an object that mediates between the material world and the mind—the principal cause of lovesickness.[26]

Plato, however, wrote about desire for absolute beauty, not for an individuated form, and even Constantine uses the abstract noun *formositas* for the sight that sends the soul into madness. In contrast, Bona Fortuna stresses the individual, singular form whose *species* provokes excessive thought. Other writers catalogue the qualities in which the beloved is thought to excel all other women: so, for example, Gerard of Berry and Peter of Spain say she is thought to be more noble, more beautiful, and better than the rest, and Bernard of Gordon adds that she is superior in the endowments of nature and culture. Nonetheless, neither they nor others use the term "individual" to denote the preeminence of the beloved in the opinion of the lover. Only Arnald of Villanova, in his *Tractatus de amore heroico*, uses *singularem* to denote the object of love. The lover's erroneous judgment, arising from the error of his estimative power, drives him to desire the object as though it were uniquely superior: *cogitur hanc rem ut singularem vehementer optare*.[27] Perhaps Bona Fortuna was influenced by Arnald's formulation. In any case, these two authors stand apart from their contemporaries in their decision to express the lover's valuation of the beloved in terms of unique individuality rather than as the sum of superior qualities. They may reflect something of the late thirteenth-century disputes on the cognition of singulars, which, as Laín Entralgo has shown, were gradually absorbed into medical thinking in the conception of an individuated patient.[28] Since, however, it is the beloved, not the patient, whose individuality is at stake here, literary sources may have exerted more influence on the semantic usage of Arnald and Bona Fortuna than philosophical debates.

## Causality

For Bona Fortuna, to define is to explain a thing's causes; in his definition of love, the concept of the *species* links the definition to the reasoned cause (*propter quid*) of the disease. He bases his account of causality on the psychology of Aristotle's *De anima* rather than on that of Avicenna, which Gerard of Berry and Peter of Spain had used. The most important difference between the two systems for the analysis of *amor hereos* is the absence of the estimative power from Aristotle's classification of mental powers. Consequently, the terms used to denote the process by which the lover values the beloved excessively, his "mis-estimation" of her worth, will require some explanation.

Bona Fortuna subordinates Constantine's "necessity to expel superfluous humor" and "sight of beauty" as coadjuvant causes to what he terms the principal cause: an external apprehension that is considered "fitting and congenial." The cause lies not in the beauty itself, but in the apprehension of it. But mere apprehension does not suffice to initiate the morbid condition. The image has to be considered *conveniens et amicum*. With these terms, Bona Fortuna continues the Platonic strain of the medical tradition of lovesickness embodied in Constantine's phrase *in sibi consimili forma conspiciat* ("it [the soul] sees a similar form within itself"). "The similar is fitting and congenial," wrote contemporary physicians, and Dino del Garbo noted in his gloss on Cavalcanti's love *canzone* "Donna me prega" (ca. 1311) that the image of the beloved, whose apprehension causes love, is perceived *sub ratione similis et convenientis* ("in the guise of the similar and the fitting").[29] As such, Bona Fortuna remarks, it pleases the patient above all things.

By defining the *species* as fitting and desirable at the moment of perception, Bona Fortuna avoids to some extent the problem of determining where in the perceptual process and how exactly the misjudgment characteristic of the disease occurs, a problem Peter of Spain had solved by declaring that the disease begins in the imagination but is completed in the estimation. Bona Fortuna, in contrast, states that the principal cause, the extrinsic apprehension, moves the *phantasia vel intellectum*, which then in turn disturbs the reason. This description is drawn from the third book of Aristotle's *De anima* (433a–34a), where the psychological causes of local motion are analyzed. Peter of Spain's comments on Aristotle's text (in his *Expositio libri de anima*) clarify why Bona Fortuna might have felt he could dispense with the traditional appeal to a damaged estimative power in favor of his slightly more cumbersome Aristotelian exposition. Peter notes that "intellect," which denotes the practical (rather than speculative) intellect, apprehends an object *per suam speciem* insofar as that object is good or bad, and hence is moved to pursue or avoid it.[30] The practical intellect is thus analogous to Avicenna's estimative power. Peter's exposition further clarifies why Bona Fortuna equates *phantasia vel intellectus*, powers generally considered distinct in most medieval classifications of the internal senses. Aristotle says there are two movers, the practical intellect and appetite. Peter agrees, if by "intellect" both "intellect" and "phantasy" or "imagination" are understood. If the name "intellect" is not used to designate both intellect and phantasy, then one has to posit three movers, intellect, appetite, and phantasy or imagination.[31] Bona Fortuna thus proposes a causal explanation based on an understanding of Aristotle's *De anima* very close to Peter of Spain's, in which the *species* plays the crucial role of moving the fantasy or practical intellect and consequently the reason to desiring and pursuing the desired object.

The concept of *species* situates Bona Fortuna's explanation firmly in contemporary thinking about *amor hereos*. We have already seen certain affinities with Dino del Garbo's explanation of how the *species* is perceived, and parallels are also evident in the *Practica* of William of Corvi (or Brescia) and in Gerard of Solo's *Determinatio de amore hereos* (ca. 1335).[32] These authors' attention to *species* situates their work within a larger contemporary problematic, that of *species in medio*, a concept at the heart of interlocking controversies in optics, psychology, epistemology and philosophy.[33] The emergence of visual *species* in causal analyses of *amor hereos* in the late thirteenth and fourteenth centuries also placed lovesickness in a fertile nexus of debates on imagination and magic in natural philosophy and theology. The language of *species*, as I have shown elsewhere, allowed a cross-fertilization among disciplines that resulted in the entry of magic, previously excluded, into academic medical writing on love.[34]

## Signs and Symptoms

It has been remarked concerning medieval pathography that, in the wake of later medieval philosophical developments, the real and concrete person became the protagonist of his story of illness.[35] The narrative and dramatic elements this development implies suggest why medicine and the arts forged such a productive alliance over the lover's malady in the later Middle Ages and the Renaissance. Of all the categories under which physicians considered lovesickness, symptomatology provided the richest field for artistic elaboration; as we have seen in chapter three, the *signa amoris* were common ground for literary, religious, and medical discourses on love.

Bona Fortuna's division of symptoms or signs into three classes allows the narrative and dramatic potential of the diagnosis of love to stand out more sharply than in the works of Gerard of Berry or Peter of Spain. Our master of medicine divides the signs of the disease of love into the following groups: 1. those taken from the external appearance of the body; 2. those taken from behavior (*ab operationibus moralibus*); 3. those taken from the parasympathetic nervous system (pulse, breathing). He has nothing new to add to the first group, drawn from Constantine and Avicenna. To the second, he adds the desire for solitude, found also in William of Corvi, who says that the lover *stat libenter solitarius* ("gladly remains alone").[36] He devotes most attention to the third class of signs, which he subdivides to include a section on signs revealing the beloved (*signa super re amata*). These are involuntary changes in pulse and breathing that occur when the beloved is mentioned. Though Constantine notes that the pulse is disordered in patients suffering from erotic love, he does not specifically allude to the pulse test as a diagnostic tool; Gerard, Egidius, and Peter of Spain omit it as well. There seems to have been little interest in it among writers on lovesickness until the later thirteenth century, when it appears not only in the *Tractatus*, but also in the works of William of Saliceto, Arnald of Villanova, William of Corvi, and Bernard of Gordon, who quotes Galen's story of a successful diagnosis of love.[37]

The popularity of the pulse test at this time is probably due to the integration of Avicenna's *Canon* into medical curricula, and was doubtless reinforced by the recovery of the pulse story in Galen's *De praecognitione* in the early fourteenth century.[38] Renewed interest in classical stories, such as Valerius Maximus' account of Antiochus and Stratonice, that narrated savvy diagnoses using the pulse test (cf. Figure 1.2) may have also contributed to its currency in medical circles.[39]

In keeping with his pedagogical and practical concerns, Bona Fortuna's description of the diagnosis of love from the pulse is the most elaborately detailed of similar accounts. From his step-by-step instructions it is but a short distance to a case history such as that by Pieter van Foreest.[40] But the distance between Bona Fortuna's instructions and Foreest's experience is the distance between late medieval and Renaissance pathography.[41] Our physician's cures come closest to bridging that gap, but even they remain firmly rooted in the intellectual world of the late Middle Ages.

Bona Fortuna introduces the section on symptoms by explaining: "Sometimes [the patients] conceal and in no way wish to reveal the person whom they love." The physician must therefore recognize the signs that involuntarily betray the identity of the beloved, since joining her with the patient is the best cure. The ideal doctor must therefore exercise his ingenuity to ferret out the patient's secret. Since the pulse, "by elucidating the passions of the soul, manifests the mind's secrets," the doctor can use changes in the pulse to determine the object of the patient's desire (Figure 7.2).[42] As Bona Fortuna says, it is impossible that the pulse *not* change when the right woman is named, thus involuntarily revealing the patient's secret.

Since the patients of academic physicians such as Bona Fortuna were generally well-to-do, and therefore likely to be acquainted with literary culture either as readers or listeners; and since some of the patients Bona Fortuna envisions farther on in the chapter are scholars and hence literate, the "code of secrecy" in the literature of *fin' amors* offered both a model for and an endorsement of Bona Fortuna's patients' reticence about naming whom they desired.

But that reticence was potentially double-edged. On the one hand it may have been part of the game of love (however seriously played), one of the "rules" by whose enactment the lover declared himself to be among the "noble hearts." On the other hand—and possibly simultaneously—social pressure of various kinds and the patient's own internalized values could render the game of love a dubious one fraught with conflict. Secrecy be-

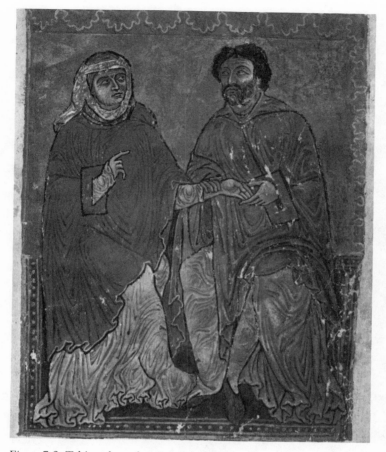

*Figure 7.2.* Taking the pulse. London, British Library, MS Arundel 295, fol. 266.

tokened not only that one loved fashionably and well, but also served as a defense against fear of disapproval, censure, familial rejection or worse. As noted in the first chapter, the specter of incest forced the lovers in antiquity to hide their passion. Bona Fortuna himself suggests in a series of "therapeutic" objections to love why a late medieval lover might refuse to admit his desires. "How will you eat? What will you drink? What will you spend? How will you live? All your goods will perish and thus you will be wretched." To these reproaches Bona Fortuna adds that this mad love will earn the lover the rejection and hate of his friends. Faced with such social censure, the patient may well have decided to "conceal and in no way reveal the beloved."

Diagnosis, then, involves two conflicts of will: between the patient and

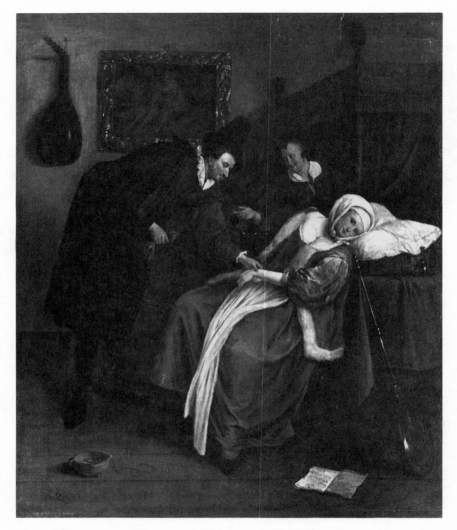

*Figure 7.3.* Jan Steen, "The Doctor's Visit," ca. 1663. The painting of Venus and her lover on the wall suggests the malady for which the doctor tests the patient's pulse. Cincinnati, The Taft Museum, Gift of Mr. and Mrs. Charles Phelps Taft (1931.396).

the family who presumably object to the desired person, and yet who are anxious to remedy the patient's languishing; and between the patient, determined not to reveal his secret, and the doctor, just as determined to find a cure. In Bona Fortuna's chapter at least, the physician intervenes in the patient's love life—recommendations of therapeutic intercourse notwithstanding—on the side of convention, order, and responsibility. As in the anecdote of the young man cured by a trumped-up charge of homicide (below), the attitudes and values of the family win out over individual desire. The other authors treated in this volume show that medical discourse on love is not always as strongly normalizing as it is in the hands of Bona Fortuna or Bernard of Gordon.[43] Yet as Bona Fortuna's therapy for suffocation of the womb shows, he is neither prudish nor theologically conservative about sexual topics in general. Significantly, then, the type of passionate love represented by *amor hereos*—a kind of emotional and social excess—appears to a physician like Bona Fortuna to require more constraint through medical intervention and social pressure than do sexual diseases, like involuntary ejaculation or suffocation of the womb, that are caused by physiological excesses. The complex social rituals of love evidently threaten the order of things more than does mere libido.

Bona Fortuna's discussion of the pulse test and of the remedies for love signal indirectly his own discomfiture with erotic love and its conflicts with normal social order. Similarly, the stories of Antiochus, Perdica, and the lovers in *Decameron* 2.8 and 10.7 illustrate the potential drama that the pulse test offered for exploring characters and values in conflict. In the seventeenth century that drama was represented visually in a genre of painting known as the "Doctor's Visit" that flourished in the Netherlands.[44] Masters like Gerrit Dou, Jan Steen (see Figure 6.4), and Gabriel van Mieris typically portray a well-to-do young woman feebly reclining in a chair or even tossing in bed, while a physician takes her pulse. His dress and bearing convey his power to reveal her secret and his authority to ordain a remedy. That love is her secret malady is sometimes indicated by the titles of the paintings ("Liebeskrankheit," "Mal d'amour") and sometimes by iconographical clues like background paintings (Figure 7.3).

## Cures

Bona Fortuna's section on cures refers to experimentation (in the medieval sense of the word) more often than those of other contemporary writers on *amor hereos*.[45] However, Bona Fortuna offers the fruits of his experience to validate and specify general therapeutic suggestions made by previous medical authorities. For example, where al-Rāzī, Avicenna, or Gerard of Berry recommend purging excessive humor (Figure 7.4) as one part of therapy, Bona Fortuna offers specific compounds and recipes for doing so. Despite Ovid's dictum that "Love is not curable by herbs" (*Remedies for Love*) Bona Fortuna instructs the physician how to compound a decoction of wild endive, honeysuckle root, dandelion, and basil, to which a little

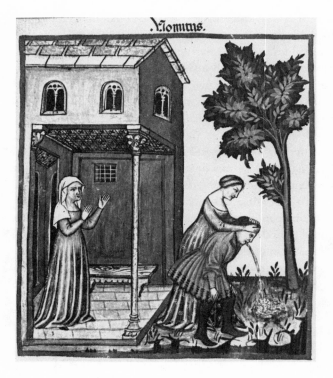

*Figure 7.4.* Purgation "upward." From the *Tacuinum sanitatis.* Vienna, Bildarchiv, Österreichische National-bibliothek, Cod. ser. nov. 2644, fol. 99v.

dodder is added after it has come to the boil. It should then boil for as long as one cooks an egg. According to both medieval and modern herbals, Bona Fortuna's empirical pharmacy, unusual in medical discussions of *amor hereos*, was probably effective for its stated purposes. The simples he lists generally have laxative, diuretic, or cathartic properties, and hence probably effected the purgation for which they were intended. Compound *ieras*, which he also recommends for lovesickness, were commonly used purgatives based on aloes.

The paragraphs on basil (Figure 7.5) at the end of the chapter on love suggest that the physician could not always predict the effects of his simples or compounds. The recipes given in this section are the "certain helps" promised at the outset of the chapter and thus are an integral part of Bona Fortuna's doctrine on lovesickness. The remedies for persistent diarrhea that he describes allay severe reactions to the purgative compounds he recommends earlier in the chapter. The basil-stuffed chicken and almond-basil crepes (*tortellos*) that he suggests are delightful culinary touches.

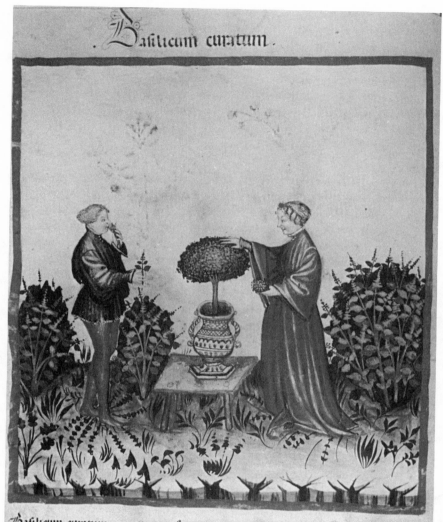

*Figure 7.5.* Basil, according to the *Tacuinum sanitatus,* "dissolves superfluities of the brain." Vienna, Bildarchiv, Österreichische Nationalbibliothek, Cod. ser. nov. 2644, fol. 39v.

As with these purgative and anti-purgative recipes, Bona Fortuna cites his own experience to confirm the recommendations of earlier authorities in his discussion of universal and particular cures. *Documenta universalia*, he explains, will work for all patients, but *documenta particularia* cure only some. No doubt prompted by Avicenna, he critiques Constantine's recommendation of songs and instrumental music by pointing out that they cheer up some patients, but plunge others into deeper sadness. Hence they are particular rather than universal cures. The doctor must, therefore, *de sua industria* (by his own efforts) find out and administer what in fact will work in a given case.

In Bona Fortuna's opinion, there are four universal cures for lovesickness: travel, litigation (Figure 7.6), business, and intercourse with other women, whose efficacy he attests by appeals to his own experience in practice. To illustrate the point that change of scenery (*mutatio regionis*) is a universal cure for lovesickness, he relates the case of a young man whom he caused, with the consent of the young man's relatives, to be charged with homicide. The man was forced to flee the country, and so was cured of lovesickness by separation from the object of his desire (Figure 7.7).[46] Bona Fortuna's particular experience with this young man thus confirms the efficacy of the traditional universal cure. Moreover, without being a case history, it nonetheless provides interesting information on the social context of treatment for lovesickness. Bona Fortuna was apparently called in by the young man's relatives, and physician and family together plotted a rather extreme, though effective, cure.

Bona Fortuna's psychotherapy is as remarkably specific as his somatic therapy. Like Bernard of Gordon, who classifies patients suffering from love as rational or irrational, Bona Fortuna divides them into the corrigible and the incorrigible. If a patient cannot respond to rational arguments, then one is to treat him with caution and gentleness. One must proceed with such a patient, he says, "just as we do with boys whom we teach ABC without blows, but with all gentleness, whom we promise nuts, apples, and other things." If, for example, the patient is a scholar, he should be promised honors and benefices.

Bona Fortuna's sensitive handling of his patients stands in sharp contrast to the violence of Bernard de Gordon, who recommends whipping unreasonable patients until they begin to stink, or of Gerard of Solo, who advocates blows with a good belt. Bernard's opinion in fact became proverbial—"Que le Medecin qui va sans Gordon, va sans baston," says Jacques Ferrand in his encyclopedia on erotic melancholy (1623), only then to distance himself from the Montpellier master's therapy.[47] In their recommendation of beating, Bernard and Gerard seem to be among the minority of

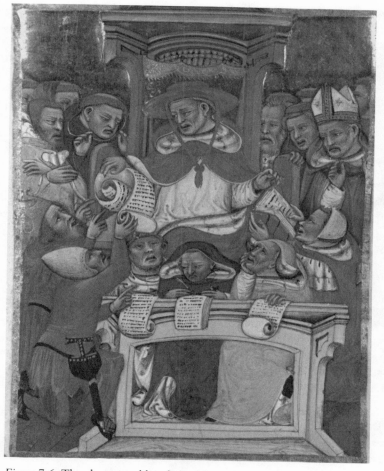

*Figure 7.6.* The clamor and bustle in this courtroom scene show why lawsuits would distract the lover from his preoccupation. Part of a leaf from the *Novellae* of Johannes Andreae. Cambridge, Fitzwilliam Museum, MS 331, detail.

writers on lovesickness. If, however, the patient is "corrigible," then Bona Fortuna follows Avicenna, Gerard of Berry, and others in advocating vilification of the beloved, a cure in which the misogyny of the "clerks" (to use the Wife of Bath's phrase for educated male intellectuals) is readily apparent.

Given Bona Fortuna's claims of practical experience in curing *amor hereos* and the striking specificity of his remedies, it is tempting to argue that lovesickness was a disease of some frequency, and that physicians in the late

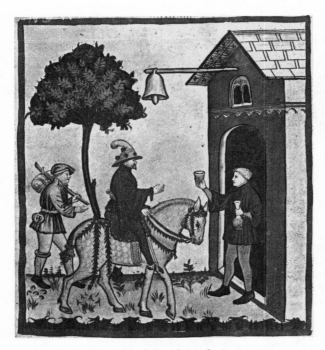

*Figure 7.7.* A rider is handed a glass of wine at a tavern or inn. From the *Tacuinum sanitatis*. Vienna, Bildarchiv, Österreichische Nationalbibliothek, Cod. ser. nov. 2644, fol. 87r.

thirteenth and early fourteenth centuries were not only ready to diagnose *amor hereos*, but did it regularly enough to elaborate semeiology and to compare the efficacy of various therapies. New *signa*, the foundation of diagnosis and prognosis, would appear to reflect the fruits of practice. For example, Bona Fortuna's claim that symptoms of a dry mouth and tongue, and bitterness in the throat, as though the patient had eaten unripe plums, signal *amor hereos* caused by adust ("burnt") humor, suggests experience with lovesick patients on the basis of which these signs have been proven accurate and reliable.

Inviting as it is to see in Bona Fortuna's chapter the traces of actual cases of *amor hereos*, we must also remember that what seems to derive from experience could be, in fact, a recasting of traditional accounts without recourse to observation. The dry and bitter tongue and throat, for instance, could be accounted for in two other ways, neither of which implies any interaction with patients. It could derive from symptoms in al-Rāzī's exposition in the *Liber continens* of *coturub vel ereos* (a conflation of lycanthropy and lovesickness), in which dryness of the tongue and throat are repeatedly mentioned. Alternatively, the symptoms could be "predicted" from the causality of *amor hereos*. As the *Viaticum* says, excessive humor can cause lovesickness. The heat of the patient's complexion, generated by insomnia, could then burn such matter, rendering it "adust" and even more malignant. This form of humor, often melancholic, is associated with dryness, bitterness, or sourness.[48] The excessive heat thought to be generated within the body in *amor hereos* could also contribute to dryness in the throat. To such symptoms "predicted" by causal theories of *amor hereos*, then, Bona Fortuna need only have added the descriptive simile *quasi pruna novella immatura* to arrive at his seemingly new, empirically derived symptom.

These considerations cast doubt on our ability to recover the realities of medieval medical practice from texts whose fundamental orientation is to theory and to authority.[49] Despite the difficulties these works present, however, careful interdisciplinary study of both texts and contexts can enlighten us about physicians' experience with lovesick patients. Medieval medicine was a social and pragmatic art, composed of *practica* as well as *theorica*, and practiced between and among historical individuals. The medical tradition of *amor hereos* was intellectually vigorous and long-lived because there was a continuing social need to which it responded. That need is the subject of the next chapter.

# RECREATING A CONTEXT FOR THE LOVER'S MALADY

> The love of melancholics is hateful, twisted, and death-carrying, like that of voracious wolves . . . They have intercourse with women but they hate them.
>
> Hildegard of Bingen[1]

On St. Valentine's Day in 1402, Gadifer de la Salle, knight errant and veteran military adventurer, was elected to the Court of Love of Charles VI. Its members met to compose and perform love poetry, but they also held jousts in honor of the ladies. Gadifer's election to the company meant that he was recognized "as a tried knight and as an established courtier, with an understanding of fashionable style and recognized literary interests."[2]

Gadifer was participating in what had become a standard set of ritual practices, regardless of whether they were organized around a Court of Love or not. Between the twelfth and the fourteenth centuries, the cultural fantasy of "noble love" evolved into a form of social behavior among the aristocracy. The thirteenth-century *Art d'amours* notes that "one who wants to begin his love affair well must pretend that he is prepared to do every service, every wish and every private duty that he can for his lady." Around 1400 Christine de Pisan warned naive young women against believing courtiers' vows of love and service. She was echoed by the wife of the Knight of the Tour Landry, who cautioned her daughters against loving "peramours."[3] "Lordes and felawes," she claims,

> saye that alle the honour and worshyppe whiche they gete and have, is comynge to them by theyre peramurs . . . but these wordes coste to them but lytell to say, for to gete the better and sooner the grace and good wylle of theyr peramours. For of such wordes, and other much merveyllous many one vseth full ofte; but how be it that they saye that

'for them and for their loue they done hit,' In good feyth they done it only for to enhaunce them self, and for to drawe vnto them the grace and vayne glory of the world.

Henry of Lancaster (d. 1361), one of the most powerful nobles in England, gives the masculine side of the story when he confesses that he persuaded go-betweens to help his plans for seduction by claiming love-sickness ("I'm a dead man unless you help me").[4] To judge from these warnings, courtly lovers talked a good line, and had to do so as part of their self-fashioning—"to enhaunce them self, and for to draw vnto them the grace and vayne glory of the world." And women had to beware of the social consequences of falling for their lines.

Late medieval art corroborates that the ideals of noble love penetrated the rituals of everyday life among the nobility. The man kneeling before his mistress in Figure 8.1 is carved atop a *gravoire*, an instrument that both sexes used to part the hair. Similar scenes are found on fourteenth-century mirror backs, small caskets, and covers for writing tablets. The images and postures of courtly love, with its inversion of men's usual "maistrie" (mastery), appeared on objects associated with moments of literal self-fashioning: grooming, adornment, and writing. These images on objects of daily use support the claim that "By 1400 courtly love had become for many not just a way of talking but a way of feeling and acting."[5]

Just as courtly love in the later Middle Ages was more than a simple literary posture, more than a set of rhetorical clichés, so too was lovesickness more than a traditional category of medical writing: it must also be understood as a form of social behavior. Recovering the circumstances of that behavior, however, is a difficult task. Though each author in this volume approaches lovesickness with different questions and concerns, as a group the commentators share a common perspective, that of literate, urban, university-trained physician-teachers—in short, that of the masculine intellectual elite. They view their subject from the vantage point of distance and authority, and their view is framed by scholastic rationalism. While that frame encloses a vision of love in the human subject conceived as a body composed of elements in a state of continuous interaction and change, it for the most part excludes direct evidence for the social setting and context of lovesickness.

How, then, may we understand the lover's malady as a socially-influenced form of medieval culture? This chapter draws together converging lines of evidence from medicine, mysticism, art, literature and magic to argue that in the later Middle Ages the lover's malady was a social and psychological response to historical contradictions in aristocratic culture. It offered a way of controlling a historically- and socially-conditioned experi-

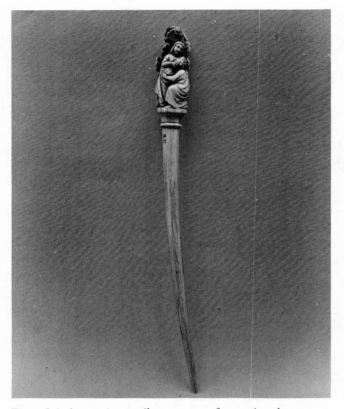

*Figure 8.1.* A *gravoire,* a toilet accessory for parting the hair. The lover kneels before the lady, caressing her hip, while she chucks his chin in affection. New York, The Metropolitan Museum of Art, Anonymous Gift in Memory of J. Pierpont Morgan, 1918 (18.71).

ence of eros that was felt to threaten the normative hierarchy of gender and power.

A theoretical problem must be addressed at the outset: how "real" was this disease? As a historian of medicine has put it: "The conservative tendency of medical literature was just too strong to rule out the possibility that writers talked about diseases they had never seen or (perhaps) on a fundamental level never really expected to see."[6] Some literary critics have also been reluctant to grant the historical reality of *amor hereos,* which is seen as a form of "courtly love." Since "courtly love" in this view never existed as a social practice or social ideology, or existed only as a set of ironic literary conventions, lovesickness is simply a literary posture, a game of poetic conventions.[7]

As the first chapter has shown, the medical tradition of lovesickness had a long history before the troubadours sang of refined love in the twelfth century. *Amor hereos* cannot in any simple fashion, therefore, be reduced to an outgrowth of medieval literary style. While there is no denying the conservative tendency of medieval medicine, the preservation of one culture's texts and ideas by another is an active appropriation, allowing for selection, modification, and amplification of what seems important and useful.[8] That the medical analysis of love survived two cultural transfers, from Greek and Latin medicine of late antiquity to medieval Islam, and from Islam to European Latin Christianity argues for its relevance to the experiences of the borrowing cultures, since medicine was, after all, a practical art. As the differences among the *Viaticum* commentaries reveal, Constantine's teaching on lovesickness was not disseminated unthinkingly, but rather was elaborated and developed through the creative efforts of generations of teacher-practitioners. The more than thirty surviving discussions of lovesickness, in the form of translations, commentaries, and chapters in new practical handbooks of medicine attest that lovesickness was as "real" for medieval physicians as melancholy, headache, baldness, and scalp lice—as real as the other diseases of the head among which *amor hereos* was classified.

My analysis therefore assumes that the doctors' investment of intellectual energy in the subject of morbid love responded to practical needs as much as to theoretical advances within the universities. In Bona Fortuna's anecdote of the lovesick young man charged with homicide, for example, we can see that patients or their families on occasion sought medical help for the lover's malady, and that physicians did their ingenious best to cure them.

## Medicine and Society

Since human subjects are open systems in constant interaction with the world, their desires, hopes, and fears bear the stamp of their place in society and history. While there may be a biochemical component to lovesickness, it is also shaped, like other mental illnesses, by social and cultural settings.[9] Because the manifestations of culturally shaped illness encode social relations, social relations can conversely be "decoded" from their inscription in the medical accounts of lovesickness.

What clues about the social context of the lover's malady can be gleaned from the medical accounts? Since medieval society had clearly demarcated gender roles (both theoretically and functionally), the relation of lovesickness and gender is significant. Though, as chapter six has shown, there was some debate about how susceptible women are to the disease, most medieval physicians claimed that men suffered from lovesickness more often. Despars summarizes general opinion on this point. The disease of love affects men more than women, he explains, because men are generally hotter, their seed more "itching," and their desire for intercourse more vehement. Moreover, they pay less attention to the counsels of modesty than women do, they are less shamefast, and they do not fear the cleverness and tricks of women as women do of men.[10]

These physiological inclinations, moreover, were particularly apt to affect men of the nobility. Arabic medical texts that were the sources of Western teaching do not mention a particular social class as more or less susceptible to the disease; the attribution of lovesickness to the nobility is peculiar to the European adaptations of these works. Already by 1100 or so, the retranslation of the *Viaticum's* chapter on love in the *Liber de heros morbo* spoke of "lordly" or "heroic" love. And as we have seen, Gerard of Berry glossed the phrase "love that is called heros" as "heroes, that is, noble men."

Nor was this assignment of the disease of love to the nobility restricted to commentaries on the *Viaticum*, which had to make sense of the text's *eros/heros/hereos*. In the early fourteenth century Gerard of Solo, commenting on al-Rāzī's chapter on lovesickness, says that it is called *amor ereos*, "that is, noble love, so called from nobility because it is a very strong love, for knights (*milites*) are more apt than others to have this passion."[11] Commentators on Avicenna, whose word for the disease (*al-ʿishq*) was transliterated into Latin as *ilisci* or *ylisci*, equated it with *amor hereos* and declared it a hazard of noble life. Jacques Despars, whose commentary on Avicenna's *Canon* dates from the middle part of the fifteenth century, explains that this insane love is called "hereos" or "hereosus" because it befalls noble men and heroic men more often than simple men of the common people. The nobles are more given to leisure and delicately nourished with meat and wine; they frequent dances and often converse with attractive ladies and demoiselles "who are like darts wounding the mind."[12] Physicians like Arnald of Villanova and William of Brescia, who wrote of lovesickness outside the framework of textual commentary, also perceived it as a disease afflicting noble men.[13]

Given the anthropological observation that "the relation of head to feet, of brain and sexual organs, are commonly treated so that they express the relevant patterns of hierarchy,"[14] it comes as no surprise that this disease of aristocratic men was thought to be located in the brain. Though physicians debated whether love was a disease of the head, the heart, or the generative organs, they all decided that it was principally an affliction of the brain.

In the physicians' view, then, the lover's malady resided at the top of three hierarchies: body, gender, and society. A social interpretation of the disease may therefore reasonably be sought within the structures of masculine aristocratic culture. Further aspects of the medical works support this localization.

In describing the dysfunction of the mental faculties caused by love, the physicians note the lovers' tendency to idealize the beloved. As Gerard of Berry says, the patient considers her better, more noble, and more desirable than other women, even though this may not really be so. The misjudgment of her desirability fixes the lover in meditation on her mental image. In medieval lyric the image of the woman, thus internalized, stood as an ideal for the self.[15] The physician William of Brescia (d. 1326) doubtless perceived the similarity between the idealization in lyric and lovesickness when he said that the patient fears to lose his love object because he believes he will be perfected by her or it.[16] Her overestimated nobility mirrors at a psychological level the lover's own social elevation, but at the same time points up a gap or distance in their relative psychological positions: in her existence as an idealized mental image, she is "above" the lover, who is sunk in depressed thoughts (*profundatio cogitationum*).

The distance between lover and idealized object becomes more apparent if we examine the social metaphors embedded in causal analyses of the disease. As shown in the third chapter, Gerard explains the disease's cause using the language of hierarchy and governance: the faculties at the top rule and give orders, those below bow and obey. This telling metaphorical language reveals that the ennoblement of the woman upsets the inner hierarchy of self-rule, threatening the lover with psychological, if not actual social, abasement. As Dino del Garbo puts it, the lover's mind loses its liberty, as it were, and becomes servile: "fit servilis in cogitationibus."[17] Or, as Arnald of Villanova says in his treatise on heroic love, the disease is called heroic—"lordly, as it were"—not only because it befalls lords, but also because the acts of such lovers toward the desired object are the acts of servants toward their lords, whom they strive to serve with faithful subjection (cf. Figure 3.7).[18]

Finally, the symptoms of the disease "unman" the lover. As a patient he is passive, helpless and vulnerable. The signs of lovesickness, as shown in chapter three, connote feminine and infantile behavior. The universally-recognized symptom of lovesickness in the Middle Ages, wasting from failure to eat, is associated, as Caroline Bynum has shown, with the feminine and the maternal.[19] Physicians also observed that the lovesick are unable to participate in normal social discourse; they are like the *in-fans*, the non-speaker. Some of the symptoms—the wasting, silence, interrupted breathing—embody prelinguistic, infantile modes of signifying.[20] And the infantile is very close to the feminine as it was construed by medieval society—uncontrolled emotion, language, and behavior. Through the *signa amoris* and the disease of love the lover's body and behavior are thus "unmanly" because feminine- or infantile-seeming. Yet at the same time, they express an identification with the unattained object of desire insofar as they are "feminine" and a return to childlike object relations insofar as they are "infantile."

The medical treatises give us, then, the following set of relations. An aristocratic man falls helplessly in love with a woman whom he idealizes. This results in a narcissistic mirroring of the noble lover in the ennobled love object; at the same time, the elevation of the object entails a loss of inner control and governance in the noble subject, a degradation of the mental faculties. This lowering is paralleled by the feminization and infantilization of the lover's body and behavior. The lover's state of disease, in other words, transgresses the usual structures of gender and power. As a "heroic lover" and noble man he is at the top of the hierarchy, yet is also somewhere "below" as a patient unmanned by love.

This tension between idealization and abjection inscribed in the medical accounts of lovesickness bears elaboration through other sources. Evidence from medieval mystical writings suggests that idealization is both linked to the maternal and tinged with ambivalence. A number of literary works and texts on magic indicate that self-abasement is a way of expressing, in displaced form, hostility toward another that cannot be expressed directly. My goal in the following analysis is to suggest that the lover's malady was a way of both expressing and coping with simultaneous feelings of desire and hostility.

## *Mystical Rapture*

From the twelfth century onwards, mystical writers described spiritual experience by its carnal analogues. Some of them tried to put the experience of ecstatic spiritual love into words by using the language of lovesickness, at first drawn from the Song of Songs ("quia amore langueo"), and then later from the medical treatises themselves. As early as Richard of St. Victor's (d. 1173) treatise on the *Four Degrees of Violent Charity*, we find that passionate spiritual and carnal love are semiotically indistinguishable. In this treatise, Richard first describes the four stages of violent charity: wounding love, binding love, love that makes the lover languish and that is satisfiable by only one object, and finally love that leads to physical and psychological disintegration ("caritas vulnerat, ligat, languidum facit, defectum adducit"). This last degree, an incurable illness, *morbus irremediabilis*, is unsatisfiable; it "often turns to madness" and "often becomes hate when nothing can satisfy mutual desire." "Thus loving they hate, and hating they love, and miraculously, or rather miserably, from desire grows hate and from hate desire." Only after describing the psychological progression of the four steps does Richard declare that they are different in divine and human affections. In spiritual desire, the higher the grade, the better; in carnal desire, the higher the grade, the worse.[21] The behavior and the symptoms associated with the grades, however, are the same.

As noted in the first chapter, other writers also used the analogy with the psychology and symptoms of lovesickness in order to clarify the nature of the mental alienation of ecstatic love. They thus appear to have perceived a single psychological dynamic underlying mystical love and lovesickness, however they differentiated good and bad loves *a posteriori* by their objects. In both modes of love unsatisfied desire for an ideal object alienates the lover from himself. God or an idealized woman is the desired other whose inaccessibility turns desire into madness ("alienatio mentis"). What does it mean, however, to say that God and an idealized woman occupy the same psychological space?[22]

Julian of Norwich's (d. after 1416) devotion to "mother Jesus" is perhaps the most famous case of the medieval perception of God's feminine and maternal qualities, but a significant number of twelfth-century men used maternal imagery to describe relations to a God usually conceived of as male.[23] Nor was this an arcane clerical tradition. As the beautiful Middle English poem of about 1400, "In the valley of restless mind," shows, the tradition of feminine imagery for God reached a vernacular audience. Christ, who throughout the rest of the poem is a masculine lover of the human soul in the tradition of the Song of Songs, speaks of himself as a nurturing mother suckling her babe in one of the last stanzas:

> My loue is in hir chaumber: holde ȝoure pees,
> Make ȝe no noise, but let hir slepe:
> My babe y wolde not were in disese,
> I may not heere my dere child wepe.
> With my pap y schal hir kepe.
> Ne mervaille ȝe not þouȝ y tende hir to;
> Þis hole in my side had neuere be so depe,
> But quia amore langueo.[24]

The poem draws such themes from affective mysticism to shape its invitation to loving union with God figured as mother.

We have already seen that some of the symptoms of lovesickness signify a childlike relation to the desired object. The story of Antiochus recounted in the first chapter, an Oedipal comedy in which the lovesick prince is cured by marriage to his father's wife (see Figure 1.3), also suggests that intense experiences of love rapture and lovesickness embody powerful desires for union with the maternal.[25] And desire for his mother causes Perdica to sicken and die (Figure 1.1). Whether carnal or spiritual, these instances of love madness and its somatic manifestations seem to express through the idealized and "feminine" objects of love a deep desire for an all-powerful, sovereign, nourishing "other" who corresponds to the image of the mother from the earliest stages of psychological development.[26]

Medieval literature is replete with traces of this desire. In Christine de Pisan's *Epistre au dieu d'amours* (1399) Cupid proclaims: "Car tout homme doit avoir le cuer tendre / Envers femme qui a tout homme est mere, / Et ne lui est ne diverse n'amere" (For each man ought to have a tender heart toward woman, who is mother to each man, and is neither different nor bitter toward him).[27] It has been argued, in fact, that courtly love "represents an institutionalized manifestation of an intense fixation on the mother . . . it is a systematic organization of interpersonal relations, the conception of which is derived from and bound together by a shared unconscious phantasy."[28]

In a number of instances that fantasy was hardly unconscious; the desire for union with the mother was scarcely, or not at all, repressed or displaced. A remarkable number of medieval stories recount examples of incest between mother and son. Hartmann von Aue's *Gregorius* (late twelfth century), for example, narrates a version of a widely circulating medieval Oedipus story, found in the *Gesta Romanorum* and elsewhere. Instead of the double tragedy of death and blinding after the discovering of incest, however, mother and son repent and pursue monastic callings.[29] Cantiga 17 of Alfonso X "The Wise" (d. 1284) tells the story, also recounted by Vincent of Beauvais, Jacques de Vitry, and Odo of Cheriton, of a woman whose son lay with her and got her with child (Figure 8.2).[30] Even a down-to-earth bourgeois like the Menagier of Paris saw in a man's desire for his wife a replaying of the child's desire for the woman who nourished and took care of him. If a woman makes sure her husband is well provided for, in a snug house, and couches him well between her breasts like a child, then she will surely bewitch him. "Chere seur, je vous pry que le mary que vous arez vous le veuilliez ainsi ensorceler et rensorceller" (Dear sister, I hope that you will bewitch the husband you will have again and again in this fashion).[31]

That men in some fashion desire their mothers and that they recreate that desire in their adult sexual relations was thus no secret to medieval

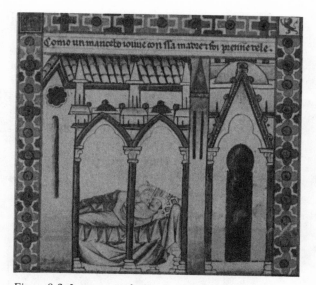

*Figure 8.2.* Incestuous desires could be represented in art as well as literature. "How a youth lay with his mother" from the *Cantigas de Santa María* of Alfonso X, the Wise. Escorial, Bibl. MS T.I.1, Cant. XVII. Photograph granted and authorized by the Patrimonio Nacional, Madrid.

writers, preachers, artists, and their audiences. The opening of a Middle English poem, "A song of great sweetness from Christ to his daintiest dam," neatly expresses the deep affective connection between maternal nurturing and adult (masculine) sexuality; articulating a long tradition in the visual arts and exegesis, it honors mother as bride (Figure 8.3):

> Surge mea sponsa, swete in siȝt,
> And se þi sone þou ȝafe souke so scheene;
> Þou shalt abide with þi babe so briȝt,
> And in my glorie be callide a queene.
> Thi mammillis, moder, ful weel y meene,
> Y had to my meete þat y myȝt not mys.[32]

Whether overt or repressed, however, a man's desire to revert to a childlike state of dependent, identifying love conflicted with the dominant social and cultural codes of masculine superiority that shaped his sense of self. The Menagier's use of "bewitch" (*ensorceler*) for a wife's method of gaining hold over her husband, though meant positively, nonetheless intimates that the

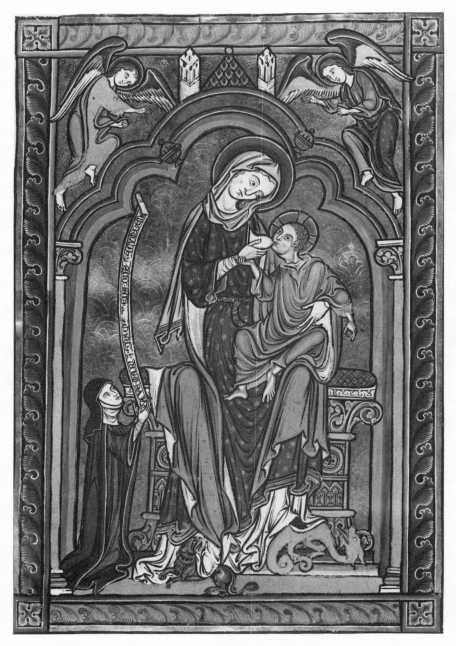

*Figure 8.3.* Mary, enthroned as Queen of Heaven, and the infant Jesus show their love for each other in gestures of nurturing, protection, and dependence. Mother and Child were depicted with increasing frequency from the 13th century on. Oxford, Codrington Library, MS All Souls 6, fol. 4r. By permission of The Warden and Fellows of All Souls College, Oxford.

desire for union with an object (God, a woman) who evokes the maternal is not simple or without conflict. As Richard of St. Victor so strikingly announces in his analysis of the fourth step of violent love, aggression and hate are inseparable from the extreme reaches of both carnal and spiritual love. Nor is Richard an isolated case; historians of spirituality have documented this affective ambivalence in other medieval authors writing on love of God.[33]

Just as love for the divine can be ambivalent, so too can love for an earthly woman. In his study of courtly love, Roger Boase has assembled texts from Arabic and European writers documenting the affinity between love and hate.[34] Because it treats the nexus of love and hate in terms that recall the physicians' analysis of *amor hereos*, Dante's "Amor, da che convien" is worth quoting at length:

> Io non posso fuggir ch'ella non vegna
> ne l'imagine mia,
> se non come il pensier che la vi mena.
>     L'anima folle, che al suo mal s'ingegna,
> com'ella è bella e ria,
> così dipinge, e forma la sua pena:
>     poi la riguarda, e quando ella è ben piena
> del gran disio che de li occhi le tira,
> incontro a sé s'adira,
> c'ha fatto il foco ond'ella trista incende.
> Quale argomento di ragion raffrena,
> ove tanta tempesta in me si gira?
> L'angoscia, che non cape dentro, spira
> fuor de la bocca sì ch'ella s'intende,
> e anche a li occhi lor merito rende.
>
>     La nimica figura, che rimane
> vittorïosa e fera
> e signoreggia la vertù che vole,
>     vaga di se medesma andar mi fane
> colà dov'ella è vera,
> come simile a simil correr sòle.
>     Ben conosco che va la neve al sole,
> ma più non posso : fo come colui
> che, nel podere altrui,
> va co' suoi piedi al loco ov'egli è morto.
> Quando son presso, parmi udir parole
> dicer: 'Vie via vedrai morir costui!'

Allor mi volgo per veder a cui
mi raccomandi; e'ntanto sono scorto
da li occhi che m'ancidono a gran torto.

[I cannot avoid her coming into my imagination any more than the thought that brings her there. My rash soul, actively working to its own harm, depicts her there with all the beauty and malice that is hers, thus giving shape to its own torment: then it gazes at her so imaged, and when it is wholly filled with the great desire that it draws from her eyes, it falls into a rage against itself for having lit the fire in which it miserably burns. What rational argument has the power to curb when such a tempest whirls within me? My anguish, which cannot be confined, pours out audibly in breath from the mouth and also gives my eyes what they deserve.

The hostile image, that remains victorious and pitiless and dominates the faculty of willing, attracted to herself, makes me go where she is in reality, as like runs toward like. Well I know that it is snow going toward the sun, but I can do nothing else: I'm as a man in another's power who goes on his own two feet to the place where he is killed. When I draw near her I seem to hear words that say: 'In a moment you will see him die!' Then I turn to see to whom I can have recourse, but in the same moment the eyes light on me which so unjustly slay me.][35]

Like writers on *amor hereos*, Dante anatomizes the psychological breakdown caused by intense erotic passion. The lover's imagination is invaded by the image of the beloved; obsessive contemplation of that image generates "great desire" (Constantine's *magna concupiscentia*). Sighs and tears, standard symptoms of the lover's malady, express his anguish.

The beloved, idealized woman is at the same time a dominatrix who rules (*signoreggia*) the lover's faculty of willing, an image that recalls Gerard of Berry's analysis. Moreover, the stanzas contain a complex sequence of direct and screened hostility. The woman is "beautiful and malicious"; she is a "hostile image, that remains victorious and pitiless"; and she inflicts psychological death on the lover. The lover, meanwhile, both desires her and rages against himself in an infernal fury of passion (fire and whirlwind). The hostility attributed *to* the woman and the anger toward self screen hostility *toward* her for not yielding to the lover's desires. The last poem in Dante's Pietra sequence symbolizes in one of its violent final images the anger born of thwarted desire. "Così nel mio parlar," filled with images of death and vengeance, culminates in a fantasy of rape in which the lover promises: "non sarei pietoso né cortese, / anzei farei com'orso quando scherza" (I would not be pitying or courteous, instead I'd do like a bear when it plays).

The literary theme of the affinity of love and hate is a commonplace because it expresses the common experience of ambivalence in erotic life.

Dante's poems depict an ambivalence born of frustrated desire. Psychologists have argued that ambivalence can also be rooted in early childhood experiences and re-emerge in severe form in adult life at times of stress or crisis. It grows out of the infant's relation to its "primary attachment figure," the mother or other caretaker who nourishes and protects it. In an early developmental stage, the infant begins to perceive the world as different from itself and to differentiate itself from the mother. Once the mother becomes an "other" who is different from the baby's self, she becomes part of the now separate and hostile world and is no longer, from the baby's point of view, under his "control." As source of food, protection, and satisfaction of needs, and yet as part of a threatening environment, the mother attracts ambivalent feelings of love and hate.[36] In the baby's internalized representations, which seem to persist through life, the mother is both "good" and "bad."

Ambivalence toward the mother is not a product of the post-Freudian twentieth century, but can be found in medieval sources (to say nothing of the literature of antiquity). The invectives against women in Book 3 of Andreas Capellanus' *De amore*, for example, read like an encyclopedic listing of the "bad mother"'s traits. She hoards and controls resources—food, wine, and money. She acts independently of masculine control; she is fickle, disobedient, rebellious, and indulges in sexual excess. Worst of all, she does not love: "No woman ever loved her husband, nor can she ever bind herself to a lover with a reciprocal bond of love. . . . she loves no man from the heart."[37] The accusations amount to a baby boy's ambivalent view of a mother whose autonomy is experienced as threatening.

Modern clinical and experimental research has shown that, in addition to the process of psychological maturation just described, the loss or threatened loss of a loved object also evokes feelings of ambivalence in later life, an interpretation supported by medieval evidence.[38] Guibert de Nogent's (d. after 1125) complex feelings for his mother illustrate this kind of ambivalent love. She gave him "a mother's special affection for her last-born" in childhood, but when she decided to retire into a convent when Guibert was about twelve, he claims she did it knowing "that I should be utterly an orphan with no one at all on whom to depend," and knowing certainly that "she was a cruel and unnatural mother."[39] Klapisch-Zuber has documented similar ambivalent feelings among Florentines abandoned by their mothers upon remarriage.[40]

Behind the desire for an idealized object lies a desire for the maternal, but that desire is ambivalent. In order, however, for psychopathological states like lovesickness to develop, more than ordinary ambivalence seems to be involved. In the view of a leading theorist of attachment,

John Bowlby, "anger and hostility directed toward an attachment figure, whether by a child or an adult, can be understood best . . . as being in response to frustration." For children the greatest source of anxiety and frustration, and thus of hostility, is "experiences of repeated separation or threats of separation." The disruption of affectional bonds in early life is thus pathogenic; it plays a role in contemporary clinical disorders including depression and chronic mourning (Freud's "melancholia").[41] "Early loss, it seems, can sensitize an individual and make him more vulnerable to setbacks experienced later, especially to loss or threat of loss," Bowlby contends.[42]

Young children in the Middle Ages faced profound threats to their emotional security. Numerous catastrophes could sever them from the figures they depended on for love as well as for the necessities of life. A child's development could be hindered at the start if its mother died in childbirth. Though statistics are hard to come by, the death rate from the complications of childbirth was doubtless high.[43] If the child survived infancy, the practice of wetnursing, a childrearing practice that began among the nobility and then spread to the middle classes, could seriously rupture its affections at a crucial developmental stage.[44] After having become attached to the wetnurse to whom it had been given shortly after birth, a year or two later the child would have had to leave her to return home to its natural parents. If Bowlby's analysis is correct, this trauma may in some cases have resulted in long-term disturbances of affective life. Whether or not a child was wetnursed, it ran a significant risk of being orphaned at an early age.[45] The early life of Peter Damian exemplifies both these perils. Rejected by his mother shortly after birth, he was rescued from the verge of death and cared for by a priest's concubine. Though his mother restored him in her affections and took him back, Peter was orphaned by the deaths of both parents while he was still a young child. In Italy children might lose their mother as a result of the dowry system: young widows left their husband's families with the dowry but without their children, who remained behind with their father's family.[46] Finally, noble boys often left home around the age of seven to be taught the aristocratic arts of war and courteous service in another household. Duby has suggested that this separation entailed a desire to regain maternal love. In his view the fabulous female creatures of romance "are probably best understood as substitutes for the knight's lost mother. . . . When they imagined themselves winning, by violent and dangerous means, these enticing, elusive, dominating fays, they must have felt they were conquering their anxieties and returning to the warm bosom of their earliest infancy."[47] Guibert de Nogent describes the trauma of separation for a boy as old as twelve.

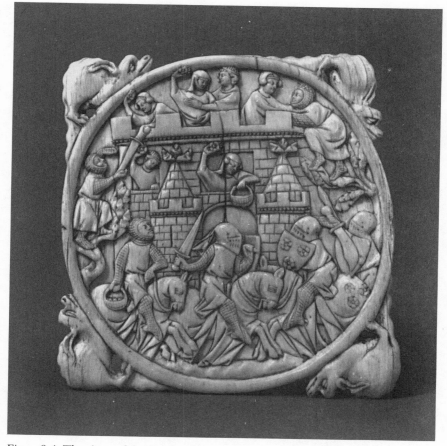

*Figure 8.4.* The siege of the Castle of Love on this ivory mirror back depicts the relation between eros and aggression in stylized and playful form. Numerous examples of the motif survive from the fourteenth century. Paris, ca. 1320–50. Seattle Art Museum, Donald E. Frederick Memorial Collection (49. 37). Photo: Paul Macapia.

All these circumstances indicate that the medieval aristocracy, the class most subject to lovesickness, was exposed to significant disruptions of the affectional bonds between children and their attachment figures, whether mothers or wetnurses. As a consequence, anxiety, anger, and hostility toward maternal figures may well have complicated their feelings of love. The conventional scene in Figure 8.4, known variously as the "assault on" or "siege of the castle of love," illustrates in light, playful fashion the current of aggression that runs throughout medieval visions of erotic relations. (One thinks, for example, of the cruel punishments in Andreas' Garden of

Love.) In pathological cases like lovesickness, exaggerated infantile and adult feelings of "lovehate" may have fused to produce the idealization and depression characteristic of the disease.[48]

Since expressing anger toward a powerful figure of attachment is difficult, such feelings are often displaced or projected. Freud argues that in melancholia the sufferer punishes and torments a loved one by means of the illness, which is resorted to so as to avoid expressing hostility openly, a theory supported by recent clinical studies.[49] In the first chapter we saw how a variety of medical and literary texts from antiquity and the early Middle Ages connected melancholy and anger, or lovesickness and anger. The connection was also evident in the later Middle Ages. "Anger engenders melancholy," claimed the Old French *Art d'amours*, and Dante wrote:

> Un dì si venne a me Malinconia
> e disse: "Io voglio un poco stare teco";
> e parve a me ch'ella menasse seco
> Dolore e Ira per sua compagnia.[50]

[One day Melancholy came to me and said: "I would like to stay with you a little while." And it seemed to me that she led with her Sorrow and Wrath for company.]

With remarkable psychological acuity, Hildegard of Bingen (d. 1179) foreshadows Freud's understanding of the connection between anger and melancholy. The love of melancholics, she says, is "hateful, twisted, and death-carrying, like the love of voracious wolves. . . . They have intercourse with women but they hate them."[51] Viewed in this framework, the depression and self-abasement characteristic of melancholy—or lovesickness—is nothing other than hostility toward the object redirected to the self.

## Sexual Magic and Revenge

"I have heard," claimed Jacques de Vitry (d. 1240), "of a certain old crone who could not convince a woman to consent to a young man's desire." The old woman said to the young man: "Pretend that you are sick (*finge te infirmum*) and convey to the woman that you are sick on account of loving her." The old woman starved her dog for three days, and then fed it mustard. She took it to the woman's house, where it began to cry because of the mustard. She then told the woman that the dog had been another woman who had allowed a youth to die of love. The gravely ill youth had exacted vengeance by magically transforming the unyielding woman into that very dog. The go-between's fiction worked, and the resisting woman agreed to take the young man as a lover (cf. Figure 8.5).[52]

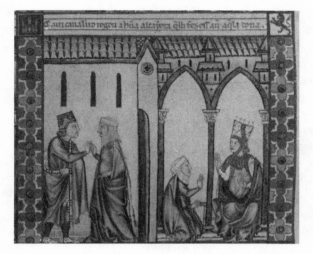

*Figure 8.5.* Love magic was practiced throughout the Middle Ages. On the left a lover hires a sorceress, and on the right she cajoles a married woman. *Cantigas de Santa María* of Alfonso X, the Wise. Escorial, Bibl. MS T.I.1, Cant. LXIV. Photograph granted and authorized by the Patrimonio Nacional, Madrid.

Told in a sermon for the people, the story is a variant of a tale widely diffused in Europe. Its motif of pretended lovesickness as a cynically effective seduction ploy means that incurring the lover's malady had a certain plausibility. More significantly, the illness is associated with a magical act of revenge against the love object. Desired one moment and transformed into a beast the next, the woman occupies a dangerous space that attracts the lover's vengeful hate as well as his desire. The exemplum couples feigned illness with a fiction of revenge against a woman who thwarts the man's desire. That revenge is both enacted and symbolized by her degradation into a dog.

Both Hippocrates and Vergil figure in similar stories of sexual revenge and degradation. In the thirteenth-century Grail romance *L'Estoire del Saint Graal*, Hippocrates falls sick with love for a noblewoman from Gaul. When he arrives at her tower for an assignation she tricks him. After hoisting him halfway to her in a basket, she leaves him dangling. When daylight comes, he incurs public ridicule, since criminals were punished in that fashion. In some versions of the story Hippocrates then takes his revenge. He culls an aphrodisiac herb, enchants it, and gives it to a hideous crippled dwarf. Any woman whom he touches with it will have no power to resist her passionate desire for him. The dwarf, who slept near the emperor's palace, touches the woman from Gaul with the herb. That night she finds her way to his bed.

Hippocrates calls the emperor to see the noblewoman in the arms of the dwarf, whereupon the emperor declares: "Voilà bien ce qui prouve que la femme est la plus vile chose du monde" (Behold well what proves that woman is the vilest thing on earth). The emperor then forces her to marry the dwarf and to become chief laundress in the palace.[53] That she is humiliated both sexually and socially suggests how closely the two are related in medieval constructions of sexuality.

The variant involving Vergil entails a different, though no less humiliating, revenge. Like Hippocrates, he falls in love with a woman who fails to return his affections, and who leaves him dangling in a basket to be mocked by the Romans. Figure 8.6 shows that scene on the left side of an ivory writing tablet from the late fourteenth century. The spatial relation between the two—woman in power above, man helpless below—echoes the symbolically charged postures of courtly love (cf. Figures 8.1, 8.8, and 3.7). After Vergil's release from the basket, he extinguished Rome's lights for three days. When the desperate Romans came to him for help, his magic arts enabled them to rekindle their candles from the part of his love's anatomy Boccaccio calls "the fury of hell."[54] The aggressively crude symbolizing of what the night in the basket deprived him is shown on the right half of the ivory. Note how the revenge/fulfillment reverses the relative position of the woman, so that now she is the one below, powerless, and violated (cf. Figure 8.7).

In these stories men wield magic arts to avenge the humiliation of their sexual desires. What happens in the inverse situation, when women are the agents? The discussion of lovesickness in the *Malleus Maleficarum* (*Hammer of Witches*, 1486), a manual for inquisitors and judges, is motivated by a masculine fear of sexual victimization. It embodies the fear that women, given the power of magic, would turn the tables and avenge *their* sexual humiliations by causing men to suffer lovesickness.

The most influential of the witchcraft treatises, the *Malleus*, though dubious evidence for the practice of witchcraft, does exemplify how anxiety and fear become objectified as magic and/or disease, and culminate in a persecuting hostility.[55] The authors declare that lovesickness (*amor hereos*) is one of the commonest forms of bewitchment, and that it affects "optimi, praelati, alii divites" and "saeculi potentes" (eminent men, prelates, other wealthy men, and secular rulers).[56] They claim that women rather than men become witches because, among other reasons, through their "disordered affections and passions" they "search for, brood over, and inflict various vengeances, either by witchcraft or by some other means. Wherefore it is no wonder that so great a number of witches exist in this sex." The motive for their vengeance becomes clear when the authors explain how witches are recruited:

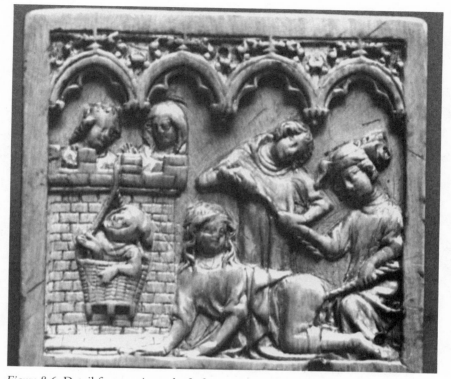

*Figure 8.6.* Detail from an ivory leaf of a writing tablet illustrating the *Lai de Vergile*. French, 14th century. Baltimore, Walters Art Gallery (71.267).

For when girls have been corrupted, and have been scorned by their lovers after they have immodestly copulated with them in the hope and promise of marriage with them, and have found themselves disappointed in all their hopes and everywhere despised, they turn to the help and protection of devils; either for the sake of vengeance by bewitching those lovers or the wives they have married, or for the sake of giving themselves up to every sort of lechery. Alas! experience tells us that there is no number to such girls, and consequently the witches that spring from this class are innumerable (part 2, q. 2, c. 1).[57]

The hyperbole invites us to consider the emotional subtext of the authors' claim rather than its empirical accuracy. Men who have power and wealth fear women who don't. Like the vision of the hapless Hukbert in Odo of Cluny's story, the *Malleus* embodies a nightmarish fantasy of women's vengeance for the ills they have suffered; retribution takes the form of witchcraft and magically caused lovesickness. The authors project onto women a psychology of revenge that we have seen at work in the stories of

Jacques de Vitry, Hippocrates, and Vergil. They cast men as the helpless victims, not of their own desires, but of the external, demonic agency of witches. The whole tenor of the *Malleus*, a blend of hair-splitting scholastic argumentation and disturbing images from collective fantasies about women, indicates that the rationalized explanation, whatever its degree of truth, screens a more general and basic fear of and anger toward women. The *Malleus* suggests, then, that medieval lovesickness may have involved displaced, somaticized forms of hostility and fear.[58]

In a mid-fifteenth-century *Dialogue between a Noble and a Rustic* the lover's malady is presented as a class-specific form of fear of women. The author explains that what the nobleman views as the "natural disease" (*naturalis infirmitas*) of lovesickness, described by Avicenna, the rustic experiences as magical attack; he considers himself "infected" and "molested by a woman's secret wiles."[59] Fear of "women's secret wiles" is displaced and objectified in the commoner's case as magical attack, in the case of the nobleman as the disease of love. The author thus articulates what is hidden from the surface of the elite medical treatises, though implied by their metaphors. The "natural infirmity" of lovesickness is an upper-class naturalization, and therefore mystification, of a fear of being victimized by "women's secret wiles."

## Lovesickness and "Courtly Love"

This analysis suggests that the social origins of lovesickness may be sought in circumstances where aristocratic men, already vulnerable to melancholia and lovesickness from precarious childhood ties, exerted an inordinate level of power over women, generating fears of reprisal. Circumstances where women temporarily or symbolically assumed power, reversing the usual hierarchical arrangement, would also generate masculine anxieties conducive to lovesickness. Indeed, the two conditions overlapped in late medieval aristocratic culture. Men like Gadifer de la Salle, the "powerful men" of the *Malleus*, and the noble men whom the physicians described—these were the men who idealized or played at idealizing women who both were inferiors in the natural hierarchy and were increasingly losing effective social power as well. Generalizations about women in the later Middle Ages and early modern periods are admittedly difficult. There is, nonetheless, an observable trend toward a tightened hold of patriarchal authority within the family and the economy.[60] It is especially evident in handbooks of conduct for women of the upper levels of society. The Knight of the Tour Landry instructed his daughters to be submissive, humble, and obedient toward men, and Philippe de Mézières advocated the same for married women of the nobility. Even Christine de Pisan, who elsewhere shows with eloquent pain the sufferings inflicted by patriarchal culture on women, advocates obedient submission to husbands who may be brutally violent in her treatise on women's conduct.[61] The sexual hierarchy was transmitted through the family, and enforced by fathers and husbands, in the worst of cases with violence as we see in Figure 8.7. A law in fourteenth-century Flanders, for example, "stipulated that the husband may beat his wife, injure her, slash her body from head to foot and 'warm his feet in her blood.'"[62]

The conventions of courtly literature, no matter how seriously enacted, could not eradicate the strong medieval sense of hierarchy in which man's place was at the top. "Who, then, reveals himself such a fool and madman as to try to obtain what forces him with oppressive serfdom to subject himself to another's dominion, and to be wholly tied to another's will in all things?" asks Andreas Capellanus.[63] Even in playing out courtly conventions the customary sexual and social hierarchy asserts itself. A thirteenth-century French "Minneallegorie," *La Puissance d'amour,* counsels the lover that when the woman seems about to grant his desires, he should remain master of himself ("sires de vous") in order to prevent her from seizing mastery. The fragmentary thirteenth-century text *On True Love* well illustrates the tension between service and hierarchy. On the one hand, a lady is advised to love below her station so that she can have the greater obedience of her lover, and a man is advised to love above his "because a lover is transformed according to what he loves." On the other hand, a woman's use of the polite plural pronoun (*vos*) to her lover, and the man's use of the familiar singular (*tu*) to her is grounded in the fact that "woman is naturally subjected to man because she was made from him."[64]

Nonetheless, to paraphrase Chaucer's Franklin, those who were to be "lords in marriage" did play at being "servants in love." The lover's abjection is perhaps most clearly expressed by Guillaume de Machaut, who wrote that his lady should not merely consider him her servant, but hold him in servility as her serf: "Eins me deves tenir en vo servage / Comme vo serf qu'avez pris et acquis" (Balade CCXXXI).[65] To the extent that the courtly conventions of service and idealization were internalized or acted out, then, they conflicted with powerful structures of masculine dominance. The strain between the two cultural models for upper-class masculine behavior was undoubtedly increased by the deep currents of antifeminism. Just as love service ran counter to men's usual precedence, so idealization of women ran counter to a long tradition of denigration. Once again Andreas provides the commonplaces: "They are prone to every evil"; "Women cannot be in full possession of outstanding character"; "So it seems that no man of sense fittingly binds himself to a woman's affection, because she

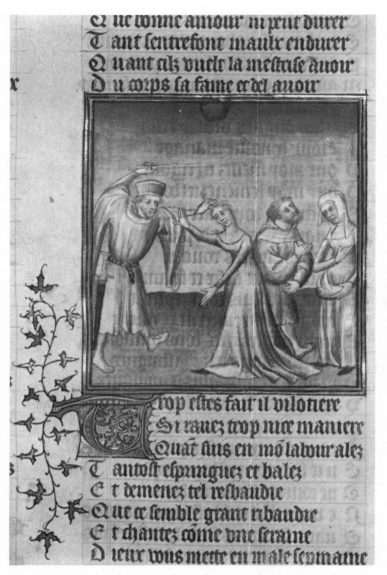

*Figure 8.7.* A husband exercises his authority by beating his wife with a stick (Paris, ca. 1405). Guillaume de Lorris and Jean de Meung, *Roman de la Rose,* fol. 54, detail. Malibu, CA, The J. Paul Getty Museum. (83.MR.177, ms. Ludwig XV 7).

never continues to reciprocate anyone's love, and she must clearly be condemned for all the strong reasons already enumerated."[66] To practice love service to an idealized woman—that is, to take the conventions seriously at whatever imaginative or active level—was to abase one's own sense of self, of masculine superiority.

Figure 8.8, a fifteenth-century parade shield depicting a knight's submission before his lady, shows how one artist symbolized the courtly lover's dilemma. A scroll bears the words "You or Death." The kneeling lover is separated from his lady by the center line of the shield. Death, much closer, occupies the same space as the lover, and even seems to touch him. Death also mirrors the lady's stance, in effect becoming her double. The scene powerfully signals the psychological threat contained in courtly love by implying that there is no choice between "You" and "Death."

Duplicity and lovesickness were two culturally sanctioned ways of dealing with this threat. As the *Art d'amours* and other works suggest, in some circles lovers had to *pretend* to serve their ladies in order "to enhaunce them self and for to drawe vnto them the grace and veyne glory of the world." Richard of Fournival warns against dissemblers who assume the posture of service without meaning it from the heart.[67] Chaucer creates a number of characters who illustrate the problem: the glib, false-hearted Diomede, rival to the lovesick Troilus; the tercelet of the *Squire's Tale* who "many a yeer his service . . . feyned"; and Jason, who in the *Legend of Good Women* is the model of deceitful lovers:

> Thow madest thy recleymyng and thy lures
> To ladies of thy statly aparaunce,
> And of thy wordes farced with pleasaunce,
> And of thy feyned trouthe and thy manere,
> With thyn obesaunce and humble cheere,
> And with thy contrefeted peyne and wo.
> There othere falsen oon, thow falsest two!
> O, often swore thow that thow woldest dye
> For love, whan thow ne feltest maladye
> Save foul delyt, which that thow callest love! (1371–80)

Jason's strategy of "contrefeted peyne" makes literary and psychological sense in cultural circles dominated in reality by men but in which love service (or talk of love service) is necessary for erotic or social success. Duplicity solves the contradiction between power and submission.

The other possible way of responding to this dilemma was lovesickness. The success of the lover's malady in the later Middle Ages as a literary pos-

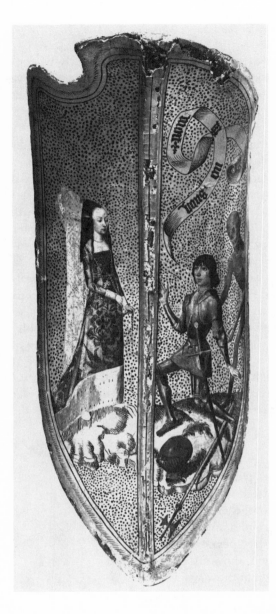

*Figure 8.8.* The scroll above the lover on this fifteenth-century Flemish parade shield says "You or Death." Reproduced by Courtesy of the Trustees of the British Museum.

ture, as a seduction ploy, and as an illness requiring treatment rested on its ability to modulate an erotic subjectivity that contravened the realities of gender roles and power relations. *Amor hereos* mediated between a perceived social ideal of desire for an idealized woman whom one served and the contradictory social and psychological reality of her inferiority. Insofar as idealized love requires a deposition of men's power, a willed vulnerability, so to speak, it may have been difficult to act out without serious disturbance of men's sense of self. A dubious desire may have seemed less threatening if alienated from its origin in the lover and expressed as the morbid though curable delusion of loving a woman "more noble" than she is in reality. The anxiety, hostility, and fear accompanying a socially problematic desire for an idealized woman could thus be displaced and objectified as the disease of love.

The *preux chevalier* Gadifer de la Salle's knightly career "gives a flavour of the violence of the times" and included charges against him of murder and abduction. He could give himself over to the amorous courtesies of the Court of Love, we may imagine, because the *mal d'amour* was a socially-recognized way of coping with love, hostility, and the inversion of gender-power relations. By suffering love as a disease, or by imagining himself to do so in poetry, the lover could alienate himself from responsibility for this dubious desire and yield himself to its most intense degree. Passion could thus become a sign of "noble love" and the "feminine" state of illness be reclaimed into a masculine sphere of value.

That reclamation was aided by a transformed sensibility concerning masculine values. The ethos of courtliness itself represented a "feminization" of aristocratic behavior and sentiment in comparison with that of the earlier Middle Ages. Suffering itself was exalted by Christianity, perhaps nowhere more so than in the later medieval cult of the wounded, broken Christ. An early fourteenth-century pietà (Figure 8.9; compare the emaciation of Perdica in Figure 1.1) shows the male body stripped, wounded, and helpless, held by a powerful female figure. The disturbing image, which deliberately echoes the iconography of Virgin and Child, contrasts with the dominant values of physical strength, autonomy, and bodily wholeness so valued by knights. Such qualities, necessary for their military exploits, were also deeply ingrained in their sense of self and of their desirability.[68]

Meditation on the Christian inversion of worldly values represented by images like the pietà and crucifixion scenes (Figure 1.5) doubtless aided men in allowing themselves the vulnerability of lovesickness. The pierced and broken body of Christ was both a culturally sanctioned image of masculine suffering for love and a psychological model for the individual. Moreover, the homiletic theme of Christ the Lover-Knight who languished for his

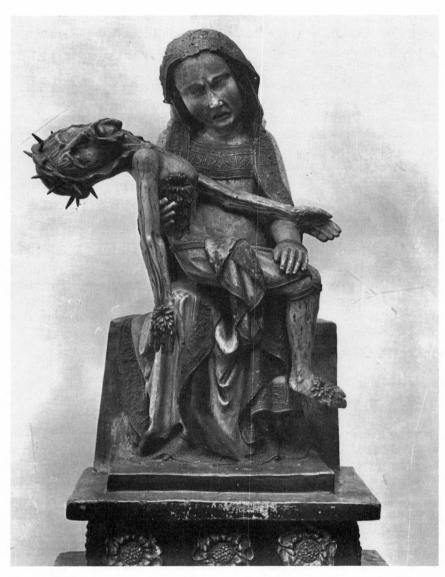

*Figure 8.9*. Pietà Roettgen. Bonn, Rheinisches Landesmuseum (Inv. nr. 24189).

bride, the human soul, further encouraged imitation of the Savior's lovesickness. If Christ himself had suffered lovesickness to the death, then his human imitators may have found it possible and strategic to do so as well.[69]

## Lovesickness as Cultural Symptom

This chapter has attempted to recreate a context in which *amor hereos* was meaningful both as a literary commonplace and as a form of behavior. We have seen how it could resolve psychological and social tensions in aristocratic male patients. Yet there is another level on which the large body of medical writing about lovesickness calls for further interpretation. What functions did it serve for the teachers and students who pored over the manuscripts of Constantine and Avicenna and who debated love's causes and cures?

Taken as a group, the medical discussions of lovesickness enabled the commentators and their students to master, through scientific discourse, powerful collective anxieties over erotic love. The physicians who wrote about love were particularly well placed to articulate this cultural strain, mediating as they did between the worlds—and worldviews—of clergy and laity. From the twelfth century onwards, medicine was increasingly secularized; it moved from the monasteries to the urban universities where it was regulated and professionalized throughout the course of the later Middle Ages. Though not secluded from the world as the monasteries ideally were, the universities were nonetheless dominated by a clerical culture hostile to women and the pursuit of passionate love.[70] As Chaucer's Wife of Bath says, "No womman of no clerk is preysed."

Yet on the other hand, the professors who wrote and argued about lovesickness were also practitioners whose clientele was the nobility and the urban well-to-do. These patients were likely either to be literate or to enjoy the literacy of clerks; they were the patrons of vernacular literary culture, and hence those most able to absorb and act out the ideals of courtly behavior. Both patients and physicians were schooled in a common literary culture of love that was stocked with the rhetoric of love as illness and countless examples of languishing lovers.

And let us not forget the audience of the masters' teaching, the young male students of the universities, the bachelors.[71] Unmarried, away from home and kin, of an age, according to the theorists, most suited to love, the students were on their own against the world, the flesh, and the Devil. They were grounded in vernacular literature and in the Latin authors who spoke of love, and yet as clerks they were theoretically bound to the ideals of continence, sobriety, and nonviolence, however lustful, drunken, and violent their actual behavior was.[72] The masters of medicine expounded their views of the disease of love to an audience of young clerks caught between the lure of secular pleasures and the ideals of their station.

While courtliness in general is an ethos of self-mastery, ritualizing and aestheticizing basic libidinal and aggressive drives, the essence of "courtly love" is its excess, its failure to remain within the bounds of normal social behavior. As the prince Arcite asks rhetorically in Chaucer's *Knight's Tale*: "Who shal yeve a lovere any lawe?" The discourse of lovesickness—articulated by men and sustained through generations of male teachers and students—allowed the psychological and somatic "riot" of femininity and vulnerability, which threatened self-control and masculine identity at the most fundamental bodily levels, to be ordered and controlled within a rational (masculine) universe of causes and cures. The corpus of European texts on lovesickness can therefore be viewed as a counterweight to the energies unleashed by the powerful idealism of love.

The entire body of medical texts, Arabic and European, available in the West from the late eleventh to the fifteenth centuries both fostered and responded to medieval views of passionate love. The Arabic texts in translation were appropriated by European intellectuals at the same time that the troubadours sang their vision of idealized love. The authority and pragmatism of the medical descriptions of lovesickness were able to assist the evolution of a cultural fantasy into social reality. "I'm dying of love" became both a cliché and a medical possibility, remote but dreadful. Once romantic ideology had become a social practice that the nobility had to reckon with, the medicalized vision of lovesickness enabled lovesick aristocrats to cope with their own erotic vulnerability.

## Women and Lovesickness: From the Middle Ages to the Renaissance

Women as loving subjects, in contrast to desired objects, have been conspicuously absent from my account. This is in part due to the fact that when medieval physicians theorized the disease of love, they understood it as a masculine ailment. As noted in the beginning of chapter six, however, in literature women were no strangers to the lover's malady, and historical women appropriated to themselves the language of mystical love-languor.[73] If, as I have argued above, a single dynamic underlies mystical love and lovesickness, how do we explain the absence of women from the academic medical tradition when they seem to appear everywhere else as subjects of lovesickness? And to complicate the problem further, why do they emerge from their obscurity in medieval medical sources to become prominent victims of love in Renaissance medical accounts? To resolve these questions properly requires another book; I shall close this one by indicating where answers may fruitfully be sought.

The relative silence of the physicians concerning women follows from, in the first instance, their preoccupation with analyzing *amor hereos* from a masculine perspective. If I am right in suggesting that the discourse of lovesickness was a way of working through collective anxieties that were particularly intense at the universities, then this self-absorbed analysis held little room for women except as desired objects or the means of cure.

Moreover, men's lovesickness needed explanation and cure because it made them "other." Its signs and symptoms feminized them, separated them from normal masculine ways of behaving. But the same signs and symptoms would only render a woman more feminine. Since they only reinforced what was perceived as her nature, they required no diagnosis or cure.

Given these reasons for women's invisibility in academic treatises, their appearance in Renaissance medical accounts of lovesickness is all the more puzzling. Historians of medicine have noted a tendency among medical writers of the Renaissance not merely to consider women subject to morbid love, but to deem them, as did Jacques Ferrand, the primary victims of the malady, or at least particularly susceptible to it.[74] Cases of lovesick women from Renaissance medical writers are often dramatic and memorable. For example, in 1565 Pieter van Foreest (Petrus Forestus) treated a young woman whose family had called him in when she fell into convulsions as the result of unfulfilled love. By testing her pulse he discovered the object of her love, and arranged with her parents to marry her to the young man in question, which cured her illness.[75] In the seventeenth century, Dutch genre painting included the remarkably popular subject known as "The Doctor's Visit" (cf. Figures 6.4, 7.3), in which a physician examines a young woman languishing from the "mal d'amour."[76] Although men still continued to suffer from lovesickness, it became, in some post-medieval medical texts, gradually identified with or considered a cause of other "female disorders" such as chlorosis, hysteria, and nymphomania.[77]

Herein lies a clue to the change. As I have suggested in chapter six, Peter of Spain's discussion of the role of gender in lovesickness opened the way for others to ponder the links among sexual physiology, pleasure, and love. In any case it is clear that a certain branch of medical writers on lovesickness began to consider it a disease linked to the sexual organs and their humors. Once connected directly to pathology of the sexual organs, lovesickness may have then become "visible" as a disease of women, since women's ailments received special notice insofar as they were related to sexual physiology.[78]

To this change within medical thinking may be added several external pressures. The recovery of ancient texts brought Galen's story of the lovesick wife of Justus to Europe in the fourteenth century. His authority may have encouraged physicians to "see" what he saw. Similarly, the humanistic study of ancient literature (on which Renaissance doctors prided themselves) enabled the physicians to ponder the famous lovesick women of antiquity: Sappho, Medea, Dido, and a host of others.

All of these factors would help account for the change in medical writing. Was there a corresponding change in the social reality of lovesickness? Did women suffer from it in actuality as well as on paper? Once again, a proper answer would entail a detailed interdisciplinary study, and only brief suggestions can be offered here. Marriageable women outnumbered eligible men in the early modern period. With marriage closed to them, and with patriarchal enforcement of female chastity, they had little hope of sexual or romantic fulfillment. Lovesickness may have been a strategy, as in the case related by Foreest, by which young women could gain the "cure" of marriage. In this case lovesickness would serve as a form of negotiation for marriage rather than mediate the masculine dilemma of dominance and submission.

Other social conditions affecting women besides a difficult marriage market deserve investigation as potential determinants of lovesickness. As Boccaccio, a master hand at setting the social stage for his stories, wrote in the *Decameron*, "melancholy ladies" had time on their hands for erotic reveries, and leisure, as the medieval doctors tell us, is one of the reasons why the nobility suffer from love. Working men are too busy to spend their time in idle obsession with erotic fantasies. Social historians of women in the early modern period may be able to clarify whether women's lovesickness was related to increasing leisure for wealthy middle-class women.

More difficult still, though perhaps more rewarding, would be to investigate the psychological consequences for women of the social restrictions of early modernity. In view of the powerful connections between melancholy, anger, and lovesickness in men's erotic life, such investigation might fruitfully consider whether the tightened grip of patriarchy was responsible for a somaticization of women's anger in the form of lovesickness. Such research would not only clarify the important question of possible gender asymmetry in the psychology of lovesickness, but also illuminate the diverse, historically contingent ways in which lovesickness reduces anxieties and mediates psychological conflicts. A study of women's lovesickness will, finally, enlarge our understanding of how the various discourses on the lover's malady condition individual, historical, and gendered experiences of eros.

# PART TWO

§§§§§§§

# *The Texts*

# CONSTANTINE THE AFRICAN, *VIATICUM* I.20

## *Manuscripts*

Of the one hundred twenty-three manuscripts of the *Viaticum* earlier than the fifteenth century discovered thus far, I have examined thirty-five in person or on microfilm.[1] This group of manuscripts contains the earliest that I know of as well as most of the twelfth-century manuscripts.[2] None of the manuscripts have been shown to issue from Montecassino and none are listed in the modern catalogue of the library at Montecassino.[3] Although these manuscripts represent only about a quarter of the extant *Viaticum* manuscripts written before 1400, this quarter is likely to be representative of the larger number.

There are four printed editions of the *Viaticum*:

Venice, 1505: *Opera Geraldi de Solo, Commentum super Viatico cum textu.*
   The commentary is that of Gerard of Berry.
Lyons, 1510: in al-Rāzī, *Divisiones.*
Lyons, 1511: in al-Rāzī, *Opera parva.*
Basel, 1536: *Opera omnia Constantini Africani.*

The printed editions are of no value in establishing the text of the chapter on lovesickness. The Basel text has been edited to "improve" the Latinity, and the others are based on late manuscripts in which glosses had crept into the text, if the printers themselves did not incorporate them.

The goal of this edition is to reconstruct the text of Constantine's chapter on love insofar as it is possible given two major limitations: the absence of early *Viaticum* manuscripts traceable to Montecassino and the lack of a critical edition of Ibn al-Jazzār's Arabic text and its Greek and Hebrew translations. Since the textual tradition is contaminated, it has not proved possible, on the basis of a collation of one chapter, to discover reliable family traditions. I have also foregone the option of attempting to establish a text of the chapter on *amor* such as Gerard of Berry might have received; to do so would have entailed the possibility of yet other versions for Egidius, Peter of Spain, and Bona Fortuna, since the variants continued to evolve through the thirteenth century. In view of the basic editorial work that still needs to be done on Constantine's entire corpus, a working edition of the chapter on love based on a limited selection of manuscripts seems justified.

I have therefore edited from a subset of the manuscripts examined. Obviously poor texts (major omissions, nonsense) were eliminated, as were most thirteenth- and fourteenth-century mss. Though *juniores non semper deteriores*, the later manuscripts offer no useful readings not found earlier. Manuscripts were included for their early date,[4] or, in the case of thirteenth-century mss, for containing readings adopted by later mss. Since the evolution of text, and particularly of the word *hereos*, is not without interest, some later manuscripts are included for the sake of their variant readings. Several fourteenth-century manuscripts exemplify the text as it circulated in the company of Gerard's gloss and as it found its way into the printed editions.

## *Edition*

The edition is based on the following manuscripts:

**B**: Bern, Burgerbibliothek, A 94 (10) (s. 11/12).
Described by Hermann Hagen, *Catalogus codicum Bernensium (Bibliotheca Bongarsiana)* (Bern, 1875; rpt. Hildesheim, 1974), p. 140. *Viaticum*, fols. 1–11 (a fragment of Book I). De amore, fols. 9v–10r.

**C**: Oxford, Corpus Christi College, 189 (s. 12).
Described by H. O. Coxe, *Catalogus codicum manuscriptorum qui in collegiis aulisque Oxoniensibus hodie adservantur* (Oxford, 1852) 2:76. *Viaticum*, fols. 8–70; De amore, fols. 14v–15r. Formerly at Christ Church, Canterbury (1284–1331). Once belonged to John Holyngborne.

**E**: London, British Library, Egerton 2900 (s. 12 late; England?).
Described in *Catalogue of Additions to the Manuscripts in the British Museum in the Years MDCCCCXI–MDCCCCXV* (London: Trustees of the British Museum, 1925), pp. 413–15. *Viaticum*, fols. 1–105; De amore qui et heros dicitur, fols. 15v–16v.

**G**: Cambridge, Gonville and Caius, 411/415 (s. 12).
Described by M. R. James, *A Descriptive Catalogue of the Manuscripts in Gonville and Caius College* (Cambridge: University Press, 1908) 2:480–82. Written in a hand "of southern aspect" (James). *Viaticum* (damaged at the beginning), fols. 1–68; De amore qui heros dicitur, fols. 7r–v.[5]

**L**: Oxford, Bodleian Library, MS Laud misc. 567 (s. 12[1]).
Described by H. O. Coxe, *Laudian manuscripts*, rev. R. W. Hunt, Bodleian Library Quarto Catalogues, 2 (Oxford: Bodleian Library, 1973), col. 406. *Viaticum*, fols. 2–50. De amore qui et eros dicitur, fols. 7r–v.

**O**: Oxford, Bodleian Library, MS Bodl. 489 (s. 12; France). Described by Falconer Madan and H. H. E. Craster, *A Summary Catalogue of Western Manuscripts in the Bodleian Library at Oxford which have not hitherto been catalogued in the Quarto Series* (Oxford: Clarendon Press, 1922) 2:1:194. *Viaticum*, fols. 1–77. De amore et qui heros dicitur, fols. 10r–11r.

**P**: Paris, Bibliothèque Nationale, lat. 6951 (s. 12). Described by E. A. Lowe, *The Beneventan Script: A History of the South Italian Minuscule*, rev. Virginia Brown (Rome: Storia e Letteratura, 1980) 2:114. *Viaticum*, fols. 105–77v. De amore qui & eros dicitur, fols. 113r–v.

**V**: Vatican, Biblioteca Apostolica, Pal. lat. 1163 (s. 12²). Described by Ludwig Schuba, *Die medizinischen Handschriften der Codices Palatini Latini in der Vatikanischen Bibliothek* (Wiesbaden: L. Reichert, 1981), pp. 120–21. Thirteenth-century glosses contain references to France. *Viaticum*, fols. 1r–114v; De amore qui hereos dicitur .i. furiosus uel irrationalis, fols. 15v–16v.[6]

**T**: Cambridge, Trinity O.1.40 (1064) (s. 12/13). Described by M. R. James, *The Western Manuscripts in the Library of Trinity College. A Descriptive Catalogue* (Cambridge, 1902) 3:45–46. *Viaticum* damaged at the beginning; (illeg.) et eros uel eros dicitur, fol. 4r–v.

In addition, variant readings from the following manuscripts have been noted when they represent common later readings not found in the manuscripts listed above:

**D**: Durham, Dean and Chapter library ms. C.IV.4 (s. 13 in.), *Viaticum*, fols. 38r–75v; de amore qui eros dicitur, fols. 42v–43r.

**Vp**: Vatican, Biblioteca Apostolica, Pal. lat. 1165 (s. 13¹), *Viaticum*, fols. 1r–39r; amor, f. 1r–v.

**M**: Bethesda, National Library of Medicine, MS 12 (s. 13), *Viaticum*; Amor, fols. 17r–18r.

**Vl**: Vatican, Biblioteca Apostolica, lat. 4425 (s. 14), *Viaticus liber Ysaac*, fols. 131r–82r; de amore qui et hereos dicitur, fols. 135r–v.

**A**: Erfurt, Wissenschaftliche Allgemeinbibliothek, F 266 (s. 14), *Viaticum cum glosulis magistri Geraldi Bituricensis*; de amore qui dicitur hereos, fols. 14r–15v.

I have referred to the Arabic version in the translation of G. Dugat and to the Greek translation printed among the works of Rufus of Ephesus. Where the Latin manuscripts disagree among themselves, the correspondence of the Arabic and Greek is of some use in making editorial decisions. I have also checked difficult passages against the *Liber de heros morbo*.

The testimony of the earlier manuscripts is weighted more heavily when the choice of readings is not obvious, though even they are not always reliable: C contains a number of omissions, as well as changes made by later hands, while B has been heavily erased and corrected. Of the twelfth-century manuscripts, P, V, and T (heavily glossed) are fairly sound; E is heavily corrected; L and O contain some idiosyncratic readings but are on the whole good. G's text is relatively poor but representative of other mss (it is closely related to Vat. pal. lat. 1158 and Oxford Laud 106). The trouble spots in the text are relatively few and well-defined. As indicated above, all the forms of *eros* and its derivatives provoked a scribal free-for-all. In addition, the syntax of lines 15–16 and 21–22, the use of the subjunctive, and the proper case after *incidere in* show a lot of variation.

Orthography generally follows B; except for *eros*, orthographical variants are not listed in the apparatus. I have, however, simplified B's double consonants (*occuli*) and restored dropped consonants (*aflictione, orribilis*) where these were likely to distract readers accustomed to lightly normalized medieval Latin. In all of the editions of Part 2, capitalization, punctuation, and paragraphing are editorial, though they are based on manuscript indications. Abbreviations are expanded silently and minor variations in word order are not noted. I have not improved Constantine's Latinity, since, as Baader's work has shown, much can be learned from a careful study of his language.

The translation aims to be as literal as possible while still making sense in modern English. In some places I have had to expand Constantine's elliptical style to give acceptable English syntax. I have retained potentially misleading cognates such as *humor* because these technical terms cannot be replaced by modern terms without distortion.

## EROS, HEROS, AND HEREOS

Because Constantine was the first to endow Arabic ʿishk with a Latin equivalent, and because the *Viaticum*'s name for the disease spurred later linguistic and conceptual developments, the verbal form he gave to ʿishk when he carried the idea of lovesickness from the Arabic world to the West is worth investigating. It can tell us about Constantine's practice as a translator, and can also clarify the convoluted path by which the Greek physicians' *eros* and the Arabs' ʿishk became the *amor hereos* and *amor heroicus* of the Christian scholastics.

Because Constantine tackled the *Viaticum* after he had worked on the encyclopedic *Pantegni* (as we know from the preface to the *Viaticum*),[7] he had by then a reasonable amount of translating experience. As Baader's study of terminology in the *Pantegni* has shown, Constantine was a linguistic innovator; many of the terms he introduced were adopted into the standard terminology of medicine.[8] Compared to the chapter on love in the *Pantegni*, however, that in the *Viaticum* is both ampler and more precise in its treatments of causes, symptoms, and cures. Perhaps this more fully conceptualized discussion seemed to call for a distinguishing label, one that would separate this *amor* from all the others. Daremberg has pointed out Constantine's desire "parler grec" in the *Viaticum*, and Jacquart and Thomasset have suggested that by defining *amor* as the one "qui et eros dicitur," Constantine gave his chapter on love an "allure hellénisante."[9] It is thus reasonable to suppose that Constantine might use *eros* as a technical term for distinguishing the illness of love from all other types of *amor*.

This hypothesis finds limited support in the evidence of the early *Viaticum* manuscripts. Since the earliest of them are one to two generations removed from Constantine's time, there is a significant chronological gap between the currently available evidence and what Constantine actually wrote, with ample time for scribal alterations to influence the manuscript traditions. Whether the distance can be bridged by cautious inference may be judged by the following.

The *Viaticum* manuscripts copied before Gerard of Berry wrote his gloss on the *Viaticum* ca. 1180–1200 contain no reliable evidence for Constantine's use of *hereos*.[10] They do, however, suggest that Constantine coined the neologism *eriosus (attested forms are *eriosis* and *eriosos*) to name the patient of lovesickness, and that he limited the meaning of *amor* by *eros*. The earliest (twelfth century) manuscripts show most agreement on the word designating the patients, *eriosis* and *eriosos*:

Quid melius *erios* adiuvat (= B): eriosos (V), ebriosos (L), eriosos (G), eriosos (P), heriosos (O), heriosos (E), eriosios (Oxford, CCC 189, s. 12), eriosos (Yale 16, ca. 1200), erios (T).

Hec est via medicine circa *eriosos* exercenda (= B): eriosos (V), otiosos (L), eriosos (G), eriosos (P), heriosos (O), heriosos (E), heriosos (Oxford, CCC 189), eriosos (Yale 16), eriseos (T).

If we add the evidence of early thirteenth-century manuscripts, the weight of the testimony indicates that *eriosos, eriosis* was Constantine's word for the patients of this disease.[11] This word may have been modelled on medical terms like *ebriosus* or *maniosus*.

*Eros* is probably the word from which *eriosus* was derived. *Eros* renders *'ishk* perfectly well, and fits the definitions of love given in context. Moreover, this Greek word would not have been hard to come by. It occurs in Greek-Latin and Latin-Greek glossaries; Constantine's mentor Alfanus was well-versed in Greek; and the very place where Constantine worked, Montecassino, had both Greek-speaking monks and Greek manuscripts.[12] Since Latin writers in the Salerno area, including Constantine himself, rarely inflected Greek technical terms, *eriosos* is readily conceivable as a neologism.[13] This limited (or non-existent) familiarity with Greek inflection also clarifies the wild variety of manuscript readings for oblique cases of *eros*. Although the evidence of the early manuscripts shows that *eros* and *heros* were rival forms for the nominative case, the uncertainty over the genitive points to *eros* as the original nominative.

The Arabic word in the following phrase means "of love" or "of the lover." If *heros*—however it came to mean "love" or "lover"—were the original form, there should have been no difficulty in arriving at the genitive *herois*, whose declensional forms are spelled out in glossaries.[14] With *eros*, however, the genitive may well have presented difficulty. The variety of forms points to a confusion that is more readily understandable for *eros* than for *heros*:

molestatio *herios* tollitur (= B): erroris (V, G, T and Yale 16), herios (L), heros (E and Oxford, CCC 189), erous (P), herois (O).

The variant *erroris* is most telling: it is improbable that it derives from a nominative *heros* or from *error*, since no manuscript attests the latter form. It is plausible that it was formed by analogy with *os, oris,* thus giving *eros* as its nominative.[15]

Whatever Constantine wrote—and I suggest that it was *eros*—there was no certainty among the scribes as to the proper terminology for the disease. Some continued to write *eros* through the fourteenth century, while others used *heros* or *hereos*. The origin of *hereos* is even more mysterious than Constantine's original term. The earliest instance I have found occurs in an Oxford manuscript (Corpus Christi College 189) from the second half of the twelfth century. *Eros* and *heros* also appear in this manuscript. The declined forms of *eros, heros,* and *herus* yield nothing that clarifies the form *hereos*. Perhaps it is a scribal back-formation from *(h)eriosis,* thus giving a nominative *\*herios*. Rather more likely, to my mind, is its origin in a confusion between genitive and nominative forms. The earliest manuscript (Bern A 94 [10]) and another twelfth-century manuscript (Oxford, Bodleian Library, MS Laud misc. 567) both contain the genitive *herios: molestatio herios tollitur*. It is possible that a scribe mistook this for an indeclinable form, especially since the following sentence in the *Viaticum* does contain an undeclined form: "Aliquando etiam eros causa pulchra est formositas considerata." Since confusion of *i* and *e* is common enough in medieval Latin (e.g. Vat. pal. lat. 1163, *hireos*), the metamorphosis of *herios* to *hereos* is an easy one.

Though the origin and meaning of *hereos* remain mysterious, the manuscripts show that it, rather than *eros*, gradually gained ascendancy as the proper name for the disease. As I view the evidence, two developments encouraged the triumph of *hereos*. The first was the appearance of a morphologically distinct form (to avoid the *eros-heros* confusion) that we see already in the Oxford manuscript. *Hereos* then won the day among Western physicians and became the standard term for the disease when its unique morphology gained the semantic support of Gerard of Berry's gloss, which explained that *heros* meant *heroes*, that is, the nobility who were more subject to the disease because of their soft lives. Henceforth physicians had a unique label for their descriptions of the disease of love.

The connection between *eros* and *hereos* was not altogether lost in the later Middle Ages. Gentile da Foligno (d. 1348), in his commentary on Avicenna's chapters on *ilisci* (*'ishk*), notes that while the Arabs call the disease of love "ilisi," it is also called "erreos, that is, erotic passion, that is, divine [passion]."[16]

## NOTAE

These notae apply to the apparatus accompanying all the editions in this volume.

*add.* = addit, –unt
*al.* = alius . . .
*cod(d).* = codex, –ices
*corr.* = correxit, –erunt, correctum
*del.* = delevit, –erunt
*eras.* = erasum . . .
*exp.* = expunxit, –erunt, expunctum
*l.* = linea . . .
*litt.* = littera . . .
*man.* = manu(s) . . .
*marg.* = margo . . .
*om.* = omittit, –unt
*rel.* = reliquit, –erunt
*scr.* = scribit, –unt; scriptus
*sp.* = spatium
*s.l.* = super lineam
*vac.* = vacuus . . .
*verb.* = verbum . . .
< > = supplevi

# Constantinus Africanus
## *Viaticum* I.20

**B**: Bern, Burgerbibliothek A 94 (10)
**C**: Oxford, Corpus Christi College 189
**E**: London, British Library, Egerton 2900
**G**: Cambridge, Gonville and Caius 411/415
**L**: Oxford, Bodleian Library, MS Laud misc. 567
**O**: Oxford, Bodleian Library, MS Bodl. 489
**P**: Paris, Bibliothèque Nationale, lat. 6951
**T**: Cambridge, Trinity College O.1.40 (1064)
**V**: Vatican, Biblioteca Apostolica, Pal. lat. 1163
**D**: Durham, Dean and Chapter Library MS C.IV.4
**Vp**: Vatican, Biblioteca Apostolica, Pal. lat. 1165
**M**: Bethesda, National Library of Medicine, 12
**Vl**: Vatican, Biblioteca Apostolica, lat. 4425
**A**: Erfurt, Wissenschaftliche Allgemeinbibliothek, F 266

### DE AMORE QUI ET EROS DICITUR

Amor qui et eros[1] dicitur morbus est cerebro contiguus.[2]
Est autem magnum desiderium cum nimia concupiscentia et
afflictione cogitationum. Unde quidam philosophi dicunt:
5  Eros est nomen maxime delectationis designatiuum. Sicut
autem fidelitas est dilectionis ultimitas, ita et eros
delectationis quedam est extremitas.[3]

---

*Tituli in prologo*:  De amore qui et heros dicitur BCE    De amore qui et (*om.* P) eros (er°os P
er°os V) dicitur LPV *deest*   TG   De amore qui et hereos dicitur O
**1** *Tituli* De amore qui et eros dicitur P   De amore qui et heros dicitur uel heros B   De amore
C   De amore qui et (*om.* GM) heros dicitur GEM   De amore et qui heros dicitur O   De
amore qui zeros dicitur L   De amore qui et hereos dicitur *s.l.* .i. furiosus vel irrationalis V
(illeg.) qui et eros uel ereos dicitur *ut videtur* T    **2** et] *om.* BLODVp      eros]
BGVDP   heros OET   *corr. in* hereos Vl   zeros L   hereos CAVp   cerebro] in c. MVl
contiguus] continguus B   conti[eras.]guus *s.l.* .i. assiduus V   contingens E   continuus *in
marg.* vel contiguus A    **3** magnum] nimium O   *s.l.* cum ista passione sunt (?) C   *om.*
A    nimia] magna PEA   *om.* D      concupiscentia] cupicentia B    **4** afflictione]
af- *et* -e *add. s.l.* E   afflictionem O    cogitationum] --is E   *om.* O      quidam] quia C
philosophi] pilosophi B   philophi C -so- *add. s. l.*   philosophorum D      **5** Eros] PVD
*corr. in* ereos CVL   *s.l.* .i. amor C   heros BEO   *corr. in* hereos TMAVp   Zeros L   heres G
est] esse Vp   *ante* dilectionis G     nomen maxime] maximum nomen G   maximi n. P
maxime n. O    delectationis] dilectionis PG   *s.l.* uel dilectionis V    designatiuum]
*post* eras. *et spat. unius uel duorum verb. vac. rel.* B   designatum P   significatiuum L    assig-
nativum D    **6** fidelitas] felicitas *s.l.* uel fidelitas uel fiducialitas C     est] *om.* G
dilectionis] delectationis O    ultimitas] extremitas G   et] *om.* G    eros] VDP
*corr. in* hereos M   *corr. in* ereos Vl   heros BGEOT   zeros L   hereos CAVp    **7** de-
lectationis] *om.* C   dilectionis PE    quedam] quidem *corr.* E    est] *add. s.l.* C
extremitas] ultimitas *corr.*  T

# Constantine the African
## *Viaticum* I.20

The love that is also called "eros" is a disease touching the brain. For it is a great longing with intense sexual desire and affliction of the thoughts. Whence certain philosophers say: Eros is a word signifying the greatest pleasure. For just as loyalty is the ultimate form of affection, so also eros is a certain extreme form of pleasure.

Aliquando huius amoris necessitas[4] nimia est nature
necessitas in multa humorum superfluitate expellenda. Unde
10    Rufus:[5] Coitus, inquid, ualere uidetur quibus nigra colera
et mania dominantur. Redditur ei sensus et molestatio
herios[6] tollitur, si etiam cum non dilectis loquatur.
Aliquando etiam eros[7] causa pulchra est formositas
considerata. Quam si in sibi consimili forma conspiciat,
15    quasi insanit anima in ea ad uoluptatem explendam
adipiscendam.[8]

Cum hec infirmitas forciora anime subsequentia habeat,
id est cogitationes nimias, fiunt eorum oculi semper
concaui, cito mobiles propter anime cogitationes,
20    sollicitudines ad inuenienda et habenda ea que desiderant.
Palpebre eorum graues, citrini ipsorum colores. Hoc ex
caloris fit motu qui ex uigiliis consequitur.[9] Pulsus
induratur neque naturaliter dilatatur neque sua percussio
secundum quod oportet custoditur.[10] Si in cogitationibus
25    profundatur, actio anime et corporis corrumpitur, quia
corpus animam in sua accione sequitur, anima corpus in sua
passione comitatur. Galenus: anime, inquit, uirtus
complexionem sequitur corporis.[11] Unde si non eriosis
succuratur ut cogitatio eorum auferatur et anima leuigetur,
30    in passionem melancolicam necesse est incidant. Et sicut
ex nimio labore corporis in passionem laboriosam incident,
itidem ex labore anime in melancoliam.[12]

---

**8** Aliquando] φa. G    causa *add. s.l.* P    necessitas] *s.l.* causa V    causa DVlVp    extremitas *s.l.* .i. principium et sic (?) est causa C    extremitas *add. in marg.* E    nimia] causa T
nimia . . . necessitas] *om.* O    *add. s.l.* P    *add. in marg.* B    nimia est *add. in marg.* E    na-
ture] *corr.* E    *om.* L    **9** necessitas] *om.* L    multa] --am G    humorum] humi-
dorum h. O    horum G    *om.* A    **10** Rufus] *s.l.* inquit C    ruffus GT    Coitus] *eras.*
E    coito A    uidetur] *om.* C    uidentur E    quibus] qui *add. s.l.* b; E    nigra] *s.l.*
.s. adusta V    colera] calida G    **11** mania] *corr.* B    ma- *post eras.* E    melancolia *in*
*marg.* vel mania A    dominantur] --atur CPOL    Redditur] --tur *post eras.* B    ei]
eis CPGVlVp    enim A    **12** herios] BL    heros *corr. in* hereos CVl    *s.l.* hereos .i. illius
amoris C    herois O    heroys A    erous *corr. in* erosis P    erroris GT    *s.l.* vel herois M    *corr.*
*in* hireos V    heros Vl *post eras.* E    erois *corr. in* erios D    hereos Vp    tollitur] *hic scrib.*
fiunt oculi *et in marg.* eorum semper concaui mobiles (ll. 18–19) G    cum] *om.* B    non]
*eras.* E    *exp.* Vl    *om.* D    dilectis] delectis V *corr.* P    loquatur] --antur CPOGAVp
*s.l.* .i. coeatur V    **13** etiam] et PLT    *om.* Vp    eros] BV *corr. in* erois P heros
GOETA    erios D    zeros L    herios *s.l.* .i. illius amoris C    hereos Vp    eteos *exp. et s.l. al.*
*man.* hereois M    *om.* Vl    **14** considerata] *corr.* V    desiderata O    si] *om.* G
in] *om.* OM    sibi] his V    *om.* Vl    *add. in marg.* Vp    consimili] in simili O    simili
L    **15** anima] *add. s.l.* E    in ea] *om.* C    eius P    mea O    uoluptatem] uolun-
tatem GLMD    explendam] expellendam C *corr.* B    complendam ipsius (*om.* Vp) EVp
ad implendam A    **16** adipiscendam] et a. ODVp    et *add. s.l.* PVl    adinspicienda *corr.*
*in* et inipiscendam C    adipiscen *add. s.l.* dam T    adipiscenda L adipiscendi BA    concupicendi
G    adipisci VM    *om.* E    **17** Cum] *om.* V    sub sequentia] *s.l.* .i. accidentia V

Sometimes the cause of this love is an intense natural need to expel a great excess of humors. Whence Rufus says: "Intercourse is seen to benefit those in whom black bile and frenzy reign. Feeling is returned to him and the burden of eros is removed, even if he has intercourse with those he does not love." Sometimes the cause of eros is also the contemplation of beauty. For if the soul observes a form similar to itself it goes mad, as it were, over it in order to achieve the fulfillment of its pleasure.

Since this illness has more serious consequences for the soul, that is, excessive thoughts, their eyes always become hollow [and] move quickly because of the soul's thoughts [and] worries to find and possess what they desire. Their eyelids are heavy [and] their color yellowish; this is from the motion of heat which follows upon sleeplessness. Their pulse grows hard and does not dilate naturally, nor does it keep the beat it should. If the patient sinks into thoughts, the action of the soul and body is damaged, since the body follows the soul in its action, and the soul accompanies the body in its passion. "The power of the soul," Galen says, "follows the complexion of the body." Thus if erotic lovers are not helped so that their thought is lifted and their spirit lightened, they inevitably fall into a melancholic disease. And just as they fall into a troublesome disease from excessive bodily labor, so also [they fall] into melancholy from labor of the soul.

consequentia Vp   accidencia subsequencia D        **18** id est] *om.* L       nimias] nimis C
--a-- *add. s.l. post eras.* B       semper] *om.* Vp       **18-19** fiunt . . . cogitationes] *om. et*
*add. s.l. et in marg.* G       **19** mobiles] mutabiles O   cogitationes] --m BVT       **20** sol-
licitudines] solliciti L   inuenienda] -as D   habenda] ᵇabenda B   adhabenda O   habentia
GD   ea] *om.* P   desiderant] --ent B   desiderat C   habere desiderant G   deside-
rantur OA   desidā E       **21** palpebre] p. sunt C       eorum] earum *corr.* G       citrini]
c. sunt C   citrinum O       ipsorum] eorum O   occulorum Vp       Hoc] *om.* EM
**22** caloris] calido OVl *corr.* VP   calore CLE   calor̄ G   colore *corr. in* calore M       motu]
motus CLE   *add.* fit D   qui] quem G   consequitur] consecuntur G       **25** pro-
fundatur] pessundatur L (*cf. Liber de heros morbo*, ll. 24-25)       quia . . . sequitur] *add. in*
*marg.* T       **26** animam] *om.* G   et a. C       accione] --em B   *add. s.l.* E   passione G
anima] et a. L   *add. in marg.* E   animam O   corpus] et c. C       **26-7** anima . . .
comitatur] *om.* G       **27** passione] actione *exp. et scrib.* passione B       **28** corporis]
*om.* COL       eriosis] BTD   eriosis *s.l.* .i. illis qui habent hanc passionem C   *exp. et s.l.*
heroisis M   eriosus P   ebriosis L   heriosis OEAVp   hireosis V   ueneriosis usus G   erosis
*corr. in* ereosis Vl       **29** succuratur] succurat C inuocatur G       ut] et V       eorum]
eius P       auferatur] c̄uferatur P       leuigetur] leuietur COV       **30** passionem] --e
BPG   melancolicam] --a BPG   melancoliam OV       necesse est] necessario L
incidant] ut incidant C   incidat P   inciderat V   incidatur OGD   incident L       **31** la-
bore] dolore et l. D       passionem laboriosam] passione est l. L   --e   --a CGPV *s.l.* .i.
febrem ethicam E       incident] inciderit C   incidant T   incidit OV   incidit homo GM   incidunt PE   incidunt homines ut in ethicam A **32** itidem] itidem et C   ita P idem G uiđe (?) L
ex] in E melancoliam] --icam GL   --ia BV

Quod melius eriosos adiuuat ne in cogitationes
profundentur nimias: uinum est temperatum et odoriferum dandum[13]
35 et audire genera musicorum; colloqui dilectissimis amicis;[14]
uersus recitacio;[15] luciferos uidere ortos, odoriferos et
fructiferos, currentem habentes aquam et claram; spatiari
seu deducere cum femina seu maribus pulcre persone.[16] Rufus:
uinum, inquit, est medicina fortis tristibus et timidis et
40 eriosis.[17] Galenus: Quicumque primitus uinum educere est
molitus de uitibus inter sapientissimos est computandus.[18]
Zenon dixit: Sicut lupinorum amaritudo tollitur si aqua
infundatur, similiter sic animi mei asperitas ebibito uino
in dulcedine est mutata.[19] Item Rufus: Non solum modo uinum
45 temperate ebibitum aufert tristiciam, sed et alia quidem sibi
similia, sicut balneum temperatum. Unde fit ut cum quidam
balneum ingrediantur ad cantandum animantur. Quidam ergo
philosophi dicunt sonitum esse quasi spiritum, uinum quasi
corpus, quorum alterum ab altero adiuuatur. Dicunt alii
50 quod Orpheus[20] dixit: Imperatores ad conuiuia me inuitant ut
ex me se delectent; ego condelector ex ipsis. Cum quo
uelim animos eorum flectere possim, sicut de ira ad
mansuetudinem, de tristicia ad leticiam, de auaricia ad
largitatem, de timore in audaciam. Hec est ordinatio
55 organicorum musicorum atque uini circa sanitatem anime.

---

**33** Quod] Quid P        eriosos] erios BT        eriosios *s.l.* .i. habentes hanc passionem C        heriosos OEAVp        ebriosos L        oxiosos *exp. et s.l.* heroisis M        **34** profundentur] --antur L
--untur V        --etur O        incidant siue profundantur T        infundantur Vp        est . . . dandum]
*om.* CO        est *om.* PD        dandum *om.* L        *in marg.* eis est V        detur E        debent nimium *exp.*
uinum *s.l.* bibere et temperatum et odorif. G        dandum est VlAVp        **35** et] *om.* T
genera] diuersa g. A        colloqui] corr. B        --ium G        dilectissimis] dulcissimis CO
dilectis P        dulcibus D        **36** versus] vesus B        -uum AL        luciferos] *corr.* B        lucidos
L        lutiferos G        odoriferos] et o. CG        **37** fructiferos] fructiferosos E        curren-
tem] --es V        habentes] CGOD        habentem P        *om.* BVTVp        habere Vl        *post* claram E
spectare L        aquam et claram] aquas et claras, --s *add. s.l.* V        **38** deducere] *corr. in*
delectari V        seu] siue BL *corr.* E        maribus] cum m. PLD        cum maribus -io- *add. s.l.*
(maioribus) C        Rufus] Rursus *corr.* T        **39** fortis] fortiter C        et[1] *om.* CGOL
et[2]] *om.* L        **40** eriosis] ebriosis L        ereosis *post eras.* Vl        heriosis COAVp        *post eras.*
E *corr.* M        timorosis GT        *s.l.* et hereosis V        Quicumque] Q. inquid G        primi-
tus] primitiis O        educere] deducere P        **41** molitus] *s.l.* .i. conatus V        uitibus]
uirtutibus B        computandus] deputandus G        **42** Zenon] Yenus B        Zenus EVVp
Zeno T        Seneca siue Z. A        amaritudo] *post eras. et spat.* B        **43** infundatur] *corr.*
B --antur OL        -itur Vp        similiter] *om.* PGCO        similiter sic] *om.* ELDVp        dulcissimis CO
ebibito] est (*om.* A) bibito EA        **44** in . . . mutata] mitigatur asperitas L dulcedine] --em
VPTODA        Item] iterum VTEM        modo] *om.* C        uinum] uino E        **45** tem-
perate] --um V        ebibitum] bibitum OVGTED        et] etiam G        *om.* BT        quidem]
quedam LP        que sunt G        sibi] *om.* LD        **46** temperatum] *om.* E ut] *om.* GD
cum] *om.* A        quidam] liquidum Vp        **47** ingrediantur] --untur L        i. tristes Vp
animantur] --entur O        aninantur B        **48** philosophi] pilosopi *corr.* B        phylosopi O

What better helps erotic lovers so that they do not sink into excessive thoughts: temperate and fragrant wine is to be given; listening to music; conversing with dearest friends; recitation of poetry; looking at bright, sweet-smelling and fruitful gardens having clear running water; walking or amusing themselves with goodlooking women or men. "Wine," Rufus says, "is a strong medication for the sad, the timid, and erotic lovers." Galen: "Whoever first strove to press wine from the vines is to be reckoned among the most wise." Zeno said: "Just as the bitterness of lupines is removed by infusing them in water, so the harshness of my spirit is changed into sweetness after drinking wine." Again, Rufus [says]: "Not only wine, temperately drunk, relieves sadness, but indeed other similar things, like a temperate bath." Thus it happens that when certain people enter a bath they are moved to sing. Therefore certain philosophers say that sound is like the spirit and wine like the body, each of which is aided by the other. Others say that Orpheus said: "Emperors invite me to banquets so that they may take pleasure in me, [but] I delight equally in them; as I wish I am able to bend their spirits from anger to mildness, from sadness to joy, from avarice to liberality, from fear to boldness." This is the regulation of music and wine for the health of the spirit.

---

sonitum] secutum G   alii s. B   quasi spiritum vinum balneum quasi corpus D        spiritum]
*s.l.* anima V        uinum] u. uero C        **49** alterum] unus C   alter LT *corr.* P        ab
altero] ablato G        adiuuatur] iuuatur G   adiuatur B        Dicunt] Dixunt V        **50** Or-
pheus] orp^heus B   orfeus PT *s.l.* .i. citarista V        dixit] dixerit O   Imperatores] Imperatos
*add.* -re- *s.l.* V        conuiuia] seruicia *s.l.* conuiuia V        **51** ego] etiam e. B   et e. VP
*add. s.l.* E        condelector] delector *s.l. add.* con V   *add. s.l.* E        ipsis] illis O        quo]
quorsum L   que G        **53** mansuetudinem] mansutudinem B        ad²] in COG
**54** in] ad PEVp        **55** organicorum] BCG   organorum PVOLTE

Quod perfectissimum sibi esse dinoscitur si boni
consocii aggregentur qui et in pulchritudine ualeant
scientia uel moribus. Dictum est enim quia maxima est
delectatio ut uinum bibatur et colloqui sapientibus.
60 Galenus: Colloqui, inquit, se amantibus laborem eicit ex
membris interioribus.[21] Quod si fiat in ortis lucentibus et
odoriferis seu fructiferis, optimum et iocundissimum fit.
Si autem non, eorum caminata ubi sessuri sunt munda sit et
lucida, apponantur rosa et mirta, salices, basilicon et
65 similia. Ab ebrietate caueant et cum oporteat dormiant.
Post somnum uero in balneo delectentur cum aqua et aere
temperato et lucido, neque eis accedat quod animus
abhorreat. Interrogatus autem quidam a philosophis quare
horribilis homo grauior eis esset quam quodlibet pondus.
70 Taliter respondisse fertur: Homo, inquit, horribile pondus
est solius animi. Alia uero pondera anime et corporis sunt
communia.[22] Hec est uia medicine circa eriosos exercenda.

---

**56** sibi] *om.* O    igitur Vp    si] est V    **57** consocii] conso[*eras.*]tii C    consortii
VIAVp    aggregentur] auggentur G    congregentur DA    et] *om.* OVGE    ualeant]
ualere G    *corr.* E    **58** scientia] aut s. uel de *exp.* moribus G    et s. L    uel] et D
uel ex Vp    quia] *om.* CGOTVp    h̄ GT    quod L    maxima] magna G    est] *om.*
C    **59** bibatur] bibitur C    bibant T    sapientibus] sapientissus L    amicis et s. A
**60** Galenus] *add. in marg.* E    se amantibus] cum se am. D    sapientibus EVTM *s.l.* uel
(*om.* V) se amantibus VT    *s.l.* uel amantibus T    se amantibus sapientibus A    laborem]
dolorem D    eicit] elicit VCOLT    ex] a GD    e POL    **61** si] *dittog.* B
*om.* G    fiat] sint G    fiati L    fit O    in ortis] mortis O    et] *om.* PGO    seu L
**62** seu] *om.* CEVp    uel L    fructiferis] *om.* CEVp    fructuosis G    et] *om.* PGO    io-
cundissimum] iocundum T    iocunde D    fit] sit CVE    est LG    **63** Si] sit C
non] *om.* BPEO    *add. s.l.* T    noñ autem̃ V    eorum] earum G    sessuri] sensuri BG
soliti sunt sedere O    munda] non m. BT    non *add. s.l.* P    *add. in marg.* M    sit] sint CT
non sᵗ Vp    **64** apponantur] --atur PG    appona'nt T    rosa] --e V    et¹] *om.* PC
salices] --e C    basilicon] et b. V    basilici C    **65** Ab] de V    ad OVl    ebrie-
tate]e. sua T    caueant] caueatur O    oporteat] *corr.* B    oportet CEOL    **66** som-
num] somnium B    uero] *om.* L    balneo] --eum ET    delectentur] --antur G    et]
*om.* BE    aere] *om.* E    **67** temperato] --a GE    lucido] --a E    eis] ad eos L
accedat] accidat C    *corr.* Vl    quod] quem L    animus] a. eorum L    **68** au-
tem] *om.* LG    a] *s.l.* .i. ex V *om.* GD    *exp.* Vl    philosophis] philosophus GVlD
**69** homo] quidam h. T    grauior . . . esset] est g. eorum C    eis] *om.* OEDVp    ei
A    esset] esse B    eis esset *add. s.l.* V    quam] *add. s.l.* E    quodlibet] colibet P
quamlibet D    quilibet Vp    pondus] alius p. L    **70** fertur] ei f. PEVTA    hor-
ribile] terribile T    **71** animi] --e GVp    pondera] ponda *corr.* C    anime] --i
Vp    corporis] --i POLA    corpus E    **72** est] *post* exercenda C    sunt VM
uia] uie VVl    circa] circo G    eriosos] otiosos L    heriosos COVp *corr.* EM    eriseos
T    hereoseos A    exercenda] *corr.* E    --e VOGTVl

[The cure] is judged most perfect if good companions are gathered who are outstanding in beauty, wisdom, or morals. For it is said that pleasure is greatest in drinking wine and talking with the wise. Galen says: "Speaking with friends casts out weariness from within." It is best and most joyous if it takes place in bright, fragrant or fruit-bearing gardens. If not, let the rooms where they are to sit be clean and bright, [and] let roses and myrtle, willow, basil, and similar things be placed there. Let them avoid drunkenness and when it is fitting let them sleep. After sleep let them take pleasure in a bath with bright and temperate water and air, and do not let anything befall them that the spirit might shrink from. A certain person was asked by philosophers why a horrible man was heavier than any weight. He is said to have responded in this way: "A horrible man is a weight on the spirit alone; other weights are common to body and soul." This is the way of practicing medicine for erotic lovers.

# GERARD OF BERRY,
# *GLOSULE SUPER VIATICUM*

## *Manuscripts*

Like the *Viaticum*, the *Glosule* is preserved in a large number of manuscripts, either in the form of a marginal commentary surrounding Constantine's text, or written out as an independent text. Of the seventy manuscripts written before the fifteenth century discovered so far, I have examined 15 in person or on microfilm, as well as the printed edition attributed to Gerard of Solo (Venice, 1505).[1] Manuscripts of the *Viaticum* such as Bethesda, National Library of Medicine 12, Cambridge, St. John's College D.24 (99), or Cambridge, Trinity College O.1.40 (1064), in which portions of Gerard's commentary have been entered by owners or readers in the margins or between the lines, were not used for the edition. The chapter on *amor* was studied in the following manuscripts:

Basel, Universitätsbibliothek D.III.6 (dated 1236); Cambridge, Trinity R.14.35 (907) (s. 13 mid); Cambridge, Gonville and Caius 117/186 (s. 13, England); Baltimore, Johns Hopkins University, William H. Welch Medical Library MS lat. 13.1 (s. 13, France; Paris?); Bethesda, National Library of Medicine, MS 11 (s. 13); Cambridge, Gonville and Caius 97 (s. 13); Montpellier 161 (s. 13); Munich, Bayerische Staatsbibliothek, Clm 13033 (s. 13); Munich, Bayerische Staatbibliothek, Clm 3512 (ca. 1300, Italy?); Vatican, Biblioteca Apostolica, Pal. lat. 1165 (s. 13[2]); Pal. lat. 1161 (ca. 1300); Pal. lat. 1149 (s. 14[1], Paris); Vat. lat. 4432 (s. 14); Vat. reg. lat. 1304 (s. 13); Erfurt, Wissenschaftliche Allgemeinbibliothek, Collectio Amploniana F 221 (s. 13/14, S. France); Collectio Amploniana F 266 (s. 14).

Again like the *Viaticum*, Gerard's *Glosule* survives in too large a number of manuscripts to use all of them for the type of edition offered here. Selection of a smaller number of manuscripts to edit from was based on the following criteria: early date (Basel D.III.6, Trinity R.14.35, Gonville and Caius 117/186), soundness of text (National Library of Medicine MS 11, Vatican Pal. lat. 1165, Munich Clm 13033), and relation to other manuscripts (T, N, V, R; see sigla below). The thirteenth-century manuscripts that I have seen do, in general, tend to have a better text than the fourteenth-century manuscripts because fewer glosses have crept in. However, because the "gloss type" of the *Glosule* circulated very widely in the fourteenth century and was used for early printed editions, I have included the earliest such MS that I have studied—T—as a representative of that group (see below for its members). This group developed as scribes compared manuscripts and incorporated alternate readings into the text. The process is visible at one point in T (see apparatus at line 40). Its value, therefore, is less for establishing the text than for documenting its transformations.[2] Given the contamination of the text, no attempt has been made to construct a stemma; however, certain general groupings are noted below.

**B**: Basel, Universitätsbibliothek D.III.6. (1236). Formerly at Amerbach. *Glosule super Viaticum*, fols. 17r–82v. Contains the "prologus maior": Cum omne elementum et ex elementis corpus generatum in materia communitatem habeant. "Amore" fols. 23v–24r. Described by Beat Matthias Scarpatetti, *Katalog der datierten Handschriften in der Schweiz in lateinischer Schrift vom Anfang des Mittelalters bis 1550: Die Handschriften der Bibliotheken von Aarau, Appenzell und Basel* (Zürich: Urs Graf, 1977) 1:164. Fol. 50r of the manuscript is reproduced in vol. 2. The earliest dated manuscript: "Expliciunt Glosule Magistri Geraldi Bituricensis super Viaticum parisius in studio compillata. Est liber expletus propter quod sum bene letus. M.CCXXXVJ Die veneris .viii. kalendis martis Laus tibi sit christe quoniam liber explicit iste" (Feb. 22, 1236). Orthography is marked by a high frequency of double consonants.

**C**: Cambridge, Gonville and Caius, 117/186 (s. 13, England?). *Gerardus super viaticum ysaac*, fols. 2–135r. Contains the "prologus minor" but lacks the biographical information and part of the *accessus* of the fuller versions: Cum omnia ex .iiii. elementis generata a medicis sint quodammodo cognoscenda. . . . "De amore qui dicitur hereos (?)" fol. 18v. A very good text. Described by Montague Rhodes James, *A Descriptive Catalogue of the Manuscripts in the Library of Gonville and Caius College*, 2 vols. and suppl. (Cambridge: Cambridge University Press, 1907–14) 1:124–26.

**M**: Munich, Bayerische Staatsbibliothek, Clm 13033 (s. 13 and 14). Formerly Ratisbon 33. "Incipiunt glose Magistri G. cremonensis super Viaticum" fol. 70r. "Amor qui hereos dicitur" fol. 77v. See *Catalogus codicum latinorum Bibliothecae Regiae Monacensis IV, tomi II pars II codices num. 11001–15028 complectens* (Munich, 1876; rpt. Wiesbaden: Harrassowitz, 1968), p. 95.

**N**: Bethesda, National Library of Medicine, MS 11 (s. 13, France?). *Super Viatico Constantini*, fols. 1r–95r. Prologus minor without biographical information. "De amore qui hereos dicitur" fol. 10r. Described in Dorothy Schullian and Francis Sommer, *A Catalogue of Incunabula and Manuscripts in the Army Medical Library* (New York: Henry Schuman, 1950), pp. 233–34; DeRicci 1:453, no. 11. Word order sometimes varies from other early mss (the scribe prefers verbs at the end of clauses, vs. more frequent S-V-O order of the other mss).

**R**: Vatican, Biblioteca Apostolica, Reg. lat. 1304 (s. 13). Prologus minor. Text of *Glosule* in the margins surrounding *Viaticum*, fol. 110r–68. "Amor qui hereos dicitur e&" fol. 117r. No modern description, only 18th c. handwritten catalogue at the Vatican. Orthography marked by frequent use of "s" for soft t/c: sirca, fasili, divisias, mensio. Text carelessly copied, but contains interesting additions (see apparatus at lines 43, 53, 55, 56).

**T**: Cambridge, Trinity College R.14.35 (907) (s. 13 mid). *Viaticus cum girando*, fols. i–215v. Prologus maior ("Cum omne elementum et ex elementis corpus generatum"). Gloss in margins; "Amor qui et hereos dicitur etc." fol. 21r. Montague Rhodes James, *The Western Manuscripts in the Library of Trinity College, Cambridge*, 4 vols. (Cambridge: Cambridge University Press, 1900–1904) 2:320. Closely related texts in the chapter on lovesickness are Cambridge, Gonville and Caius, 97; Erfurt, Wissenschaftliche Allgemeinbibliothek, Collectio Amploniana Q 221 (prol. maior) and F 266; Munich, Bayerische Staatsbibliothek, CLM 3512 (prol. maior); Vatican, Biblioteca Apostolica, Pal. lat. 1146 (prol. maior); Venice, 1505 edition (both prologues). T was chosen as the earliest and best representative of this group.

**V**: Vatican, Biblioteca Apostolica, Pal. lat. 1165 (s. 13²). Prologus maior. "Exposicio magistri Geraldi super viaticum Constantini" fols. 41r–82r ("expliciunt Glose viatici"). "Amor qui heros dicitur" fol. 46v. Described in Ludwig Schuba, *Die medizinischen Handschriften der Codices Palatini Latini in der Vatikanischen Bibliothek* (Wiesbaden: Ludwig Reichert, 1981), pp. 122–24.

## PROLOGUS MINOR AND MAIOR

Gerard's *Notuli* or *Glosule* were prefaced by two distinct albeit related prologues, called in some manuscripts "prologus maior" or "minor."[3] Both can be found, differing somewhat from manuscript versions, in the edition of Venice, 1505. Common to both are the following major divisions: 1) Necessity for physician to understand the elements and their interactions; 2) division of medicine into theoretical and practical sides, and classification of *Viaticum* as practical medicine; 3) origin of *Glosule* at Parisian colleagues' request; 4) *accessus ad auctorem*. The "prologus maior" considerably amplifies the first two sections. What appears as a single sentence in the shorter version ("Cum omnia ex quattuor elementis generata quodammodo sint agnoscenda, hec vero tanquam inutilia et corrumpentia, illa vero tanquam adiuvantia et necessaria, quorumdam sicut inutilia per accidens cognitio est necessaria, aliquorum sicut iuvantium proprie et per se") occupies nearly a page in the longer version. The same ideas are developed at greater length and with greater theoretical sophistication. Similarly, in the *prologus maior* Gerard goes into greater detail on the division of theoretical and practical medicine, and on Constantine's place within practical medicine.

## *Edition*

The editorial principles are, in general, the same as for the *Viaticum*. Trouble spots are again few, and tend to be at the most technical points, places where scribes would understandably be confused (lines 13–16), and at abbreviations (l. 10: m. = meliorem/mulierem?). The morally and socially problematic recommendation of therapeutic intercourse generated a variety of sometimes euphemistic and sometimes explicit variants: consorcium, consilium, colloquium, empcio, and defloratio. Orthographical variants are not noted, except in the case of *heros/hereos* and where the spelling could give rise to significant ambiguity (e. g., *intentio/intensio* but not *circa/sirca*). **B** has been used as the base manuscript.

# Gerardus Bituricensis
## *Notule (Glosule) super Viaticum*

**B**: Basel, Universitätsbibliothek D.III.6, fols. 23v–24r (1236).
**C**: Cambridge, Gonville and Caius 117/186, fols. 18v–19r (s. 13).
**M**: Munich, Bayerische Staatsbibliothek, Clm 13033, fols. 77v–78r (s. 13).
**N**: Bethesda, National Library of Medicine, 11, fol. 10r–v (s. 13).
**R**: Vatican, Biblioteca Apostolica, Reg. lat. 1304, fol. 117r–v (s. 13).
**T**: Cambridge, Trinity R.14.35, fols. 21r–22r (s. 13 mid).
**V**: Vatican, Biblioteca Apostolica, Pal. lat. 1165, fols. 46v–47r (s. 13²).

*Amor qui heros dicitur.* Hec passio dicitur apud
auctores[1] sollicitudo melancolica. Est enim plurimum similis
melancolie, quia tota intentio et cogitatio defixa est in
pulchritudine alicuius forme uel figure desiderio
5  coadiuuante.

Que sit causa huius passionis qua uirtutes impediantur
difficile est uidere. Causa ergo huius passionis est error
uirtutis estimatiue[2] que inducitur per intentiones sensatas
ad apprehendenda accidencia insensata[3] que forte non sunt in
10  persona. Unde credit aliquam esse meliorem et nobiliorem et
magis appetendam omnibus aliis.[4] Quod est ideo: quia aliquod
sensatum aliquando occurrit anime ualde gratum et
acceptabile, unde estimat cetera sensata non esse consimilia,
unde si qua sunt sensata non conueniencia occultantur a non
15  sensatis intentionibus anime uehementer infixis.[5] Estimatiua
ergo, que est nobilior iudex inter apprehensiones ex parte
anime sensibilis,[6] imperat imaginationi ut defixum habeat
intuitum in tali persona. Ymaginatiua uero concupiscibili,
unde concupiscibilis hoc solum concupiscit, quia sicut
20  concupiscibilis ymaginatiue obedit, ita ymaginatiua
estimatiue, ad cuius imperium cetera inclinantur ad personam

---

*Tituli*] Amore B De amore qui dicitur hereos (*transp.* N) CT *om.* R   **1** qui] *om.* C
*heros*] ᵇe. N et h'eos T h'cos C hereos MR   dicitur] *om.* N d. et cetera TR
**2** auctores] actores N auīc̄ VR actores grecos T a quibusdam M plurimum]
quamplurimum T ut pl. M similis] simul C   **3** cogitatio] c. eorum B de-
fixa] fixa T est] *om.* NM e. plurimum V   **4** pulchritudine] --em CT ali-
cuius] illius V forme] persone uel f. R formei R   **5** coadiuuante] adiuuante T
**6** sit] fit V autem s. R qua] que BCT et que VM est eque R uirtutes] uirtus
*post* que M *corr.* R impediantur] --atur M   **7** ergo] *om.* B autem R
huius] *om.* N error] h'er'o M   **8** intentiones] intensiones C   **9** ad
apprehendenda] adprehendendum R accidencia] alia a. R insensata] non sensata
BC   **10** credit] credet R non c. B forte c. T aliquam] unam N aⁱam V
esse] *om.* C *post* magis M magis e. appetendam et V meliorem] mulierem M *om.*

# Gerard of Berry
## *Glosses on the Viaticum*

LOVE THAT IS CALLED HEROS. This disease is called a melancholic worry by medical authors. It is indeed very similar to melancholy, because the entire attention and thought, aided by desire, is fixed on the beauty of some form or figure.

It is difficult to understand what the cause of this disease is, by which the faculties are hindered. The cause, then, of this disease is a malfunction of the estimative faculty, which is misled by sensed intentions into apprehending non-sensed accidents that perhaps are not in the person. Thus it believes some woman to be better and more noble and more desirable than all others. Thus it is, for sometimes some sensed object appears very pleasing and acceptable to the soul, so that it judges other sense objects to be dissimilar [i.e., not pleasing]. Any unfitting sensations are, as a consequence, obscured by the non-sensed intentions [i.e. that the person is more noble, better, etc.] deeply fixed in the soul. The estimative [faculty], then, which is the nobler judge among the perceptions on the part of the sensible soul, orders the imagination to fix its gaze on such a person. The imaginative [faculty orders] the concupiscible, in fact, so that the concupiscible desires this one alone, for just as the concupiscible [faculty] obeys the imaginative, so the imaginative [obeys] the estimative, at whose command the others are inclined toward the person whom the estimative judges to be

VR    mulierem omnibus aliis N    .m. esse nobiliorem T        et¹] *om.* CNRM        nobilio-
rem] *om.* C    *post* appetendam V            **11** omnibus aliis] *om.* T        quia] quod
BC    **12** aliquando] *post* quia N    *om.* B        anime] *om.* M        ualde] delectabile M
**13** cetera] et(?) c. C        sensata] non s. VMR        non] *om.* TR        consimilia] similia   CNT            **14**    sunt] sint VR        non²] *om.* TR    a ꞁ a sensatis B    aut V
**15**    sensatis] sensatu C        intentionibus] intensionibus R        anime] *om.* R        uehe-
menter] ualde V        infixis] defixis T            **16** ergo] uero M        nobilior] melior C
melior et n. R        apprehensiones] --iuas N    a. anime CT            **17**    anime] *om.* C
imaginationi] --iue TMV        ut] et N        defixum] --is N            **18** intuitum] i. et
aspectum R        Ymaginatiua] --tio NR        uero] nō V        concupiscibili]--is V    imperat c. T        **19** unde] *om.* M        hoc] hic C        solum] solet RN        quia . . .
concupiscibilis] *om.* R            **20** ymaginatiue] --tioni C            **21** estimatiue] e. obedit R

quam estimatiua iudicat esse conuenientem, licet non sit.[7]
Ymaginatiua autem uirtus figitur circa illud propter malam
complexionem frigidam et siccam que est in suo organo, quia
25 ad mediam concauitatem ubi est estimatiua trahuntur spiritus
et calor innatus ubi estimatiua fortiter operatur.[8] Unde
prior concauitas infrigidatur et desiccatur, unde remanet
dispositio melancolica et sollicitudo.[9] Ubi autem
concupiscibilis sit sita non determino.
30 　　Signa autem istius passionis quedam sumuntur ex parte
anime, quedam ex parte corporis. Ex parte anime
sunt profunde cogitationes et sollicitudines, ut si aliquis de
aliquo loquatur, uix intelliget, si autem de eodem, statim
mouetur.[10] Ex parte uero corporis sunt signa: profundatio
35 oculorum, quia secuntur spiritus currentes ad locum
estimatiue. Item siccitas oculorum et priuatio lacrimarum
nisi adueniat fletus ex parte rei desiderate. Motus adest
continuus palpebrarum, unde de facili ridet et de facili de
fletu ad risum mouetur.[11] Sed tamen flet cum audit amoris
40 cantilenas et precipue si fiat mentio de repudio et de
separatione rerum dilectarum. Omnia membra eius arefiunt.[12]
Pulsus eius inordinatus, quia aliquando frequens et uelox
dum res consimiles rei dilecte commemorantur.
　　Morbus iste perfecte non curatur nisi per coniunctionem
45 et permissionem legis et fidei.[13] Tunc enim redeunt uirtutes
et corpus ad naturalem dispositionem. Antequam ergo
confirmetur, considera an sit humoris adustio; quod si
est, euacua. Deinde administra sompnum longum,
humectationem et nutrimentum laudabile et balnea aquarum

---

**22** iudicat] indicat BM　et dicat C　esse] *om.* N　**23** autem] *om.* N　uero B
uirtus] *om.* NR　figitur] figura N　**24–25** quia . . . concauitatem] *dittog.* C
quia] que R　**25** estimatiua] --tio TC　**26** innatus] naturalis C　estimatiua]
--tio NCT　**27** concauitas] *om.* N　unde]et ideo R　**28–29** Ubi . . . deter-
mino] *om.* V　autem] añ M　**29** concupiscibilis] uirtus c. T　concupis R
sit sita] sic sica R　**30–32** Signa . . . ut] *om.* V　autem] *om.* M　istius] huius
CTR　sumuntur] sunt M　ex] a CT　**31** ex] a CT　corporis] cordis R
Ex] a CT　sunt] *dittog.* T　*om.* R　**32** profunde] --da R　cogitationes] --tio R
et] *om.* M　sollicitudines] --tudoR　**33** aliquo] alio B　aliqua re T　alia re R
intelliget] --git T　attendit V　intelligi N　intelligit et atendit R　autem] aliquis C　*om.* V
eodem] e. uel re dilecta R　**34** uero] *om.* N　**35** quia] que R　currentes]
occurrentes B　concurrentes R　**37** ex] a C　**38** unde] u. et T　u. etiam BMR
de . . . ridet] *om.* C　facili] fasili R　ridet] rident R　et] unde B　cito etiam M
unde cito R　de facili²] *om.* RM　**38–39** de fletu ad risum] de risu ad fletum TV
**39** ad] in R　mouetur] --entur R　Sed] *om.* R　tamen] enim *post* flet M　*om.* R
cā C　flet] *om.* CBN　f. autem R　**40** cantilenas] --a R　precipue] maxime
TVR　repudio] tripudio *i. marg.* .in al'. de repudio T　rupudio *corr.* C　**41** sepa-

fitting, though this may not be so. Moreover, the imaginative faculty is fixated on it on account of the imbalanced complexion, cold and dry, that is in its organ, for the *spiritus* and innate heat are drawn to the middle ventricle [of the brain], where the estimative faculty functions intensely. The first ventricle therefore grows cold and dries out, so that there remains a melancholic disposition and worry. Where the concupiscible power is located, however, I will not decide.

Now, some of the signs of this disease are drawn from the soul's part, some from the body's part. From the soul's part are depressed thoughts and worries, so that if someone talks about something, [the patient] scarcely understands; if, however, he speaks of the beloved, he is immediately moved. From the body's part are the signs: sunken eyes, since they follow the *spiritus* racing to the place of the estimative [faculty]; also, dryness of the eyes and lack of tears unless weeping occurs on account of the desired object. There is a continual motion of the eyelids, so that he laughs easily and is easily changed from tears to laughter. But nevertheless he weeps when he hears love songs and especially if mention is made of rejection and separation of beloved objects. All his members dry out. His pulse is disordered, for sometimes it is frequent and swift when he recalls something similar to the beloved object.

This disease cannot be perfectly cured without intercourse and the permission of law and faith. For then the faculties and the body return to their natural disposition. Before it is established, therefore, consider whether there may be burning of humor; if there is, purge it. Then administer lengthy sleep, humectation, and good nourishment, and freshwater baths.

---

ratione] desperatione V    dilectarum] delectarum CN    Omnia] o. enim R    eius] enim V    arefiunt] arescunt N    rarefiunt *corr. in* arescunt T    **42** eius] e. est VRT quia] *om.* N    nam R    aliquando] a. est R    et] aliquando N    **43** consimiles] *om.* B    dilecte] delecte N    dulce C    commemorantur] rememoratur N    considerantur V    --atur et ei occurrunt. tardus autem est pulsus et rarus dum desperat de re dilecta habenda.    Cum autem sperat uelox et frequens R    **44** iste] autem i. T    perfecte] *om.* N    curatur] c. secundum Avicenna T    **45** permissionem] per visionem C periussionem M    intensionem R    redeunt] redentur N    **46** et] ad C ad] et ad C    ergo] *om.* R    igitur M    **47** considera] consid'i V    an] utrum N et antequam R    adustio] uitio uel a. T    adustio . . . si] *om.* C    quod] et TR que M    **49** humectationem] et h. CBR    ad humectandum uel ad h. T    balnea] --um C    aquarum] aque C    aq. B

50  dulciarum.[14] Fac eos occupatos circa res diuersas ut ab eo
    quod diligunt diuertantur. Ad hoc autem multum ualet
    consilium uetularum ut narrent uituperationes multas et
    fetidas dispositiones rei desiderate.[15] Ualet etiam
    consorcium et amplexus puellarum, plurimum concubitus
55  ipsarum, et permutatio diuersarum.[16] Prodest etiam uenatio
    et species diuerse ludorum.
          *amor qui heros.* heroes dicuntur uiri nobiles qui
    propter diuicias et mollitiem uite tali pocius laborant
    passione.[17] *cerebro contiguus.* id est assiduus propter
60  assiduam cerebri occupationem circa rem dilectam et
    a cerebro nocumentum ad omnia membra corporis
    transfertur. *fidelitas.* qui enim intime diligit alium
    omnia secreta sibi reuelat et si qua reuelata sunt sibi
    celat.[18] *delectationis extremitas.* quia cum aliis delectetur,
65  in illo tamen potissime et extreme. *aliquando huius amoris.*
    amorem non uerum hic tangit, qui non est nisi ad deponendas
    superfluitates. *aliquando etiam hereos.* hic tangit ueri
    amoris causam.[19] *in consimili.* quia cum uidet consimilem rei
    desiderate magis mouetur et insanit. *corpus anime sequitur*
70  *actionem.* tanquam instrumentum et artificem.[20] *anima corpus.*
    quia secundum diuersas complexiones naturales et
    accidentales anima mouetur ad diuersas operationes. Dicit
    enim Philosophus quod innatus est anime amor uegetandi
    corpora.[21] Unde in hiis gaudet que conseruant eam in corpore
75  et contristatur ab hiis per que a corpore separatur, sicut

---

50 dulciarum] dul. T  dī R  dulcis CB  dulcium VM      Fac] et f. R      occupatos] --ri
R      ab eo] habō M  ab ea R      **50–51** ab . . . diuertantur] ad hoc quod diuericantur
diligunt C      **51** quod] quam R      diligunt] --gant R      diuertantur] --santur N
diuersentur sive divertantur T  quoquomodo d. R      autem] iterum BCMT  multum a.
N      multum ualet] neque C      **52** uetularum] uetutularum R      ut] ut uidelicet
T      narrent] --ant N      uituperationes multas et] uituperia multa ut R      **53** de-
siderate] considerate V  d. ut dicendo quod fetet et quod est scabiosa et duo uel tria deffert
conauteria (?) propter multitudinem sordisiei et quod cotidie patitur materia (?) et consimilia R
ualet] m *ut uid.* N      **54** consorcium] cons(c)ilium BR  empcio V  defloratio M  colloquium p. et amplexus earum T  et amplexus] *om.* R      plurimum] et pl. BCT  plu-
rimi concubituꝛ M      concubitus] c. plurimus *post* ipsarum R      **55** ipsarum] earum
TBC  et i. R      diuersarum] ipsarum B  prodest d. C  ita quod odie alias et cras alias R
Prodest] ualet R      **56** ludorum] ut squaquorum et aliarum et talorum et cetera R  l.
multum prosunt T      **57** heros] he. N  hereos R  et cetera C  heros dicitur B  et
h'eos dicitur TR      heroes] h'eos N  h'eos C  h'eos siue h'iosi T  hereos R      qui]
*ante* tali R      **58** et . . . uite] *om.* C      mollitiem] mollities N  uite m. atque delicias
T  m. et suauitatem et delicationem R      uite] *om.* B      **59** *contiguus*] continuus NT
continguus M      **60** assiduam] continuam M      cerebri] c. et R      rem dilectam]
*om.* BV  illud *add. in marg.* quod diligit assiduam C  d. creatur illud T      et] assiduus
est N      **61** omnia] o. tocius N      **62** transfertur] transferatur B  defertur T

Occupy the patients with various things, so that they are distracted from what they love. In this, moreover, the counsel of old women is very useful, who may relate many disparagements and the stinking dispositions of the desired thing. Also useful is consorting with and embracing girls, sleeping with them repeatedly, and switching various ones. Hunting and various types of games also help.

*Love that [is called] heros:* Heroes are said to be noble men who, on account of riches and the softness of their lives, are more likely to suffer this disease. *contiguous to the brain:* that is, incessant, because of the incessant preoccupation of the brain with the beloved thing, and the damage is transferred from the brain to all the parts of the body. *loyalty:* for whoever intimately cherishes another reveals all his secrets to him, and conceals whatever has been revealed to him. *the extreme form of pleasure:* for though he may delight in others, nevertheless in that one [he delights] most powerfully and extremely. *sometimes of this love:* he touches here on false "love," which is nothing but getting rid of superfluities. *sometimes also hereos:* he touches here on the cause of true love. *in a similar:* for when he sees something similar to the desired thing, he is more greatly moved and grows mad. *the body follows the action of the soul:* like tool and craftsman. *the soul the body:* for the soul is moved to various operations according to various natural or accidental complexions. For the Philosopher says that innate in the soul is a love of animating bodies. Thus it rejoices in those things that preserve it in the body and grows sad from those that separate it from the body, such as

---

intime] legitime T    intime et uero animo R         alium] aliquem T   *om.* R           **63** om-
nia] *om.* C        secreta] *om.* C    s. sua N    sua s. R        sibi¹] ei VR         reuelat . . . qua]
*om.* R        sunt] fuerint NMR        sibi] *om.* R    *add. sup. lin.* N    *ante* revelata T
**64** *delectationis*] dilectio N    dellectatio B    dilcō C    delectio R    dilectionis V    *extremitas*]
*om.* RV        aliis] in a. NM        delectetur] --entur R    --antur T         **65** illo] alia N
tamen] tunc T  est (?) V        potissime] potentissime NC        extreme] extra modum M
**66** tangit] --unt C        qui . . . superfluitates] *om.* V        deponendas] --dum R    dispo-
nendas C        **67** superfluitates] --te T    uel solum causa libidinis R         *hereos*] heros
N    tangit] t. maxime C    etiam t. M    magis t. R        ueri] magis u. T        **68** amoris]
magis a. BT        causam] --as M        cum] non M        consimilem] rem c. NR
**69** desiderate] dilecte uel d. T        magis] *om.* BCVR    tunc mouetur m. T        mouetur]
*om.* M    *corpus anime*] animam corpus T        sequitur] *om.* M        **70** actionem]
accō N    --nes R    *om.* T        et] *om.* BVMR        **71** complexiones] c. corporis V
**72** accidentales] --lis C        operationes] o. uel opiniones T        **73** enim] *om.* R
quod] quia C    qui B        amor] amore B        uegetandi] --do T        **74** corpora] corpus VMT        gaudet] congaudet R        conseruant] seruant C        eam] em R
**75** contristatur] tristatur C    --antur R    hiis] eis T    per] *om.* TM    a corpore] ab
eo N    eam a c. M        separatur] separant M

sunt superuenientes passiones. *Galenus inquit uirtus anime.*
id est, operatio uirtutis. *complexionem sequitur* etc. quia
secundum complexionem corporis mouetur anima ad operandum.
Naturaliter dico, quia aliter secundum mores acquisitos
80   a philosophia uel a conuictu, quia secundum complexionem
colericam mouetur ad iram et sic de aliis.[22] *sonitum esse*
*quasi spiritum.* sonitus organorum musicorum anime
comparatur, quia in eis maxime delectatur anima, unde ad
corpus transfertur, quia corpori ualde amicatur. Quia ergo
85   in amore leditur tam corpus quam anima, ideo docet utrique
communia remedia. *uinum bibat.* uinum enim moderatum corpus
humectat.

---

**76** superuenientes] supernenientes C        **77** id est] uel N        uirtutis] u. anime T
*complexionem*] c. corporis T      etc.] *om.* T        **78** secundum complexionem] *om.* M
corporis] corpus M     mouetur] mouet M     **79** quia] quod C    quod si T        secundum mores] sermones C   est sermones T     acquisitos] --as C        **80** a[2]] *om.* CR
conuictu] communi uictu uel usu T   conuicto R **81** colericam] calidam c. T      sic] similiter
R     *esse*] *om.* CT        **82** sonitus] id est s. T        organorum] organicorum B
**83** comparatur] --antur CR      eis] hiis T     anima] natura R     unde] uerumtamen
R   Uinum M        **84** ualde] maxime M     amicatur] amitaitur N   --antur R
**85** amore] graui a. T     ideo] idcirco BVMR     utrique] uterque C   uirtusque coniuncta
uel communia R     **86** *uinum*] *om.* M   *bibat*] quasi corpus T   *om.* MR   moderatum]
temperatum B   temperat C   moderate sumptum T

overwhelming emotions. *Galen says: the faculty of the soul*: that is, the function of the faculty. *follows the complexion etc.*: for the soul is moved to acting according to the complexion of the body. [It acts in this way] according to nature, I mean, for otherwise [it acts] according to habits acquired from philosophy or conviction, since a choleric complexion moves it to wrath, and similarly for the others. *sound like spiritus*: the sound of musical instruments is compared to the soul, for the soul delights most greatly in them, whence the delight is transferred to the body, for it is closely allied to the body. Because, therefore, the body suffers in love as well as the soul, he thus teaches a common remedy for both. *let him drink wine*: for temperate wine moistens the body.

# GILES, *GLOSE SUPER VIATICUM*

The text is preserved in a single manuscript at least one remove from the original text: Gerona, Archivo Capitular, Codex (78) 20,e,11. 145 fols. 29 cm. Saec. 14 (?). Gothic cursive. Amor hereos = fol. 1 verso.

The contents of the manuscript are:
1. Glose egidii super Viaticum, fols. 1–25v. Inc.: "Queritur de capillis. auctor distinguit . . ." Expl.: "sicut caliditas."
2. Glose super librum de febribus Isaac. fols. 26r–57v. Inc.: "Secundum quod dicit philosophus secundo phisicorum et quarto methetorum (ubi natura deficit ars incipit?)" Expl.: "inflat febrilem effectionem."
3. Glose dietarum universalium ysaaci. Fols. 58r–73v. Inc.: "Ut dicunt auct. mediana est ad hoc . . ." Expl.: ". . . omne motum ad motum altius cicius movetur."
4. Fols. 74r–77r: "Queritur de cibo per quam virtutem nutriat . . . Expl.: ". . . adducitur complexione calida quam frigida sicut visum fuit superius et sic solvitur."
5. Fols. 78r–79r: "Questio est que complexio sit longioris vite . . ." Expl.: "quod in vita non contingit dicere maxime ? mulieris."
6. Fols. 79r–79v: "Queritur de fluxu et refluxu maris . . ." Expl.: ". . . et non solum sicut apparentiam."
7. Jean de St. Amand, *Glose super librum regimen acutorum ypocratis.* Fols. 81r–104v. Inc.: "Ut testatur averroix elementa sunt propter mixtum" Expl.: ". . . magis est secundum intentionem actoris" (TK² 1624).

The remaining items are from a booklet of different origin bound together with the preceding:
8. Arnald of Villanova, *Parabolae aphorismi sive canones vel regulae,* 105r–12v (TK² 999).
9. Arnald of Villanova, *Flebotomia,* 113r (TK² 988).
10. Pseudo-Hippocrates, *Astrologia ypocratis,* 113r–16r (TK² 1379).
11. Gerard, *De modo medendi,* 116v–45r (TK² 327).

Because the arguments of Egidius and Peter of Spain often depend on equivocal senses of terms like *passio, amor, maior,* and so on, translating their Latin poses a number of challenges. Where the argument depends on it, I have tried to preserve ambiguity; but when attempting to retain the equivocation would have been misleading, I have substituted other terms. Particularly troublesome is the pair *morbus* and *passio*. Sometimes *passio* is a straightforward synonym for *morbus*, meaning "disease," "illness." Sometimes *passio* is used (as the antonym of *actio*) to denote an undergoing or "suffering" in the philosophical sense. And sometimes it is used of the mind that has undergone the disturbance of emotion, "suffering" the *passiones* or *accidentia animae*. Rendering these distinctions into English is complicated by the fact that our "passion" means yet something else, and does not convey the meanings of Latin *passio* crucial for Egidius' and Peter's arguments.

I have emended the text in two places where wrongly expanded abbreviations have marred the sense.

# Egidius
## *Glose super Viaticum*

AMOR QUI ET HEROS DICITUR MORBUS EST ETC.
Queritur: auctor determinat de egritudinibus capitis; de morbis non
dicit quod sint <capitis>. Queritur propter quid istud
5 dicat de isto morbo.

Preterea passio que non est capitis non debet determinari
inter passiones capitis. Hereos non est passio capitis ergo
inter passiones capitis non debet determinari.

Preterea odium est passio cordis ergo eius contrarium
10 est passio eiusdem.[1]

Ad hoc dicendum quod heros non dicitur morbus nisi
gratia ipsius associati sive gratia eius quod consequitur,
quia sequitur profundatio cogitationum.[2] Unde quia ista
profundatio est in ipso cerebro et non videbatur propter hoc
15 magis dicit quod sit passio capitis quam de aliis egritudinibus
ipsius capitis.

Preterea queritur de cura istius egritudinis. Ille enim
docet administrare vinum. Sed contra: nihil quod mentem
percutit debet administrari in hac egritudine. Vinum est
20 huiusmodi, ergo non debet administrari in hac egritudine.[3]

Preterea Ysaac dicit in dietis particularis quod vinum
accuit cognitionem et profundat.[4] Sed nihil quod profundat
debet administrari herosis. Vinum est huiusmodi, ergo vinum
in eis non est administrandum.

25 Preterea Ovidius in remedio amoris dicit quod vinum non
debet administrari amantibus, ergo etc.[5]

Solutio ad hoc dicendum quod vinum inducit leticiam
<quando> est mediate sumptum. Unde quando dicitur quod vinum
mentem percutit, hoc non est intelligendum universaliter,
30 sed particulariter ut in febricitantibus.

Ad aliud dicendum quod vinum profundat mentem
sapientibus, hoc est illis qui sunt sane mentis, unde
versus: Cum bene sum potus circa versibus influo totus, cum
sim ieiunus, sim de peioribus unus.[6] Unde vinum

---

**4** <capitis>] caliditatis; *suppl.*     **6** capitis] caliditatis *del. et* capitis *add. s. l.*     **7** capitis[2]] caliditatis *del. et* capitis *add. s. l.*     **9** contrarium] passio *expunc. ante* c.
**13** Unde] quia *expunc. ante* U.     **23** herosis] est huiusmodi *expunc. post* h.     **27** ad]
primum *expunc. post* a.     **28** <quando>] quare; *suppl.*

# Giles
## *Gloss on the Viaticum*

LOVE THAT IS CALLED HEROS IS A DISEASE ETC. It is inquired: [In the first book] the author discusses illnesses of the head, [but] he does not say [explicitly] that the diseases are of the head [i.e., located in the head]. It is inquired why he says that concerning this disease [i.e., that love is a disease of the brain].

A passion that is not of the head ought not to be discussed among the passions of the head. Hereos is not a passion of the head, therefore it ought not to be discussed among them.

Furthermore, hate is a passion of the heart, therefore its contrary is also a passion of the same.

To this it must be said that heros is not called a disease except by virtue of its symptoms or by virtue of what follows, for depressed thoughts follow. Therefore, since this depression is in the brain itself and is not evident, on account of this he says—with better reason about it than about other diseases of the head itself—that it is a passion of the head.

Furthermore, there is a question about the cure of this disease, for he teaches that wine ought to be administered. Yet on the contrary, nothing that disturbs the mind ought to be administered in this disease. Wine is of this nature; therefore it ought not to be administered in this disease.

Moreover, Isaac says in *Particular Diets* that wine sharpens thinking and deepens it. But nothing that deepens [thought] ought to be given to sufferers of *heros*. Wine is of this nature; therefore wine is not to be given them.

Moreover, Ovid says in *Remedies of Love* that wine ought not to be given to lovers, wherefore etc.

Solution. To this it must be said that wine brings on happiness when it is taken in moderation. Thus, when it is said that wine disturbs the mind, this is not to be understood universally, but particularly, as in feverish patients.

To the other [argument] it ought to be said that wine deepens the mind in wise people, that is, those whose minds are healthy. Thus the verses: "When I'm well soused, in poetry I'm doused; When I'm athirst, I'm one of the worst." Thus wine stirs up sluggish thought. Because sufferers of

35   cogitationem sopitam commovet. Unde cum in herosis non est
cogitatio sopita imo profundata et non est profundata in
bono sed in malum, vinum vero affert cogitationes malas,
letificat enim animam et propter hoc competit heriosis.

heros do not have sluggish thought, but rather "deepened," and not "deepened" in a positive sense but rather in a negative one [i.e., depressed], wine will truly carry away bad thoughts, for it cheers up the soul, and because of this it is beneficial for sufferers of heros.

# PETER OF SPAIN, *QUESTIONES SUPER VIATICUM*
## (Version A)

## *Manuscripts*

Version A survives in two manuscripts:

**E**: Erfurt, Wissenschaftliche Allgemeinbibliothek, CA 212 (s. 14 in., Montpellier). *Questiones super Viaticum*, fols. 1–107; *amor hereos*: fols. 18r–19r. Described in Schum 1887, 468–69.

*Inc.*: "Quoniam quidem ut ait Tullius in rethoricum. [text] Hic queruntur XV, primum utrum medicina theorica sit nobilior." *Expl.*: "utrum ibi competat coitus."

The title stems from Amplonius Ratinck in the fourteenth century: "Item glose et questiones optime Petri Hispani super libro Viatici Constantini." There seems to be no reason to doubt the attribution. The rest of the manuscript contains other medical works by Peter.

**K**: Krakow, Biblioteka Jagiellońska, Rps BJ 781 (1334, Montpellier?). *Questiones super Viaticum*, fols. 158r-204v; *amor hereos*: fols. 168v-69r. Described in: *Catalogus codicum manuscriptorum bibliothecae universitatis Jagellonicae Cracoviensis* (Krakow, 1877–81) 2:232.

*Inc.*: "Quoniam quidem ut ait tullius in rethoricis. hic queruntur xv. primo utrum medicina theorica sit nobilior." *Expl.*: "simplicis medicine operetur ergo et cetera."

The manuscript contains a list of contents that designates Peter's work as: "Scriptum super Viatico Constantini, cum Questionibus pulcris, et totus liber bonos [sic] est."

## *Edition*

The edition is based on the more carefully executed manuscript E, with a few emendations from K. Omissions common to both E and K indicate that they descend from a common ancestor. Orthography follows E, except that I have uniformly used "v" for consonantal "u" in keeping with the practice of previous editors of Peter's writings.[1] In E the letters *c* and *t* are particularly hard to distinguish; moreover, the scribe freely interchanges

-ti- and -ci-. Where I have expanded abbreviations, I have opted for -ti-. In several places I have emended the text where the manuscript readings are obviously deficient and can be easily remedied. I have not, however, been able to make sense of the passage marked with asterisks in line 71.

Some of the ambiguities in Peter's terminology that can be misleading in translation are noted in the introduction to the edition of Egidius' commentary. In this text *magis* and *maxime* also seem to be deliberately equivocal, especially when they modify some form of the verb 'to be' (*magis est* = "is more [frequent? intense?]"). Peter's scholastic Latin is, in addition, both highly formulaic and studded with numerous particles that reflect the emphases of his classroom delivery but that are difficult to render into English. Although it is tempting to prune and update Peter's style, translating it into a less stilted contemporary idiom, I have chosen to remain as faithful as possible to the Latin text. Every translation is perforce an interpretation, but one that is contemporary and idiomatic would, in this case, overinterpret the text in hand. I have preferred to give a plain rendering that leaves the reader the freedom to decide the meaning of problematic or ambiguous passages. The one apparent exception to this policy is the translation of *profundatio cogitationis* as "depressed thought." The English phrase, however, was not so much dictated by contemporary clinical usage as by the metaphors of depth and sinking implied by *profundare* and *profundatio*.

# Petrus Hispanus
## *Questiones super Viaticum* (Version A)

**E**: Erfurt, Wissenschaftliche Allgemeinbibliothek, CA 212
**K**: Krakow, Biblioteka Jagiellońska, Rps BJ 781

AMOR QUI HEREOS DICITUR MORBUS EST CEREBRI.
Hic queruntur .14. Primo cuius virtutis amor hereos sit passio.
Secundo cuius membri sit passio. Tertio in qua complexione maxime
generetur. Quarto in quo sexu. Quinto in qua etate. Sexto
5 utrum exire a patria competat in amore hereos. Septimo utrum
turpes mulieres sint adducende coram <pati>entibus amorem
hereos. Octavo utrum pulchre mulieres sint adducende coram
illis. Nono utrum ebrietas competat in amore hereos. Decimo
queritur de dictis in littera. . . .[1]

10     Circa primum argumentum. Morbus est passio illius virtutis
cui infert sensibile nocumentum.[2] Sed amor hereos infert
nocumentum ymaginative. Ergo amor est passio virtutis
ymaginative.

    Sed videtur quod sit cogitative, quia amor hereos fit cum
15 assiduitate cogitacionum secundum Constantinum. Ergo est
passio cogitative.[3]

    Contra: in amore hereos est defectus iudicii de formis vel
de rebus insensatis. Ergo est passio illius virtutis cuius
est apprehendere formas insensatas, cuius est estimativa
20 secundum Avicennam in libro *De anima*.[4] Ergo est passio
estimative.

    Sed videtur quod sit fantasie, quia amor hereos est
passio illius virtutis cuius est conferre unum obiectum alio
obiecto. Cum in amore hereos sit defectus iudicii quod fit
25 in iudicando aliquam mulierem vel pulchriorem omnibus aliis
vel unum obiectum esse melius alio, ut iam videbatur,
<obiectum confertur obiecto>.[5] Sed fantasia est virtus
conferens obiectum obiecto.[6] Ergo amor hereos est passio
fantasie.

---

**1** HEREOS] yreos K      **2** Primo] *om*. K     virtutis] virtus K      **3** membri]
cerebri K     maxime] magis K      **6** turpes] turpe K     <pati>entibus] adducentibus EK
**7** hereos] yreos K      **8** hereos] yreos K      **10** argumentum] sic arguitur K
**11** cui infert] cuius insunt K     hereos] hereseos K      **12–13** Ergo . . . imaginative]
*om*. K      **15** Ergo] *om*. E      **17** hereos] *om*. K      **18** insensatis] --as K

# Peter of Spain
## *Questions on the Viaticum* (Version A)

LOVE THAT IS CALLED HEREOS IS A DISEASE OF THE BRAIN. Here 14 questions are raised. First: of which faculty is love a disease? Second: of which bodily member is it a disease? Third: in which complexion is it generated most often? Fourth: in which sex? Fifth: in which age? Sixth: whether leaving the country is useful in lovesickness? Seventh: whether ugly women are to be brought before lovesick patients? Eighth: whether beautiful women are to be brought before them? Ninth: whether drunkenness is useful in lovesickness? Tenth: inquiries concerning the text. . . .

Concerning the first argument. A disease is a suffering of that faculty to which it brings sensible harm. But lovesickness harms the imaginative faculty. Therefore love is a disease of the imaginative faculty.

But it seems to be [a disease] of the cogitative [faculty], since, according to Constantine, lovesickness occurs with incessant thought. Therefore it is a disease of the cogitative [faculty].

On the contrary: in lovesickness there is a failure of judgment concerning non-sensed forms or things. Therefore it is a disease of that faculty whose task is to apprehend non-sensed forms, which is that of the estimative [faculty], according to Avicenna in *De anima*. Therefore it is a disease of the estimative [faculty].

But it seems to be [a disease] of the fantasy, because lovesickness is a disease of that faculty whose task is to compare one object with another. Since, in lovesickness, there is a failure of judgment that occurs in judging either some woman more beautiful than all others or one object better than another, as already has been seen, <one object is compared with another>. But the fantasy is the faculty that compares one object with another. Therefore lovesickness is a disease of the fantasy.

---

**19** insensatas] mixtas K        **20** in] *om.* E        **23** conferre] *om.* E        alio] alii E
**24** hereos] herereos K        **25** iudicando] videndo K        **27** <obiectum confertur ob-
iecto>] *om.* EK; *suppl.*

30     Dicendum quod amor hereos est passio virtutis estimative, quia morbus est passio illius virtutis cui infert nocumentum primo et per se et immediate. Sed amor hereos primo et immediate infert nocumentum virtuti estimative, cum in amore hereos sit defectus iudicii de formis vel rebus insensatis,

35     cuiusmodi sunt amicicia et inimicicia et sic de aliis. Et virtuti estimative sit apprehendere formam insensatam, quod sic intelligitur. In amore hereos estimat virtus estimativa aliquam mulierem an aliquam aliam rem esse meliorem vel pulchriorem omnibus aliis cum non sit ita, et tunc inperat

40     virtuti cogitative ut profundet se in formam illius rei. Et sic in amore hereos est profundacio cogitationis. Et tunc virtus ymaginativa ymaginatur illam rem, et eam <mandat?>[7] virtuti irascibili et concupiscibili, que sunt virtutes motive inperantes in corde existentes. Et tunc huiusmodi virtutes

45     inperantes inperant virtuti motive que est in nervis ut moveant membra ad prosecucionem illius rei.[8] Et sic patet quod amor hereos primo et per se et immediate <estimative infert nocumentum et tunc>[9] estimativa infert nocumentum aliis virtutibus. Per hoc patet solutio racionum, quia bene

50     concedimus quod amor hereos infert nocumentum ymaginative, cogitative et fantasie, non tamen immediate immo mediate sicut patet ex iam dictis. Et ideo amor hereos debet dici passio estimative et non cogitative vel ymaginative vel fantasie.

55     Circa secundum sic. Opposita nata sunt fieri circa idem ut scribitur in *Predicamentis*.[10] Sed amor et odium sunt contraria. Ergo nata sunt fieri circa idem. Sed odium est passio cordis. Ergo et amor. Quare et cetera.

     Item omnia accidencia anime sunt passio cordis, quoniam

60     omnia accidencia anime consequuntur cor ut dicit Haly super *Tegni*.[11] Sed amor hereos est accidens. Ergo est passio cordis.

---

**31** illius] *om.* K      **33** virtuti] --is K      **34** rebus] de r. K      **36** virtuti] --is K      formam insensatam] forma insensatus E    formam sensatam K    quod] et K
**38** aliquam mulierem] *dittog.* K   aliam] *om.* K      **40** virtuti] --em K      **41** cogitationis] --um K      **42** <mandat>] *om.* EK; *suppl.*      **43** motive] motē E   motiē K
**45** inerant] inperavit E      **47–48** <estimative infert nocumentum et>] *om.* EK; *suppl.*
**48** estimativa] *om.* E      **52** hereos] *om.* E      **59–60** sunt . . . anime] *om.* K
**60** ut] sicut K (*et passim*)    **61** accidens] cordis anime *scrib. et* cordis *del.* E

It must be said that lovesickness is a disease of the estimative faculty, since a disease is a suffering of that faculty which it harms first and in itself and directly. But lovesickness harms the estimative faculty first and directly, since there is, in lovesickness, a failure of judgment about non-sensed forms or things, such as friendship and enmity and similarly other things. And it is the estimative faculty's [task] to apprehend a non-sensed form, which is understood thus: in lovesickness, the estimative faculty judges some woman or some other thing to be better or more beautiful than all the rest, even though it might not be so, and then it orders the cogitative faculty to plunge itself in the form of that thing. And thus in lovesickness there is depressed thought. And then the imaginative faculty imagines that thing, and <sends> it to the irascible and concupiscible faculties, which are faculties located in the heart that control movement. And then these controlling faculties order the faculty of movement, which is in the nerves, to move the limbs in pursuit of that thing. And thus it is obvious that lovesickness first and in itself and directly <harms the estimative faculty, and then> the estimative faculty harms the other faculties. In this the answer to the arguments is evident, since we readily concede that lovesickness harms the imaginative and cogitative faculties and the fantasy, not, however, directly but rather indirectly, as is evident from what has been said. And therefore lovesickness ought to be called a disease of the estimative faculty, and not of the cogitative, or of the imaginative, or of the fantasy.

Concerning the second, thus: contraries must exist in the same type of subject, as it is written in the *Categories*. But love and hate are contraries. Therefore they must exist in the same thing. But hate is a passion of the heart. Therefore love also is. Wherefore, etc.

Moreover, all the emotions of the soul are a suffering of the heart, since all the emotions of the soul follow the heart, as Haly says in the *Tegni*. But lovesickness is an emotion. Therefore it is a suffering of the heart.

Contra: eiusdem rei sunt actus et potentia.[12] Sed actus
amoris scilicet coitus est passio testiculorum, ergo et potentia.
65  Ergo videtur quod amor hereos sit passio testiculorum.

Item morbi denominantur a sua materia ut patet in febribus.[13]
Sed materia amoris hereos vel coitus est sperma. Ergo amor
hereos denominatur a spermate. Sed sperma est in testiculis.
Ergo amor hereos est passio testiculorum.

70  Item in cura cuiuslibet morbi in quo competunt emplastra
membro *cicius ille morbus passio.*[14] Sed in cura amoris
hereos applicantur emplastra vel mulieres ad testiculos.
Ergo amor hereos est passio testiculorum.

Sed videtur quod sit passio cerebri, quoniam amor hereos
75  est passio similis melancolie secundum auctor in littera.[15] Sed
melancolia est passio cerebri. Ergo et amor hereos.

Item amor hereos est sollicitudo melancolica cum
profundatione cogitationis. Sed omnia ista sunt cerebri et
non cordis vel testiculorum. Ergo amor hereos est passio
80  cerebri et non cordis vel testiculorum. Ad idem sunt Avicenna
et iste auctor determinantes de amore hereos inter passiones
cerebri.

Dicendum quod de amore hereos est loqui dupliciter, uno
modo in quantum est amor et sic est passio cordis, sed hoc modo
85  non est morbus. Alio modo est loqui de amore hereos in
quantum est circumstantionata istis circumstanciis que sunt
sollicitudo melancolica cum profundatione cogitationis et
corrupcione estimative iudicantis aliquam rem omnibus aliis
prevalere et hoc modo est passio cerebri et hoc modo est
90  etiam morbus.[16] Et per hoc solvitur prima ratio, quia bene
concedimus quod amor est passio cordis, cuiusmodi amor non
est morbus, sed defectus vel corruptio estimative iudicantis
unum prevalere omnibus aliis ratione cuius amor hereos est
morbus et passio ipsius cerebri.

---

**64** scilicet] est *exp. et* .s. *add. s. l.* E     **67** amoris] amor E     **69** amor] et a. K     est]
debet esse K     **70** in¹] *om.* K     cuiuslibet] cuius K     **71** cicius] cuius K
**74** sit] *om.* E     quod . . . cerebri] *dittog.* E     **77** Item amor hereos] *om.* K
**79** est] sunt E     **80** Ad] et K     sunt] est E     **84** in] *om.* K     sed hoc
modo] et sic K     sed *bis et exp.* E     **86** circumstanciis] substantiis E     **88** cor-
rupcione] —nis K     iudicantis] vidi^tis K     **90** etiam] *om.* K     Et] *om.* K
**91** amor] a. hereos K     **92** defectus] defectio K     iudicantis] videntur K
**93** amor] ipse a. K     **94** morbus et] *om.* K

On the contrary: action and potential belong to the same thing. But since the action of love, namely coitus, is a suffering of the testicles, so also its potential. Therefore it seems that lovesickness is a suffering of the testicles.

Also, diseases are designated by their substances, as is apparent in fevers. But the substance of lovesickness or intercourse is seed. Therefore lovesickness is designated according to seed. But seed is in the testicles. Therefore lovesickness is a suffering of the testicles.

Also, in the cure of whatever disease in which plasters benefit a member, *that disease quickly a suffering.* But in the cure of lovesickness, plasters or women are applied to the testicles. Therefore lovesickness is a suffering of the testicles.

But it seems to be a suffering of the brain, since lovesickness is a suffering similar to melancholy, according to the author in the text. But melancholy is a suffering of the brain. Therefore so [is] lovesickness.

Also, lovesickness is a melancholic worry with depressed thought. But all these are of the brain and not of the heart or of the testicles. Therefore lovesickness is a suffering of the brain and not of the heart or the testicles. Avicenna and this author agree, discussing lovesickness among the sufferings of the brain.

It must be said that lovesickness can be spoken of in two ways: first, insofar as it is love, and thus it is a suffering of the heart, but in this way it is not a disease. The second way is to speak of lovesickness insofar as it is accompanied by these circumstances, which are melancholic worry with depressed thought and a damaged estimative [faculty], which judges something to surpass all others, and in this way it is a suffering of the brain and is also a disease. And thus the first argument is solved, since we readily concede that love is a suffering of the heart, which type of love is not a disease. But a failure or damaging of the estimative [faculty], which judges one thing to be superior to all others, is the reason why lovesickness is a disease and a suffering of the brain itself.

95        Ad aliud dicendum quod omnia accidentia anime consequuntur
ipsum cor tanquam principium remotissimum.[17] Verumptamen
sunt passio ipsius cerebri.

        Ad aliud dicendum quod coitus vel potentia coeundi non
sunt morbus in amore hereos, sed defectus estimative cum
100    profundacione cogitacionis, que sunt passiones cerebri et
non testiculorum. Per hoc solvitur alia racio.

        Ad aliud dicendum quod duplex est cura amoris hereos.
Una est cura per se, et hoc modo curatur amor hereos per
cantilenas et aspectum pulchrarum formarum. Alia est cura
105    accidentalis ipsius amoris hereos et hoc modo curatur per
applicationem emplastrorum et mulierum ad testiculos.
Argumenta probantia quod sit passio cerebri concedo.

        Circa tertium sic. Amor hereos est passio melancolica
secundum actorem in littera.[18] Ergo maxime generatur in illa
110    complexione in qua maxime habundat melancolia, cuiusmodi est
complexio melancolica. Ergo amor hereos maxime habet esse in
complexione melancolica.

        Item actores medicine docent evacuare melancoliam in amore
hereos.[19] Sed hoc non esset nisi fieret ex melancolia que
115    maxime habundat melancolicis. Ergo amor hereos maxime habet
esse in complexione melancolica.

        Contra: amor hereos maxime habet esse in illa complexione
in qua magis reperitur stimulacio ad coitum, quia stimulacio
ad coitum est maxime causa amoris hereos secundum Avicennam
120    in tertio.[20] Sed stimulacio ad coitum maxime habet esse in
complexionibus calidis, cum calidum stimulet ad coitum
secundum Galienum in *Tegni*.[21] Ergo amor hereos maxime habet
esse in complexionibus calidis.

        Quod concedo, quia stimulacio ad coitum est maxime causa
125    amoris hereos secundum Avicennam in tertio et huiusmodi
stimulacio maxime habet esse in complexionibus calidis—in
colericis et sanguineis. Et causa huius est quia in
colericis et sanguineis est calor stimulans ad coitum et
iterum in eis est sufficiens materia spermatica replens
130    testiculos, cuius repletio stimulat ad coitum.

---

**95** consequuntur] consequunt E        **96** principium] principalis K        **97** passio]
passi K        **100** cogitacionis] --um K    passiones] passio E        **103** Una] *dittog.*
E      curatur] cura E        **106** emplastrorum] --arum E        **110** maxime] magis K
cuiusmodi] cuius K        **113** docent] dicunt docent K        **118** quia] sed E        **122** he-
reos] *om.* K        **124** ad coitum] *om.* K        **126** maxime] *om.* K        **127–8** Et
causa . . . sanguineis] *om.* K        **130** cuius] cuiusmodi K

To the next argument it must be said that all emotions of the soul follow the heart itself as if the most remote origin. Truly, they are a suffering of the brain itself.

To the next it must be said that intercourse or the ability to have intercourse is not a disease in lovesickness, but rather the failure of the estimative [faculty] accompanied by depressed thought, which are sufferings of the brain and not of the testicles. Thus the other argument is solved.

To the next it must be said that the cure of lovesickness is twofold. One is the cure *per se*, and in this way lovesickness is cured through songs and the sight of beautiful forms. The other cure is of the accompaniments to lovesickness, and in this way it is cured through the application of plasters and women to the testicles. I concede the probative arguments that it is a suffering of the brain.

Concerning the third, thus: Lovesickness is a melancholic disease according to the author in the text. Therefore it is generated most in that [humoral] complexion in which melancholy most abounds, which is the melancholic complexion. Therefore lovesickness occurs most in the melancholic complexion.

Also, medical authors recommend purging melancholy in lovesickness. But this would not be unless it were caused by melancholy, which most abounds in melancholics. Therefore lovesickness is found most in the melancholic complexion.

On the contrary: lovesickness occurs most in that complexion in which is found more stimulation to intercourse, for stimulation to intercourse is the greatest cause of lovesickness according to Avicenna in the third [book of the *Canon*]. But stimulation to intercourse occurs most in hot complexions, since heat stimulates intercourse, according to Galen in the *Tegni*. Therefore lovesickness occurs most in hot complexions.

Which I concede, since stimulation to intercourse is the greatest cause of lovesickness according to Avicenna in the third [book], and this kind of stimulation occurs most in hot complexions—in the choleric and the sanguine. And the reason for it is that in the choleric and the sanguine there is a heat that stimulates intercourse, and moreover in them there is sufficient seminal matter filling the testicles, whose fullness stimulates intercourse.

Ad primum argumentum dicendum quod amor hereos est
profundacio cogitationis cum forti ymagine et corrupcione
estimative ut in passione melancolica. Vel dicendum quod
amor hereos non dicitur passio <melancolica> eo quod fiat ex
135 melancolia, sed quia augmentat melancoliam. Quare et cetera.

Ad aliud dicendum quod actores non docent evacuare
melancoliam naturalem in cura amoris hereos sed melancoliam
innaturalem generatam per adustionem, cuiusmodi melancolia
maxime habundat in complexione calida et non in frigida
140 melancolia. Quare et cetera.

Circa quartum sic. Debilitas spei est causa amoris hereos.
Sed mulieres sunt debiliores spei quam viri ut scribitur
octavus *De animalibus*.[22] Ergo amor hereos magis habet esse in
mulieribus quam in viris.

145 Contra: in amore hereos est fortis inpressio alicuius
dilecte in ymaginativa. Sed huiusmodi fortis inpressio magis
est in viris quam in mulieribus, cum viri habeant cerebella
sicciora quam mulieres, et quod inprimitur in sicco
fortius inprimitur quam quod inprimitur in humido.[23] Ergo
150 amor hereos maxime habet esse in viris.

Dicendum quod amor hereos cicius et frequencius generatur
in mulieribus propter debilitatem spei in eis et quia
frequencius stimulantur ad coitum, licet non ita fortiter.[2]
Sed in viris est difficilioris cure, eo quod inpressio
155 alicuius forme dilecte in cerebro viri est fortior et
difficilioris irradiacionis quam inpressio forme in cerebro
mulieris, eo quod vir habet cerebrum siccius quam mulier et
inpressio facta in sicco est difficilioris eradiationis
quam facta in humido. Per hoc patet solutio rationum.

160 Circa quintum sic. Amor hereos aliquando generatur ex
humoribus adustis. Sed adustio humorum magis est in
iuvenibus cum sint calidiores et sicciores quam in aliis.[25]
Ergo amor hereos maxime habet esse in iuvenibus.

Contra: in amore hereos est profundatio cogitationis cum
165 ymaginacione alicuius forme dilecte. Sed ista duo maxime
reperiuntur in pueris. Ergo amor hereos maxime habet esse
in pueris.

---

**132** ymagine] ymaginacione K    **133–4** Vel . . . passio <melancolica>] *om.* K    **134**
<melancolica>] hereos E    **137** melancoliam[1]] *om.* K    **138** cuiusmodi] cum K
**141** spei est] spei in K    amoris] minoris K    **147** habeant] habent K    **148**
mulieres] --ibus E    **149** quod] illud quod K    **154** cure] *om.* K    **156** irra-

To the first argument it must be said that lovesickness is depressed thought with a strong image and damaging of the estimative [faculty], as in melancholic illness. And it must be said that lovesickness is not called a melancholic disease because it originates from melancholy, but because it increases melancholy; wherefore etc.

To the second it must be said that the authors do not recommend purging natural melancholy in the cure of lovesickness, but unnatural melancholy generated by burning, which sort of melancholy most abounds in a hot complexion, and not in cold melancholy; wherefore etc.

Concerning the fourth, thus: Weakness of hope is the cause of lovesickness. But women are less hopeful than men, as it is written in the eighth book *On animals*. Therefore lovesickness occurs more in women than in men.

On the contrary: in lovesickness there is a strong impression of some beloved in the imaginative [faculty]. But this kind of strong impression is greater in men than in women, since men have drier brains than women do, and what is imprinted in the dry is more strongly imprinted than what is imprinted in the moist. Therefore lovesickness occurs most in men.

It must be said that lovesickness is more quickly and frequently generated in women on account of their weak hope and because they are more frequently stimulated to intercourse, although not so strongly. But in men it is more difficult to cure, because the impression of any desired form in the brain of a man is stronger and harder to erase than the impression of a form in the brain of a woman, because a man has a drier brain than a woman, and an impression made in the dry is harder to erase than that made in the moist. In this the answer to the arguments is evident.

Concerning the fifth, thus: Lovesickness is sometimes generated from burnt humors. But the burning of humors is greater in youths since their humors are hotter and drier than in others. Therefore lovesickness occurs most in youths.

On the contrary: in lovesickness there is depressed thought with the imagination of some desired form. But these two things are found most in boys. Therefore lovesickness occurs most in boys.

---

diacionis] cure i. K      **157** vir] *om.* K      siccius] cicius K      **158** eradiationis]
*corr. ex* irradiationis E      **162** sint] *om.* K      calidior et siccior] ca. et si. E      cal'i et
sicci K      **164** in] *om.* K      **166–7** hereos . . . pueris] et cetera E

Quod concedo, quia in pueris est maxime profundacio
cogitacionum et ymaginacio formarum et defectus vel
170 occupatio alterative que sunt in amore hereos. Alia causa
est quia secundum Avicennam in tertio stimulacio ad coitum
est maxima causa huius passionis.[26] Sed in pueris et maxime in
fine puericie incipiunt homines primo coire. Unde in eis
est primus coitus qui maxime est delectabilis, quare maxime
175 appetunt coitum.[27]

Ad primum argumentum dicendum quod non valet, quia
defectus estimative qui est maxime in pueris plus valet ad
generationem amoris hereos quam humores adusti qui sunt
in iuvenibus. Quare et cetera.

180 Circa sextum sic. Videre loca amena maxime competit in amore
hereos secundum Avicennam in tertio.[28] Sed exire a patria est
videre loca amena. Ergo exire a patria competit in amore
hereos.

Contra: nichil augmentans profundationem cogitacionum et
185 malam suspicionem competit in amore hereos ut per se patet.
Sed exire a patria est huiusmodi quia paciens in huiusmodi
passione semper timet amittere suam amasiam et ne aliquis
alius eam diligat.[29] Quare et cetera.

Dicendum quod a patria exire competit in amore hereos quia
190 talis exitus facit videre res pulcras et loca amena et in
quibus paciens figit suam cogitationem. Et per consequens
retrahit ymaginationem suam a sua amasia et facit patientem
oblivisci sue amasie, quod maxime competit in cura amoris
hereos. Quare et cetera.

195 Ad argumentum suppositum dicendum quod minor fuit falsa.
Non enim timet amittere amasiam quia non cogitat de ipsa
sed de rebus quas videt. Quare et cetera.

Circa septimum sic. Omnis cura per contrarium ut scribitur
in *Tegni*.[30] Sed mulieres turpes contrariantur amasie
200 patientis amorem hereos, cum illa sit pulcra secundum
estimationem ipsius. Ergo visus turpium mulierum competit
in amore hereos. Quare et cetera.

---

**169** ymaginacio] —tionem E      et] *om*. E      **170** que] qui E      **172** maxima] —e
K      **173** primo] *om*. K      **174** delectabilis] debil. E      **178** generationem]
digestionem K      **179** quare et cetera] *om*. K      **182** patria competit] patria est
videre loca competit K      **187–8** ne aliquis alius] vel aliquis K      eam] cum K
**191** figit] *om*. K      **193** quod] *dittog*. E      **194** et cetera] *om*. K      **195** sup-
positum] *om*. E      **197** sed de rebus quas] quam K      Quare et cetera] *om*. K
**200** amorem] —e K

Which I concede, since the depressed thought and imagination of forms, and failure [of judgment] or altering preoccupation that occur in lovesickness are greatest in boys. Another reason is that, according to Avicenna in the third [book], stimulation to intercourse is the greatest cause of this disease. But people first begin to have intercourse in child[hood], and especially at the end of childhood. Thus the first sexual encounter happens to them, which is most pleasurable, wherefore they desire intercourse most greatly.

It must be said that the first argument is not valid, because the failure of the estimative [faculty], which is greatest in boys, contributes more to the generation of lovesickness than do the burnt humors that are in youths; wherefore etc.

Concerning the sixth, thus: According to Avicenna in the third [book], seeing beautiful places is most beneficial in lovesickness. But to leave one's country is to see beautiful places. Therefore leaving one's country is beneficial in lovesickness.

On the contrary: Nothing that increases depressed thought and harmful suspicion is beneficial in lovesickness, as is self-evident. But leaving one's country is of this sort, since the patient in this kind of disease always fears losing his beloved and fears lest someone else love her; wherefore etc.

It must be said that leaving one's country is beneficial in lovesickness, because such travel causes one to see beautiful things and pleasant places, upon which the patient fixes his thought. And consequently he withdraws his imagination from his beloved, and it makes the patient forget his beloved, which is most beneficial in the cure of lovesickness; wherefore etc.

To the proposed argument it must be said that the minor premise was false. For he does not fear to lose his beloved, because he does not think of her, but of the things that he sees; wherefore etc.

Concerning the seventh, thus: Every cure is by a contrary, as it is written in the *Tegni*. But ugly women are contrary to the beloved of the lovesick patient, since she is beautiful in his estimation. Therefore the sight of ugly women is beneficial in lovesickness; wherefore etc.

Contra est Avicenna in tertio.[31] Quod concedo, quia
opposita iuxta se posita magis elucescunt secundum
205 Aristotelem.[32] Et ideo si mulieres adducerentur coram
paciente amorem hereos, videtur quod sua amasia esset
pulchrior quam essent et tunc magis profundaret suam
cogitationem et intentionem in formam ipsius quam prius,
quod est valde malum ut patet ex dictis.

210 Ad primum argumentum dicendum quod cura non fit per
quodcumque contrarium sed per contrarium alterans vel
evacuans.[33] Sed turpes mulieres non sunt contrarie
pulchrioribus loquendo de contrario <alterante> vel
evacuante. Quare et cetera.

215 Circa octavum sic. Simile adveniens suo simili ipsum
facit furere ut scribitur super *Afforismos*.[34] Sed si pulchre
mulieres adducerentur coram paciente amorem hereos simile
adderetur suo simili, cum sua amasia sit pulchra. Quare
et cetera.

220 Contra est Avicenna in tertio. Dicit quod pulchre
mulieres sunt adducende coram paciente amorem hereos.[35]

Quod concedo, quia quando paciens amorem hereos videt
aliquas res pulchriores quam sit res dilecta, tunc profundat
intentionem suam vel ymaginacionem vel cogitacionem in
225 huiusmodi res pulchras et per consequens retrahit
cogitacionem suam a re quam prius diligebat, quod competit
in amore hereos. Quare et cetera.

Ad primum argumentum dicendum quod non valet, quia illa
auctoritas intelligitur de simili in complexione et non
230 de simili in colore, et tu obicis de simili in colore, quare
et cetera.

Circa nonum sic. Nihil stimulans ad coitum competit in
amore hereos. Ebrietas est huiusmodi quia in ebriosis sunt multe
superfluitates replentes testiculos. Quare et cetera.[36]
235 Ad idem est Ysaac.[37]

Contra: omne auferens profundam cogitationem competit in
amore hereos. Sed ebrietas est huiusmodi cum ebrietas sit
causa oblivionis. Ergo ebrietas competit in amore hereos.

---

**204** iuxta] maxime E          **206** quod] cum K          esset] esse K          **208** in] et K
**209** dictis] predictis K          **211** sed per contrarium] *om.* K          **213** contrario] —ia K
<alterante>] contrarietate EK; *suppl.*          **214** et cetera] *om.* E          **216** si] *om.* K
**218** suo] *om.* K          **220** Dicit] dicens K          **222** quando] *om.* K          **225** huius-
modi] has K          **226** cogitacionem suam] cogitaciones K          prius] *om.* K

Avicenna says the contrary in the third [book]. Which I concede, since opposites placed next to each other are more illuminating, according to Aristotle. And therefore if women are brought before the lovesick patient, it seems that his beloved is more beautiful than they are, and then he will plunge his thought and attention in this form more than before, which is very bad, as is evident from what has been said.

To the first argument it must be said that a cure is not achieved by just any contrary, but by a contrary that alters or purges [the body's humors]. But, speaking of an altering or purging contrary, ugly women are not contraries of more beautiful women; wherefore etc.

Concerning the eighth, thus. Like added to like makes it rage, as it is written on the *Aphorisms*. But if beautiful women are brought before the lovesick patient, like is added to like, since his beloved is beautiful; wherefore etc.

Avicenna says the opposite in the third [book]; he says that beautiful women are to be brought before the lovesick patient.

Which I concede, since when the lovesick patient sees some things more beautiful than the beloved object, then he will plunge his attention or imagination or thought in these kinds of beautiful things, and consequently he will withdraw his thought from the thing that he loved before, which is beneficial in lovesickness; wherefore, etc.

It must be said that the first argument is not valid, because that authoritative statement is understood with respect to what is similar in [humoral] complexion and not with respect to what is similar in outward appearance, and you argue about similarity in appearance, wherefore etc.

Concerning the ninth, thus: Nothing that stimulates to intercourse is beneficial in lovesickness. Drunkenness is of this sort, since the drunk have many superfluities filling the testicles; wherefore etc.

Isaac agrees.

On the contrary: Everything relieving depressed thought is beneficial in lovesickness. But drunkenness is of this sort, since it causes oblivion. Therefore drunkenness is beneficial in lovesickness.

---

**230** et . . . colore] *om.* K      **231** et cetera] non valet ratio K      **237** amore hereos]

coitu E      ebrietas] --tatis K

Dicendum quod duplex est ebrietas: una que est tanta quod
240 penitus impedit operationes omnes sensitivas secundum sensum
communem, fantasiam, et estimationem et alios sensus communes
et hec competit in amore hereos, cum sit causa oblivionis
rei dilecte. Alia est ebrietas que non penitus impedit
discretionem et estimacionem sed solum ipsas perturbat, et
245 talis ebrietas non competit in amore hereos, quia amor
hereos provenit ex perturbacione vel corrupcione predictarum
virtutum sicut patet ex dictis.[38] Quare et cetera. Et
per hoc patet solucio racionum.

Circa decimum sic. Rasi dicit quod in amore hereos competit
250 ieiunium et Avicenna dicit in tertio quod in amore hereos
competit cibum temperatus.[39] Ergo sunt contrarii.

Item dicit actor in littera quod res dilecta debet
vituperari coram paciente amorem hereos.[40]

Contra: huiusmodi vituperium facit patientem amorem hereos
255 rememorari rei dilecte. Nullum tale competit in amore hereos
ut patet ex iam dictis. Quare et cetera.

Contra est actor.

Dicendum quod in amore hereos sunt duo: videlicet materia
spermatica stimulans ad coitum, et quantum ad hoc competit
260 ieiunium in amore hereos, quia per ieiunium consumuntur
superfluitates in corpore existentes et sic intelligitur Haly.[41]

Item ibi est habitudo tenuis vel macilenta et quantum ad
hoc competit ibi cibum non quicumque sed temperatus, quia talis
cibum generat humores subtiles et laudabiles et non generat
265 superfluitates que sunt cause erectionis virge. Et hoc modo
intelligitur Avicenna, cum dicit quod in amore hereos debet
exhiberi cibum temperatus.

Ad aliud dicendum quod quamvis vituperium faciat patientem
rememorari sue amasie, verumptamen retrahit mentem vel
270 cogitationem patientis a re dilecta. Quare et cetera.

---

**239** quod] et K     **245** ebrietas] *om.* E     **247** patet] *om.* K     dictis] predictis K
**248** racionum] predictarum r. K     **254** amorem] habere a. K     **263** non . . . tem-
peratus] temperato K     **266** quod] *om.* K     **267** exhiberi] dari K

It must be said that there are two sorts of drunkenness: one that is so great that it deeply hinders all the sensitive functions following the common sense, fantasy, estimation, and the other common senses—and this is beneficial in lovesickness because it causes the beloved object to be forgotten. The other [type of] drunkenness does not deeply hinder discretion and estimation, but only disturbs them, and this drunkenness is not beneficial in lovesickness, since lovesickness arises from disturbance or damaging of the aforesaid faculties, as is evident from what has been said. Wherefore etc. And thus the solution to the arguments is evident.

Concerning the tenth, thus: al-Rāzī says that fasting is beneficial in lovesickness, but Avicenna says in the third [book] that temperate food is beneficial in lovesickness. Thus they contradict each other.

Also, the author says in the text that the beloved ought to be scorned before the lovesick patient.

On the contrary, this sort of scorn will make the lovesick patient remember the beloved. Nothing of this sort is beneficial in lovesickness, as is evident from what has already been said. Wherefore etc.

The author says the opposite.

It must be said that there are two things in lovesickness: namely, seminal matter that is sexually stimulating, and as far as this is concerned, fasting is beneficial since through fasting superfluities in the body are consumed, and thus Haly is to be understood.

Also, there is a feeble appearance or emaciation, and as far as this is concerned, food is beneficial; not just any, but temperate, since such food produces subtle and beneficial humors, and does not produce superfluities that cause erection. And in this way Avicenna is to be understood when he says that temperate food ought to be given in lovesickness.

To the next it must be said that although scorn makes the patient remember his beloved, in fact it withdraws the mind or thought of the patient from the beloved object. Wherefore etc.

# PETER OF SPAIN, *QUESTIONES SUPER VIATICUM*
## (Version B)

## *Manuscripts*

The B version survives in four manuscripts. In chronological order they are:

**M**: Madrid, Biblioteca Nacional, 1877 (13th c. [1255?], Siena).[1] Fols. 142r–205r. "Amor qui hereos dicitur etc.," fol. 146r–v. *Inc.*: "Capillus est ex fumo adusto et cetera. Circa allopiciam duo queruntur. Primum est de generatione capillorum." *Expl.*: "sed hec de questionibus supra viaticum secundum magistrum Petrum Hyspanum ad presens sufficiant. Deo gracias amen." Described in *Inventario General de Manuscritos de la Biblioteca Nacional* (Madrid: Ministerio de Educacion Nacional, 1959) 5:305–06; Schipperges 1967; Grabmann 1979 [1928] 1:480–96.

**V**: Vatican, Bibliotheca Apostolica, Pal. lat. 1166 (s. 13/14, S. France). Fols. 2r–94r. "Amor qui et hereos dicitur etc.," fol. 8r–v. Described by Schuba 1981, 124–25. *Inc.*: "Capillus ex fumo grosso etc. Dividitur iste liber primo in duas partes, in quarum prima determinat Ysaac de omnibus morbis particularibus." *Expl.*: "[incomplete] modicum deficit."

The text is incomplete. Fol. 1v contains the notation *Lectura super Viaticum*; fol. 2: *Super Viaticum Ysac exposicio*. The manuscript was among those bequeathed by Kurfürst Ludwig III in 1436 to the Heilig-Geist Kirche in Heidelberg.

**P**: Vatican, Bibliotheca Apostolica, Pal. lat. 1085 (s. 13/14). Fols. 68r–153v. "Amor qui et ereos," fols. 75v–76v. Described by Schuba 1981, 14–16. *Inc.*: "Capillus ex fumo. Circa allopiciam duo sunt inquirenda. Primum est de generatione capillorum." *Expl.*: "Expliciunt questiones magistri petri hispani supra viaticum."

**A**: Erfurt, Wissenschaftliche Allgemeinbibliothek, CA 221 (s. 14 in., S. France). Fols. 25–66. "Circa capitulum de amore qui dicitur hereos .vi. inquiruntur," fols. 30v–31r. Described by Schum 1887, 477–78. *Inc.*: "Dividitur iste liber in duas partes, in quarum prima determinat Ysaac de omnibus membris particularibus." *Expl.* "et dico quod competit."

This manuscript also contains Gerard of Berry's commentary on the *Viaticum* immediately preceding Peter of Spain's.

Version B circulated in several forms; an unknown number of manuscript copies have been lost. The earliest manuscript, M, stands apart from the other three stylistically. As the investigations of Alonso, Schipperges, and da Cruz Pontes have shown, Peter's commentary on Isaac's *De urinis*, his commentary on Aristotle's *De anima*, and his commentary on Aristotle's *De animalibus* all circulated in earlier and later versions.[2] The earlier version of the *De animalibus* commentary survives in M, Madrid 1877, an early collection of Peter's works.[3] It is likely that Madrid 1877 offers an early version of the *Viaticum* commentary as well, whose later revision survives in PVA.

I have chosen to follow the later revision in PVA in order to print a readable text containing the most complete version of Peter's ideas possible. Though P, as the best manuscript of this group, has been chosen as the base for the edition, I have added a section from V (the *lectura*, lines 1–55) not found in the other two manuscripts.[4] I have not been able to resolve the difficulties of the manuscript reading in line 37, which I have marked with asterisks. Since V elsewhere shows a number of omissions, it is possible that something has dropped out at this point.

Orthography generally follows P. In this manuscript *c* and *t* are unusually hard to distinguish; both represent -ti-. In expanding abbreviations (e.g. cog[nes]), I have used -ti-.

# Edition

## Petrus Hispanus
### *Questiones super Viaticum* (Version B)

**A**: Erfurt, Wissenschaftliche Allgemeinbibliothek, CA 221, fols. 30v–31r.
**M**: Madrid, Biblioteca Nacional, MS 1877, fol. 146r–v.
**P**: Vatican, Biblioteca Apostolica Pal. lat. 1085, fols. 75v–76v.
**V**: Vatican, Biblioteca Apostolica Pal. lat. 1166, fol. 8r–v.

AMOR QUI ET HEREOS DICITUR ET CETERA. Circa capitulum istud quintum sunt determinanda. Primum est de diffinitione amoris. Secundum est de causis. Tertium est de signis. Quartum est de cura. Quintum de questionibus incidentibus.

5   Circa primum sic procedimus et potest ab Avicenna talis diffinicio extrahi: Amor est melancolica sollicitudo mentis cum profunditatione cogitacionum in qua figitur mens propter pulchritudinem et dispositionem ad effectum.[1] Et dicitur melancolica propter accidencia in quibus comitat cum

10  melancolia. Vel aliter et diffinitur sic: Amor est mentis insania qua vagatur animus per inania crebris doloribus permiscens gaudia.[2] Constantinus autem in *Pantegni* sic diffinit in capitulo de melancolia libro xx°: Amor est confidencia anime suspicionis in re amata et cogitacionis in

15  eadem assiduitas.[3]

Notandum autem quod amor intrat per sensus ad interiorem virtutem, scilicet ad fantasiam, et a fantasia usque ad virtutem estimativam cuius est cognoscere de amicicia et inimicicia sicut dicit Avicenna et preter illam

20  omnibus rebus.[4] Et ita fit hec passio que amor hereos vocatur ab heremis, id est nobilioribus quia maxime solent incurrere istam passionem.[5]

Circa secundum sic proceditur, scilicet de causis huius passionis. Causa materialis huius passionis est habundancia

25  multi spermatis, sicut accidit in illis qui vivunt in occio et quiete et deliciis corporis.[6] Sumuntur etiam cause huius a parte rerum desideratarum et a parte desiderii et a parte frequencie cogitacionum que sunt in virtute estimativa et in memorativa.[7]

---

**1–55** *om.* MPA

# Peter of Spain
## *Questions on the Viaticum* (Version B)

LOVE THAT IS ALSO CALLED HEREOS ETC. In this chapter there are five things to determine. The first is about the definition of love. The second is about its causes. The third is about signs. The fourth is about the cure. The fifth is about relevant questions.

Concerning the first we proceed thus, and this definition can be drawn from Avicenna: Love is a melancholic worry of the mind with a depression of thought in which the mind is transfixed because of beauty and an inclination toward the beloved. And it is called "melancholic" because of the symptoms that associate it with melancholy. Or it could also be defined thus: Love is a sickness of the mind in which the spirit wanders through emptiness, mixing joy with frequent sorrows. Constantine, however, defines it thus in chapter 20 on melancholy in the *Pantegni*: Love is a hopeful belief of the fearful soul in the beloved and a continual preoccupation with the same.

It must also be noted that love enters through the senses to the interior faculty, namely to the fantasy, and from the fantasy [it progresses] to the estimative faculty, whose function is to recognize friendship and enmity, as Avicenna says, and beyond that in all things. And thus this disease, which is called *amor hereos*, is formed from *heremis*, that is, from the nobility, since they are most accustomed to contracting this disease.

Concerning the second point, namely the causes of this disease, we proceed thus: The material cause of this disease is an abundance of much seed, as occurs in those who live in leisure and quiet and bodily pleasures. Its causes are also taken from the desired objects, and from the desire itself, and from the frequency of thoughts that are in the estimative faculty and in the memory.

30      Item sicut dicit Haly, ad cohitum .iiii. concurrunt:
Mala complexio calida stimulans; ymaginacio rei dilecte et
nimia eius discrecio; et ventositas elevans virgam. Quarta
causa est copia spermatis.[8]

      Circa tertium sic proceditur: Signa ergo huius
35  passionis sunt hec: profunde cogitaciones; citrina facies;
tristicia sine causa; oculi profundi et mobiles; suspiria
profunda quando fit *sine cum* dilecta; pulsus durus et
velox et debilis quando cogitaciones profundantur. Item dicit
Avicenna quod teneatur pulsus et vocentur puelle suspecte
40  vel nominentur;[9] et quando nominantur elevatur pulsus et
fortificatur et fit deformis pulsus et inordinatus. Et hec
passio dicitur ab Avicenna sollicitudo melancolica propter
accidencia que secuntur; nisi enim tangant rem amatam
efficiuntur post modum colerici.[10] Infrigidatur enim cerebrum
45  et fit melancolicum.

      Circa quartum sic proceditur: Dicit Avicenna quod
melior cura est iacere cum re dilecta.[11] Precipit autem
Rasy quod dicantur verba sagacia et fabule et frequenter
intrat balneum dulcis aque; exeat autem a patria; audiat
50  cantilenas, et sit letus et bibat vinum bonum, et purgetur
humor melancolicus cum medicina competenti.[12] Iste enim
morbus est materia et dispositio ad melancoliam nisi
curetur.

      Circa quintum sic procedimus circa questiones
55  incidentes et circa amorem sex queruntur. Primum est cuius
membri sit passio amor. Secundum est cuius virtutis anime.
Tertium est cui magis accidat hec passio, utrum sexui
masculino aut feminino. Quarto quis eorum in coitu plus
delectetur. Quintum est de signis huius passionis. Sextum
60  vero de cura.

      Circa primum sic proceditur: Queritur cuius membri
passio sit amor et ostenditur quod testiculorum. Prima ratio
ad hoc talis est: Illius membri est passio ad quod spectat
eius operatio.[13] Sed operatio amoris per se spectat ad
65  testiculos. Ergo amor passio est testiculorum.

---

**37** *sine cum*] *ut videtur*; sino(?) cū (eū?) V     dilecta] a *exp. et* e *add. s. l.* V     **54–5**
Circa . . . queruntur] Amor qui hereos dicitur et cetera.    Circa partem istam vi. inquiruntur
M   Amor qui et ereos.    Circa hoc capitulum de amor qui dicitur ereos sex queruntur P
Circa capitulum de amore qui dicitur hereos .vi. inquiruntur A    **54** procedimus] p.
scilicet V     **56** est] *om.* MA    anime] a. sit passio V     **57** est] *om.* M    cui]
cuius M   quibus V   qui A    accidat] sit M    sexui] sexus M     **58** masculino]

Also, as Haly says, four things work together for intercourse: an imbalanced warm complexion that stimulates; imagination of the desired object and excessive appraisal of it; and windiness elevating the penis. The fourth cause is copious seed.

Concerning the third we proceed thus: The signs of the disease are these: depressed thoughts; a yellowed face; sadness without cause; sunken and mobile eyes; deep sighs when it happens . . . with the beloved; the pulse is hard and quick and weak when thoughts are depressed. Also, Avicenna says that the pulse should be held and the suspected girls be called or named; and when they are named, the pulse will be elevated and strengthened and it will become an irregular and disordered pulse. And Avicenna calls this disease a melancholic worry because of the symptoms that follow, for unless they embrace the beloved object, they later become choleric. For the brain grows cold and becomes melancholic.

Concerning the fourth, we proceed thus: Avicenna says that a better cure is to lie with the beloved object. Al-Rāzī moreover instructs that wise words and stories be recited, and that [the patient] frequently enter a freshwater bath, also travel from his country, listen to songs, and be happy and drink good wine, and be purged of melancholic humor with a fitting medicine. For this disease is the matter of and disposition toward melancholy unless it is cured.

Concerning the fifth we proceed thus about the relevant questions, and inquire six things concerning love. The first is, of which member love might be a disease. The second is, of which faculty of the soul. The third is, whom does this disease befall more, the masculine or the feminine sex? Fourth, which of them takes more pleasure in intercourse? The fifth is about the signs of this disease. The sixth is about the cure.

Concerning the first we proceed thus: It is inquired of which member love might be a disease, and it is shown to be of the testicles. The first argument is this. A disease is of that member to which its action pertains. But the action of love as such pertains to testicles. Love is therefore a disease of the testicles.

---

--ni M     feminino] --ni M     quarto] quartum est V    q. queritur A      eorum] *om.*
V     in] *om.* MA     coitu] *om.* M       **59**    delectetur] delc'te M    dessicetur V
delectatur A     est] *om.* V      **60**    vero] *om.* M    est V       **62**    prima ratio] *om.*
M     **63**    ad hoc] *om.* MVA     talis] *om.* M     est] *om.* MVA      **64** operatio[1]]
o. per se V

Secunda ratio est hec: Duplex est appetitus:
universalis, qui est in cerebro, et particularis, et ille
divisus est per membra particularia.[14] Cum in amore sit
appetitus rei amate, necesse est hoc desiderium et hunc
70  appetitum ad aliquod membrum particulare pertinere; hoc non
est nisi testiculi. Ergo passio in amore est testiculorum.

Tertia ratio est hec: Cuius est actus, eius est
potentia.[15] Sed actus amoris est in testiculis; ergo et
potentia amoris erit in testiculis. Ergo inpotentia respectu
75  huius actus et passio proveniens ex eius impotentia erit
passio testiculorum.

Ad oppositum sunt rationes. Prima talis est: Omnis
passio consistens in profunditate et inordinatione
ymaginationis est passio cerebri in quo vigent cogitationes
80  et ymaginationes. Sed amor qui dicitur ereos est huiusmodi
quia dicitur sollicitudo melancolica. Ergo amor est passio
cerebri.

Secunda ratio: Si amor esset passio testiculorum,
numquam esset non habentibus testiculos. Nunc autem videmus
85  quod inest castratis et non potentibus cohire. Non est
igitur passio testiculorum sed magis cerebri.[16]

Ad hoc dicendum quod amor est passio cerebri et non
testiculorum. Ad rationes respondeo et dico quod in amore
duo sunt. Unum est inordinatio et profundacio cogitationum
90  circa rem quam omnibus aliis prefert, et sic est passio
cerebri. Hoc enim principium est formale. Aliud vero est in
amore, scilicet stimulacio cohitus et hec est duplex. Quedam
est animalis propter fortem impressionem rei dilecte factam
in virtute estimativa, et hec est a cerebro. Quedam est
95  naturalis, et hec est duplex: aut fluens, et sic est ab
epate. Ponit enim Constantinus quod desiderium in coitu
venit ab epate.[17] Quedam autem est naturalis fixa in uno
membro et hec est in testiculis, et per hoc solvuntur rationes.

---

**66** est hec] *om.* MVA    **67** universalis] naturalis M    ille] iste V    **68** divisus est
per] dividitur in V    Cum] c. ergo V    **68–70** Cum . . . pertinere] et habet aspectum
ad aliquod membrum particulare M    **69** est] *om.* A    **70** particulare] *om.* A
non] autem n. M    **71** est²] proprie e. V    passio . . . testiculorum] amor est passio
t. M    **72** est hec] *om.* MVA    **73** et] *om.* VA    **74** erit] est MV    tes-
ticulis] ipsis V    **75** et] est V    **77** prima talis] *om.* M    est] *om.* MVA    **78** con-
sistens] existens V    profunditate] p. cogitacionum V    **79** ymaginationis] ipsius y.
V    **79–80** in quo . . . ereos] *om.* V    **80** ereos] hereos MA    est] et e. V
**81** quia] que V    **83** Secunda ratio] Item M    esset] est MA    **84** numquam]

The second reason is this. Appetite is double: universal, which is in the brain, and particular, and that one is divided among the individual members. Since love entails an appetite for the beloved object, this desire and this appetite necessarily pertain to some particular member; this is nothing other than the testicles. Therefore the disease in love is of the testicles.

The third argument is this. "The subject of actuality is identical with that of potentiality." But the act of love is in the testicles; therefore the potential of love will also be in the testicles. Therefore inability with respect to this act, and the disease resulting from inability, will be a disease of the testicles.

There are opposing reasons. The first is this. Every disease consisting of depressed and disordered imagination is a disease of the brain, where thoughts and imaginings flourish. But love that is called *ereos* is of this sort, since it is called a "melancholic worry." Therefore it is a disease of the brain.

The second reason: If love were a disease of the testicles, it would never occur in those without testicles. Now we see, however, that it befalls the castrated and those not able to have intercourse. It is not, therefore, a disease of the testicles, but rather of the brain.

To this it must be said that love is a disease of the brain and not of the testicles. I respond to the reasons and say that there are two [things] in love. One is the disorder and depression of the thoughts about a thing that is preferred above all others, and thus it is a disease of the brain. This is the formal origin. There is indeed another thing in love, namely the stimulation to intercourse, and this is double. One aspect is mental, on account of the strong impression of the beloved object made in the estimative faculty, and this is from the brain. One aspect is natural, and this is double: either flowing, and thus it is from the liver. For Constantine asserts that sexual desire comes from the liver. The other, however, is natural and located in one member, and this is in the testicles, and thus the reasons are solved.

---

non M     esset] essent P     non] in non MV     **85** quod] quoniam V     inest . . . cohire] est in castratis et in hiis qui non possunt *in marg.* cohire M     Non] nec M     **86** magis] passio M     **87** dicendum] d. est V     et] *om.* M     **88** rationes] —em V respondeo et dico] dicendum MA     **89** profundacio] profunditas M     **91** Aliud] at M     **93** animalis] materialis V     fortem impressionem] fortitudinem impressionis M     factam] *om.* M     **94** est²] *om.* M     **95** hec] *om.* V     **96–7** Ponit . . . epate] quia desiderium venit ab epate M     provenit enim quidem (*exp.*) desiderium in (*exp.*) coitu (*add.* -s) venit (*exp.*) ab epate P     provenit Constantinus quod desiderium in coitu venit ab epate A     **97** venit] veniī M     Quedam] *om.* A     autem] aut A

Secundo queritur causa huius: Cum sit appetitus cibi in
100 stomacho et appetitus cohitus in testiculis, propter quid
frigida complexio intendit appetitum cibi in stomacho, sicut
patet per Galienum in *Tegni*, remittit autem appetitum
cohitus?[18] Calida vero complexio operatur contrarium.

Ad hoc dicendum quod appetitus cibi in stomacho est
105 propter inanitionem membri desiderantis repleri. Appetitus
vero cohitus est membri pleni desiderantis evacuari et
inanire. Et quia frigidum comprimit et ita inanit, ideo
generat appetitum in stomacho. Et ipsum caliditas dilatat,
et sic inducit repletionem et aufert appetitum in stomacho.

110 Frigidum vero comprimit virgam et sperma, et sic prohibet ne
sperma veniat ad virgam; sed calidum ipsum dissolvit, et
facit ipsum fluere et stimulat naturam ut se exhonoret et
illud emittat. Et ideo appetitus stomachi non viget per
calidum, appetitus vero virge viget; minuitur vero a

115 frigido; appetitus vero stomachi augmentatur.

Tertio queritur cum per villum vigeat appetitus in
stomacho, propter quid in appetitu stomachi irrigidatur
villus per frigiditatem, in appetitu vero cohitus
irrigidatur membrum per caliditatem?

120 Ad hoc dicendum quod quedam irrigidantur per
extensionem sicut virga et talis irrigidatio fit per
caliditatem. Et hoc fit in cohitu et in appetitu cohitus.
Alia autem est irrigidacio per frigidum et per contractionem et
hec irrigidacio facit inanicionem.[19] Inanitio vero movet

125 stomachum ad appetendum. Dicit enim Galienus quod stomachus
senciens inanitionem appetit repleri etc.[20]

Quarto queritur propter quid appetitus stomachi vigeat
per frigidum, appetitus matricis vigeat per calidum cum
tamen tam stomachus quam matrix appetat repleri?[21]

**101** complexio] c. in qua V      **102** remittit] et r. A      autem] eciam M      appetitum]
—us V      **103** operatur] *om.* V      **104** dicendum] d. est V      cibi] *om.* M      est]
et A      **106** desiderantis] volentis V      **107** ita] *om.* M      **108** Et ipsum] vel V
caliditas] *spat. 8–9 litt. ante* c. PA      calificat M      dilatat] dilata V      **109** inducit] *om.* V
**110** sperma] sic s. M      **113** emittat] —it V      **113–14** per . . . viget] *om.* V
**114–15** a frigido] frigidum A      **115** vero] *om.* V      augmentatur] augetur V
**116** vigeat] vigerat M      **117** in] *om.* V      irrigidatur] irrigiatur P      erigebatur V
irrigatur A      **118** appetitu vero cohitus] coitu vero appetitus V      **119** irrigidatur]
—etur P      irrigatus A      **120** dicendum] d. est V      per] propter P      **121** sicut
virga] *om.* V      **122** appetitu] exitu V      **123** Alia autem] aliud V      a. a. fit M
irrigidacio] irrigacio A      frigidum] *om. cum spat.* V      contractionem] constrictionem A
**124** hec] *om.* M      irrigidacio] arrigacio A      vero] enim M      **125** appetendum]

Second, we inquire the cause of this: since appetite for food is in the stomach, and appetite for intercourse in the testicles, why does a cold complexion increase appetite for food in the stomach, as Galen says in the *Tegni*, but decrease appetite for intercourse? A hot complexion indeed works the opposite.

To this it must be said that appetite for food in the stomach is on account of the emptiness of a member desiring to be filled. Appetite for intercourse is of a full member desiring to be evacuated and emptied. And since cold constricts and thus empties, it therefore generates appetite in the stomach. And heat expands it, and thus induces fullness, and relieves appetite in the stomach. Cold indeed compresses the penis and seed, and thus prohibits the seed from reaching the penis. But heat dissolves it and causes it to flow, and stimulates nature to relieve itself and emit it. And therefore appetite of the stomach does not grow through heat, [but] that of the penis does. [But] that is reduced through cold, [while] appetite of the stomach is increased.

Third, we inquire: since appetite in the stomach increases by means of the villus, why does the villus grow rigid with cold in the stomach's appetite, [but] in appetite for intercourse, the member grows rigid with heat?

To this it must be said that certain things, like the penis, grow rigid through extension, and this rigidity occurs through heat. And this happens in intercourse and in the desire for intercourse. There is, moreover, rigidity through cold and through contraction, and this rigidity causes emptying. Emptying in fact moves the stomach to hunger. For Galen says that the stomach, feeling its emptiness, desires to be filled, etc.

Fourth, it is inquired why the stomach's appetite grows through cold, [and] the appetite of the womb grows through heat, since both stomach and womb desire to be filled?

---

appetitum M     enim] *om.* V     stomachus] *om.* V     **126** etc.] *om.* V
**127** vigeat] vigerat M    viget V     **128** matricis] vero m. M    tamen m. V    in arteria *exp. et* m. *add. in marg.* P     vigeat] *om.* M     **129** tamen] *om.* MV     cum A
appetat] --ant M    --it A     repleri] *om.* V

130      Ad hoc dicendum quod matrix calida plus appetit cohitum
quam frigida et non solum consistit eius appetitus in
receptione, sicut dicetur postea,[22] sed etiam in expulsione
superfluorum cum sit repleta quodammodo sicut et virga. Et
quia calidum replet, ideo matrix calida plus delectatur et
135  plus appetit quam frigida et eius appetitus viget per
calidum. Sicut dicit Avicenna quod movetur matrix ad virgam
introducendam,[23] non movetur autem sine calido; immo
calidum velociter mobile, sicut dicit Philaretus.[24] Ergo ad
appetitum eius iuvat calidum et non frigidum sicut dicitur.
140      Circa secundum sic proceditur: queritur cuius virtutis
sit passio amor, et ostenditur quod sit passio virtutis
ymaginative. Prima ratio est talis: Illius virtutis passio
est amor cuius operatio leditur per se et impeditur per
amorem. Sed sicut dicit Avicenna amor provenit ex corrupta
145  ymaginatione.[25] Ergo amor est passio virtutis ymaginative.

      Secunda ratio est talis: Illius virtutis passio est
amor cuius organi vel membri deservientis substantia
patitur. Sed sicut dicit Avicenna, pars prima capitis
movetur in amore et desiccatur.[26] Sed in illa parte est
150  virtus ymaginativa tanquam in organo. Ergo amor est passio
virtutis ymaginative.

      Ad oppositum sunt rationes et est prima talis: Illius
virtutis est amor passio cuius est apprehendere formas non
sensatas ad quas sequitur delectacio vel tristicia. Sed hec
155  virtus est estimativa. Ergo amor est passio virtutis
estimative, quia fit amor non propter calorem vel odorem sed
propter bonitatem vel maliciam que consequuntur ad hoc. Quia
ut dicit Avicenna in libro *De anima*, amicicia et tristicia
sunt in virtute estimativa.[27] Ymaginatio enim apprehendit
160  formas sensibiles sed virtus ista estimativa apprehendit
intentiones formarum sensibilium.

---

**130** dicendum] d. est V      **131** consistit] sistat P      **132** postea] post M    possit V
sed] *om.* V      **133** superfluorum] superfluitatum M      **137** autem] *om.* M
immo] omne *add. s. l.* P      **139** eius] *om.* M    non] *om.* V      **140** queritur] et q.
MV      **141** ostenditur] videtur M    sit passio] *om.* M      **142** Prima ratio] *om.*
M    est] *om.* MVA    talis] *om.* MA    **144–5** provenit . . . ymaginatione] est
corrupcio ymaginative V      **146** est talis] *om.* MVA      **148** prima] *add. s. l.* P
anterior M    *om.* A      **152** et est] *om.* MVA    prima talis] *om.* M      **155** es-
timativa] 5–6 *litt. illeg. ante* e. A    virtus e. V      **156** estimative] ymaginative *exp.* A
fit] *om.* V    calorem] calidum M    odorem] propter o. A      **157** consequuntur]
secuntur V      **159** enim] vero V      **160** sensibiles] apprehensibiles M    estima-
tiva] apprehensiva A      **160–3** apprehendit . . . estimativa] *om.* V

To this it should be said that a hot womb desires intercourse more than a cold one, and its appetite does not consist solely in reception, as will be discussed later, but also in the expulsion of superfluities when it is filled in a manner similar to the penis. And since heat fills, a hot womb therefore takes more pleasure and desires more than a cold one, and its appetite grows through heat. As Avicenna says, the womb is moved to introduce the penis; it is not moved, however, without heat. Indeed, heat is quickly mobile, as Philaretus says. Therefore heat aids its appetite, and not cold, as is said.

Concerning the second [question], we proceed thus: it is inquired of which faculty love might be a disease, and it is shown to be a disease of the imaginative faculty. The first argument is this. Love is a disease of that faculty whose action as such is injured and impeded by love. But love, as Avicenna says, originates from a damaged imagination. Love is therefore a disease of the imaginative faculty.

The second reason is this. Love is a disease of that faculty whose organ or subservient member's substance suffers. But as Avicenna says, in love the first part of the head is moved and dries out. But the imaginative faculty is in that part as though in an organ. Love is therefore a disease of the imaginative faculty.

There are opposing arguments, and the first is this. Love is a disease of that faculty whose function is to apprehend non-sensed forms upon which follow pleasure or sadness. But this faculty is the estimative. Therefore love is a disease of the estimative faculty, since love happens not because of heat or smell, but because of goodness or evil which follow these things. For, as Avicenna says in *On the Soul*, friendship and sorrow are in the estimative faculty. The imagination apprehends sensible forms, but the estimative faculty apprehends the intentions of sensible forms.

Secunda ratio talis est: Amor est passio illius
virtutis que cum apprehendit operatur. Sed virtus estimativa
in amore est huiusmodi; ergo amor est passio eiusdem. Minor
165 patet quia dicit Avicenna quod virtus ymaginativa
apprehendit et non operatur; virtus vero estimativa cum hoc
quod apprehendit operatur.[28]

Ad hoc dicendum quod virtus estimativa patitur in amore
et mandat suum desiderium ad memorativam.[29]
170 Ad rationes autem dicendum quod in amore est quedam
comprehensio secundum formas sensibiles que sunt album cum
rubeo.[30] Et hec virtus comprehendens talia est inicialis in
amore. Sed consequenter sequitur delectatio vel tristicia per
accidentia que per virtutem estimativam iudicantur. Dicendum
175 igitur quod amor est passio virtutis ymaginative quantum ad
suum inicium et motum inicialem; quantum vero ad
complementum est passio virtutis estimative et sic solvuntur
rationes.

Circa tertium sic proceditur et queritur quibus magis
180 accidat hec passio et quibus minus, et ostenditur quod magis
accidat melancolicis.[31] Ratio talis est: Illis maxime accidit
hec passio quibus magis assimilatur. Sed melancolici sunt
huiusmodi; ergo melancolicis plus accidit. Quod enim plus
assimiletur melancolicis patet quia sicut dicit Avicenna,
185 amor est melancolica sollicitudo.[32]

Ostenditur autem quod non maxime accidit senibus, sed
videmus quod maxime iuvenibus accidit. Sed iuvenes sunt
minime melancolici, senes magis.[33] Ergo videtur quod amor non
sit passio melancolica vel non magis accidat melancolicis.
190 Tamen dicit Avicenna quod amor est sollicitudo melancolica.

Ad hoc dicendum quod morbus quandoque denominatur a
materia, quandoque vero ab accidentibus.[34] Et amor dicitur
esse melancolica sollicitudo non propter materiam sed
propter accidentia consimilia melancolie.

---

**162** talis est] *om.* MA      **164** eiusdem] eius M      **166** vero] *om.* M      **168** Ad hoc
dicendum] Et dicendum est (*om.* A) ad hoc VA      **169** mandat] commendat M      non dat
P      memorativam] memoriam M      memoracionem A      **170** autem] in contrarium
M      dicendum] d. est V      quedam] *om.* P      **173** Sed consequenter] si consen-
tit M      **175** igitur] est ergo MV      amor] maior *exp. et a. add. s.l.* P
**176** motum] quantum ad m. M      **177** estimative] ymaginative *exp. et e. add. s.l.* P
**179** proceditur] –mus V      **180** quibus] *om.* A      ostenditur] videtur M      magis]
*om.* M      maxime V      **181** accidat] *om.* M      ratio . . . est] *om.* M      accidit] –at
*corr. in* –it P      **182** hec] illa M      magis] maxime M      **183** enim] *om.* M

The second reason is this. Love is a disease of that faculty which, when it perceives, acts. But the estimative faculty does this in love; therefore love is a disease of this faculty. The minor [premise of the syllogism] is evident since Avicenna says that the imaginative faculty apprehends and does not act; the estimative faculty, in fact, acts upon that which it apprehends.

To this it must be said that the estimative faculty suffers in love and transfers its desire to the faculty of memory.

To these reasons it must be said that in love there is a certain perception according to sensible forms, which are white with red. And the faculty perceiving such things is the initiating one in love. But consequently delight or sadness ensues through the accidents that are judged by the estimative faculty. It must be said therefore that love is a disease of the imaginative faculty as far is its origin and originating motion are concerned; concerning its completed form, it is a disease of the estimative faculty, and thus the arguments are solved.

Concerning the third question we proceed thus and inquire whom this disease befalls more and whom less, and it is shown that it befalls the melancholic more. The reason is this. This disease befalls those most whom it resembles more. But melancholics are of this sort; it therefore befalls melancholics more. That it resembles melancholics more is evident, since Avicenna says that love is a melancholic worry.

It is shown, moreover, that it does not befall old people the most, but we see that it befalls the young most. But the young are the least melancholic; the old, more so. Therefore it seems that love is not a melancholic disease, or that it does not befall melancholics more. Nonethless, Avicenna does say that love is a melancholic disease.

To this it must be said that a disease is sometimes named from its matter and sometimes from its symptoms. And love is said to be a melancholic worry not because of its matter, but because of its symptoms similar to melancholia.

plus²] magis M          **184** sicut] *om.* M          **185** amor] quod a. M          **186** acci-
dit] --at P          **187** accidit] --at A          Sed] autem M          **188** senes] et s. V
**189** magis] maxime V          accidat] --it V          **190** Tamen] cum A          sollicitudo] passio P          **191–92** a materia . . . vero] *om.* M          **193** materiam] naturam V
**194** consimilia] --les A

195     Circa quartum sic proceditur: Queritur cui sexui magis
accidat hic appetitus cohitus et in quo sexu maior est
delectatio, et ostenditur quod in maribus. Ratio talis: Cum
quattuor concurrant ad cohitum, sicut dicit Haly—ymaginatio
rei dilecte, et mala complexio stimulans, ventositas

200    elevans, et copia spermatis—hec omnia concurrunt magis in
masculis quam in feminis.[35] Ergo maior est appetitus cohitus
in masculis quam in feminis.

     Ad oppositum est hec ratio: Ubi maior est delectacio
habite rei, ibi est maior appetitus eiusdem si non habeatur.

205    Sed dicit Constantinus quod maior est delectatio cohitus a
parte femine quam a parte viri.[36] Ergo maior est appetitus
cohitus et maior est amor et intensior in feminis quam in
viris.

     Secunda ratio est hec: Sexus femineus magis

210    precipitatur in amorem sicut vult Constantinus quam
masculinus.[37] Ergo sexus femineus magis appetit et cohitum
et amorem quam sexus masculinus.

     Ad hoc dicendum secundum quosdam quod femine plus
diligunt quam mares, sed nos credimus contrarium. Unde

215    dicimus quod intensior est amor a parte maris quam a parte
femine, tamen maior est delectatio, sicut vult Constantinus,
a parte femine. Et causa est secundum illum quod in
emittendo et recipiendo delectantur femine; viri autem solum
in emittendo. Et quantum ad hoc plus viget amor in

220    mulieribus. Item cicius vincuntur et falluntur propter
parvitatem sui intellectus sicut dicit Rasy.[38]

     Secundo queritur propter quid est tanta delectatio in
cohitu.[39]

     Ad hoc dicendum quod huiusmodi quattuor sunt cause:

225    Prima est dispositio membrorum que sunt valde sensibilia
quia nervosa. Secunda causa est a parte sue operationis quia
quelibet virtus delectatur in propria operatione; etiam
expulsiva virtus fetum delectatur in sua operatione. Tertia
causa est discursus humiditatis spermatice per membra;

---

**195** proceditur] --imus V     Queritur] et q. M     **196** hic] *om.* MVA     cohitus]
*om.* A     maior est] magis sit M     **197** ostenditur] videtur M     maribus] masculis M     Cum] *om.* A     **198** ad cohitum] *dittog.* M     sicut] *om.* V     **199** et]
*om.* V     **200** hec] et h. M     in] *om.* M     **201** in] *om.* MA     cohitus] *om.*
M     **203** est hec ratio] *om.* M     **207** cohitus] *om.* M     est] *om.* A     *add. s.l.*
M     **209** est hec] *om.* MA     **210** precipitatur] precipitur PA     amorem] amore
MA     **211** masculinus] --neus PA     et] *om.* V     **213** dicendum] d. est V
**214** mares] viri M     nos] non A     **216** femine] femelle M     **216–17** tamen

Concerning the fourth question we proceed thus. It is inquired which sex the desire for intercourse befalls more often, and in which sex pleasure is greater, and it is shown that [desire is greater] in men. The reason is this. Since four things work together for intercourse, as Haly says—imagination of the desired thing, an imbalanced complexion that stimulates, elevating windiness, and copious seed—all work together more in men than in women. Therefore the desire for intercourse is greater in men than in women.

On the contrary is this reason: Where pleasure is greater when something is had, appetite for it is greater if it is not had. But Constantine says that pleasure in intercourse is greater on the part of the woman than on the part of the man. Therefore the desire for intercourse is greater, and love is greater and more intense in women than in men.

The second reason is this. The female sex is rushed into love more than the male sex, as Constantine says. Therefore the female sex desires both intercourse and love more than the male sex.

To this it should be said that according to some, women love more than men, but we believe the opposite. Whence we say that love is more intense on the part of the man than on the part of the woman, but that pleasure is greater, as Constantine says, on the part of the woman. And according to him the reason is that women take pleasure in emitting and receiving, but men in emitting alone. And thus as far as this is concerned, love flourishes more in women. Also they are more quickly conquered and deceived because of the smallness of their understanding, as al-Rāzī says.

Second, it is inquired why there is so much pleasure in intercourse.

To this it should be said that there are four causes of it: The first is the disposition of the members, which are extremely sensitive because they are filled with nerves. The second cause is on the part of its action, since each faculty delights in its own action; even the faculty expelling the fetus takes pleasure in its action. The third cause is the passage of seminal moisture through the member, for it induces a certain tickling and pleasurable mo-

. . . femine] *om.* V        **217** femine] f. quam a parte maris M        illum] *om.* M    Avicenna V        **218** delectantur femine] delectatur femina V    viri] vir V        autem] *om.* M        **219** et] *om.* V        **220** mulieribus] m. quam in viris M        Item] *om.* V        **221** dicit] vult M        **226** quia] et M    sue] ipsius M        **227** delectatur] operatur V    in propria] in sua M    sua propria V    operatione] delectatione A    **227–28** etiam . . . operatione] *om.* MV        **228** fetum] fetus A        **229** spermatice] s. et hoc temperate V

230 inducit enim quandam titillationem et motum delectabilem.
Quarta causa est confricatio membrorum nervosorum ad invicem[40]
ex qua provenit calor temperatus, et iste sunt cause
delectationis in cohitu. Quintam etiam causam assignant
aliqui a parte finis dicentes quod magnam posuit deus
235 delectationem in opere tali ne propter eius immundiciam
ab animalibus abhominaretur et sic deficeret generatio.[41]

Tertio queritur quis sexus plus delectetur in cohitu,
et videtur quod masculinus sexus hac ratione. Membrum
masculini est maioris sensus.[42] Sed ubi maior est sensus rei
240 delectabilis est maior delectatio. Ergo in maribus maior est
delectatio.

Contrarium dicit Constantinus in libro *De cohitu*.[43]

Ad hoc dicendum quod sicut credimus maior est
delectatio in maribus quam in feminis. Et patet quia plus
245 emittunt et plus consumuntur in cohitu.[44] Sed a parte femine
est duplex delectatio in emissione et in receptione; et
tamen non est tanta qualitate.[45]

Circa quintum sic proceditur: Queritur de signis et
queritur utrum oculi plus paciuntur in amore et ostenditur
250 quod sic. Prima ratio talis: Quanto aliquod membrum habet
maiorem colliganciam cum cerebro, tanto magis sibi
compatitur in suis passionibus. Sed oculi sunt huiusmodi
ut dicit Philosophus.[46] Ergo oculi plus debent in amore pati.

Secunda ratio est hec: Oculi sunt magis passibiles et
255 fluxibiles quia sunt aquose substantie.[47] Ergo oculi magis
compaciuntur et dissolvuntur et diminuuntur.

Contrarium dicit Constantinus quod omnia membra preter
oculos attenuantur et oculi ut dicit magnificantur.[48]

---

**230** enim] in membris V     **231** est] *om.* V    membrorum nervosorum] nervorum A
ad invicem] *om.* V     **233** delectationis] --um V    etiam] *om.* A     **234** fi-
nis] fetus M     quod] *om.* V    magnam] maximam M    *om.* V    deus] *om.* A
**235** opere] operatione P     **236** abhominaretur] abhoreretur M     **237** sexus] *add.*
*s.l.* P    delectetur] --atur A     **238** masculinus] masculus M    sexus . . . mem-
brum] *om.* M     **239** masculini] masculi MV    est] enim sunt M    sensus] sexus
*corr. in* sensus P    est²] *om.* M     **240** delectabilis] delectationis M    maior] ibi
m. V     **243** dicendum] d. est V    credimus] concedimus V     **244** et patet]
*om.* M et hoc p. V     **245** plus] *om.* M     **246** et¹] scilicet et V    emissione]
emixtione A    in²] *om.* M    et²] sed V     **246–47** et . . . qualitate] *om.* M
**247** est] *om.* V     **248** proceditur] --imus V    Queritur] et q. M     **249** pa-
ciuntur] --antur V     **250** Prima . . . talis] *om.* M    talis] t. est V    aliquod]
aliquid A    membrum] organum V     **251** maiorem] *om.* M *add. s.l.* P    col-
liganciam] convenienciam V    colimiᵃ PA     **252** passionibus] compassionibus A    operationibus *exp. et* compassionibus *add. s.l.* P      **253** ut . . . Philosophus] *om.* M

tion. The fourth cause is the rubbing of sensitive members against each other, which results in a temperate heat, and these are the causes of pleasure in intercourse. Some assign a fifth, final cause, saying that God created a great pleasure in such an action lest, because of its uncleanness, animals abominate it and thus procreation would perish.

Third, it is inquired which sex takes greater pleasure in intercourse, and it seems that it is the masculine sex, for this reason: the masculine member is more sensitive. But where there is greater sensation of a pleasurable thing, there is greater pleasure. Therefore pleasure is greater in men.

Constantine says the opposite in *On Intercourse*.

To this it must be said that, as we believe, pleasure is greater in men than in women. And this is evident because they emit more and are more consumed in intercourse. But pleasure is double on women's part (in emitting and receiving), yet it is not of such a quality.

We proceed thus concerning the fifth question: it is inquired about symptoms, and it is inquired whether the eyes suffer more in love, and it is shown that they do. The first reason is this. The greater connection any member has with the brain, the more it suffers in the brain's illnesses. But the eyes are of this sort, as the Philosopher says. Therefore the eyes ought to suffer more in love.

The second reason is this. The eyes are more passible and fluxible because they are of a watery substance. Therefore the eyes suffer more and are dissolved and diminished.

Constantine says the opposite, that all the members except the eyes are attenuated, and the eyes, as he says, are enlarged.

**254** est hec] *om.* MVA     **255** aquose] magis a. A     **256** compaciuntur] paciuntur
MV     et¹] *om.* V     **258** et] *om.* MVA     oculi . . . magnificantur] *om.* V

Ad hoc dicendum quod quando facies crescit et
260 impinguatur oculi minuuntur id est videntur minui. Sed
quando facies decrescit caverne oculorum secundum
apparentiam elevantur et oculi apparent maiores. Vel aliter
dicunt quod in amore est multa vigilia et ideo vapores multi
elevantur ad oculos et sic distenduntur oculi et
265 magnificantur.

Circa sextum queritur de cura et queritur an ebrietas
competat in hoc morbo, et ostenditur quod sic. Prima ratio
talis: Dicit Ovidius in libro suo *De remedio amoris*: aut
nulla ebrietas aut tanta sit ut tibi curas eripiat.[49] Ergo
270 videtur per auctoritatem Ovidii quod competat.

Secunda ratio est hec auctoritas Rasy dicentis quod
ebrietas cura est talium.[50]

Ad oppositum est hec ratio: Nichil quod operationes
perturbat animales confert ad curam amoris. Sed ebrietas est
275 huiusmodi; ergo non confert.[51]

Ad hoc dicendum quod in cura amoris duo competunt. Unum
est reductio virtutis estimative ad rectitudinem et
ordinatam dilectionem, et quantum ad hoc non competit
ebrietas. Aliud est ablatio et ereptio cure et
280 sollicitudinis, et sic procedit Ovidius et duo dicit, primum
quantum ad primum et secundum quantum ad secundum.

Secundo queritur utrum balneum competat et ostenditur
quod non. Ratio talis: Nichil quod cohitum augmentat
competit. Sed balneum et cibi laudabiles sunt huiusmodi quia
285 carnem fovent et delectant. Ergo balneum non competit.

Contrarium dicit Rasy et Serapion.[52]

Ad hoc dicendum quod hec competunt in amore, scilicet
balneum et cibi laudabiles, et hoc est quia distanciam habent
cogitationem et auferunt sollicitudinem melancolicam.

---

259 dicendum] d. est V       facies crescit] fauces crescunt M       260 impinguatur] impingatur VA   impingantur M       minuuntur] minuantur M       id est] et M 261 facies decrescit] fauces decrescunt M       262 oculi] *om.* M       263 dicunt] *om.* MPA       266 an] utrum M       267 ostenditur] videtur M       Prima . . . talis] *om.* M       268 suo] *om.* MV       amoris] *om.* M       269 sit] *om.* M   s. tibi A eripiat] etc. V       270 per . . . Ovidii] *om.* M       auctoritatem] actorem A       quod] q. ebrietas V       271 ratio . . . auctoritas] auctoritas est ratio M       hec] *om.* MV 272 cura est] aufert curas V       273 est hec ratio] *om.* M   est A       274 perturbat] *om.* M       275 confert] c. ad curam V       276 dicendum] d. est V       amoris] a. hereos A       Unum] qm̄ *exp. et* u. *add. s. l.* P       279 ereptio] extorsio M 280 procedit] processit V       Ovidius] ob'o V       281 et] *om.* MVA       283 ratio talis] *om.* M       287 dicendum] d. est V       hec] *om.* V       288 laudabiles] delectabiles P       est] *om.* PA

To this it must be said that when the face grows and fattens the eyes grow smaller, that is, they appear smaller. But when the face grows thinner, the hollows of the eyes appear to increase and thus the eyes appear larger. Or they say otherwise that in love there is much insomnia, and therefore many vapors rise to the eyes, and thus the eyes are distended and enlarged.

Concerning the sixth [question], it is inquired concerning the cure, and it is inquired whether drunkenness is useful for this disease, and it is shown to be so. The first reason is this. Ovid says in his book *Remedies of Love*: Let there be no drunkenness or so much that it takes away your cares. Therefore it seems to be useful, on the authority of Ovid.

The second reason is this, namely the authority of al-Rāzī, who says that drunkenness is a cure for this disease.

On the contrary is this reason. Nothing that perturbs the actions of the mind helps to cure love. But drunkenness is of this sort; therefore it does not help.

To this it must be said that two things are useful in the cure of love. One is returning the estimative faculty to rightly ordered love, and as far as this is concerned, drunkenness does not help. The other is the taking away and removal of care and worry, and thus Ovid proceeds. And he says two things, the first concerning the first, and the second concerning the second.

Second, it is inquired whether baths are useful, and it is shown that they are not. The reason is this. Nothing that increases intercourse is useful. But baths and good food do this, because they soothe and delight the flesh. Therefore baths do not help.

Al-Rāzī and Serapion say the opposite.

To this it must be said that these things, namely baths and good food, are useful in love, and this is because they are far from thought, and relieve melancholic worry.

290     Tertio queritur utrum alicui pacienti amorem competat videre formas turpes et ostenditur quod sic. Curatio per contrarium.[53] Ergo cum aliquis diligit pulcram formam debet ei representari forma turpis.

    Contrarium dicit auctor.[54]

295     Ad hoc dicendum quod non debet ei presentari mulier turpis, tanto enim forcius arderet in amore mulieris pulcre que sibi pulcherrima videbatur. Sed si sibi presentetur mulier pulcra, tunc placabitur animus eius et sic remissior efficietur passio et eius desiderium remittitur.

300     Sunt autem in hoc capitulo in precedentibus et consequentibus questiones, scilicet utrum amor sit morbus nec ne; et si est, utrum sit consimilis vel officialis, et huiusmodi alie questiones.[55] Sed non est causandum de hiis.

---

**290** queritur] *om.* A      **291** per] fit p. M     est p. V      **293** turpis] deformis V **294** dicit auctor] dicunt auctores VA      **295** dicendum] d. est V      presentari] repre- sentari M      **296** arderet] ardet A      **297** si sibi] sibi M    si VA      presentetur] representabitur M      **299** efficietur] —itur M      passio] eius p. A      remittitur] *om.* MVA      **300** in] *om.* V      precedentibus] precedentes V      **301** consequen- tibus] subsequentes V      questiones] communes q. VA     scilicet] et M      **302** est] sit V     sit] *om.* MA      **303** est] *om.* V      causandum] cān̄ V      **304** de hiis] *om.* PV

Third, it is inquired whether it helps any patient suffering from love to see ugly forms, and it is shown that it does. Curing is by contraries. Therefore when someone loves a beautiful form, an ugly form ought to be shown him.

The author [i.e. Constantine] says the opposite.

To this it must be said that he ought not to be shown an ugly woman, since he will burn in love so much the more for a beautiful woman who will seem most beautiful to him. But if a beautiful woman is shown to him, then his mind will be pleased and his disease will become milder and his desire will abate.

There are also in this chapter questions about things which precede and follow, such as whether love is a disease or not; and if it is, whether it is a consimilar or official disease, and other similar questions. But we will not discuss them.

# BONA FORTUNA,
## *TRACTATUS SUPER VIATICUM*

### *Manuscripts*

Bona Fortuna's *Tractatus super Viaticum* is preserved in two manuscripts, both from the fourteenth century.

**P**: Paris, Bibliothèque Nationale, lat. 15373. Bona Fortuna, *Tractatus super Viaticum*, fols. 44r–162r. *Inc.*: "Capillus ex fumo grosso. . . . (text) Nota primo quid est allopicia." *Expl.*: ". . . et postea calidiusculas et deinde calidiores. Explicit tractatus super viaticum magistri bone fortune." *Amor hereos*: fols. 13v(56v)–14r(57r).

BN lat. 15373 is composed of two originally separate manuscripts that have been bound as the present volume. Folios 1–43, the first MS, contain Richard FitzRalph's treatise on the poverty of Jesus Christ, written in *anglicana* script. Folios 44–162r (1–109 = the second MS) contain Bona Fortuna's treatise on the *Viaticum*, into which portions of other treatises have been interleaved.[1] The MS ends with two short medical works, Bernard of Gordon's *Compendium regiminis acutorum* and the Salernitan *De adventu medici ad aegrotum*.[2]

Since Bernard de Gordon composed the *Compendium regiminis acutorum* in 1294, the manuscript can be no earlier.[3] On palaeographical grounds, M.-T. D'Alverny has dated it to the first part of the fourteenth century.[4] If Bona Fortuna is indeed Bernard de Bona Hora, the MS would be nearly contemporary with his lectures on the *Viaticum*. Evidence for the place of origin is inconclusive.[5] Bona Fortuna translates the Latin *cimex* as *pimes* in French, a type of louse. In another place he glosses the Latin *kulinge* or *kulenge* as *loches*, or loach. Both glosses suggest an audience for whom the French terms would be useful. However, he also offers glosses in German, Slavic, and "Chaldean," so that no firm conclusions can be drawn as to his audience or place of teaching from linguistic evidence.[6]

The composition of the medical portion of BN 15373 tells us that for at least one early fourteenth-century physician, Bona Fortuna's *Treatise on the Viaticum* was a focus for organizing academic yet practical medical knowledge.[7] As the central text in a small anthology it provided comprehensive, up-to-date coverage of standard medical topics, supplemented, however, by portions of more specialized works. The extensive and systematic marginal annotations show that Bona Fortuna's work was carefully read, perhaps by readers at the Sorbonne, where the manuscript was located in the later fourteenth century, probably arriving there after 1338.

**R**: Rouen, Bibliothèque municipale A 176 (formerly 983) S. 14. Bona Fortuna, *Tractatus super Viaticum*, fols. 1–72. *Inc.*: "Capillus ex fumo grosso . . . (text) Hic nota primo quid est allopicia." *Expl.*: ". . . calidiusculas et deinde calidiores. Explicit tractatus magistri bone fortune super viaticum." *Amor hereos*: fols. 10r–11r. Described by Henri Omont, *Catalogue général des manuscrits des Bibliothèques Publiques de France. Départements*. Vol. 1: Rouen. Paris, 1886.

A single scribe copied the work. The date of origin is probably the mid-fourteenth century and the MS may have been written in northern France or by a northern-trained copyist.[8] Spaces were left for initials that were never executed. Frequent blanks occur where either the scribe could not read his exemplar or where the exemplar itself was blank. There are marginal corrections throughout in a number of hands, some contemporary with the text, others later. The text is preceded by a table of contents in a fifteenth-century hand.

Formerly at the abbey of Fécamp (no. 67). The water damage, severe in places, especially the upper margins, most likely happened when the abbey library suffered neglect during the sixteenth century.[9]

Both texts derive from a common defective source. Both R and P share a number of omissions that may or may not be marked by blank spaces and that leave grammar or sense deficient. If the text derives from a *reportatio*, as some of its internal characteristics seem to indicate, the omissions may stem from difficulties of classroom reporting that were not edited out by the master. If so, R and P may be first-generation copies from a faulty exemplar. This would explain why P, though corrected, is not "correct."

The edition of Bona Fortuna's chapter of *amor hereos* is based on R. R was chosen as the base manuscript because it contains significantly less haplography than P, fewer omitted lines or passages, and a greater number of grammatically or stylistically preferable readings. In some cases I have replaced R's readings with those of P where R is clearly mistaken or where P gives better sense. In several cases I have ventured to supply the sense of the text where both R and P are deficient.

## *Edition*

# Bona Fortuna
## *Tractatus super Viaticum*

**P**: Paris, Bibliothèque Nationale, lat. 15373
**R**: Rouen, Bibliothèque municipale, A 176 (983)

*AMOR QUI ET HEREOS DICITUR ET CETERA.* Superius determinat auctor de multis passionibus capitis seu cerebri. Quia igitur ista passio que amor hereos dicitur habet principium a cerebro, ideo hic determinat de ista passione.[1] Circa

5  illud capitulum nota tria: primo de morbo, secundo de signis, tercio de cura. De morbo nota duo: primo de eius diffinitione, secundo de eius causis. De signis sunt etiam duo notanda: primo de signis que signant egritudinem, secundo de hiis que signant rem de qua est egritudo. De cura

10  notanda sunt duo: primo notanda sunt quedam ex parte corporis, secundo quedam ex parte anime. Deinde etiam dicemus quedam adiutoralia ad istam passionem.

Circa primum. Nota quod amor hereos est incitatio cogitationum circa speciei humane formam et figuram

15  individualem sive singularem sollicitudini melancolice persimilis, adiuvantibus desiderio et concupiscentia inexpletis, que si explerentur, hereos tolleretur.[2] In hac diffinitione notatur morbus et forma eius. Item notatur causa morbi. Item notatur forma curationis morbi.

20  Forma morbi notatur in hoc quod dicitur *Incitatio cogitationum et cetera.* In eis enim incitate sunt cogitationes per hoc quod dicit *circa speciei* et cetera. Tangit propter quid est ista species vel passio[3] effective sicut patebit in causis. *Coadiuvantibus desiderio et*

25  *concupiscentia.* Nisi enim illa essent nullo modo pateretur talem insaniam. *Inexpletis.* Si enim explerentur tunc cessaret morbus. *Sollicitudini melancolice persimilis.* Hoc dicitur propter duo: tum quia isti sunt illis similes in essentia, tum quia quando non curantur fiunt melancolici

30  vel manici.

---

**1** *et*[1]] est et *expunc.* P      **3** ista] hec P      amor] *om.* P      **5** illud] istud P
**12** adiutoralia] adiutoria P      **14** speciei] ɸ ōi P      **16** persimilis] similis P

# Bona Fortuna
## *Treatise on the Viaticum*

LOVE THAT IS CALLED *HEREOS* ETC. The author treats of many diseases of the head or brain above. Because this disease, which is called "amor hereos," originates in the brain, he therefore treats of this disease here. Concerning this chapter, note three things: first, about the disease; second, about the signs; third, about the cure. Concerning the disease, note two things: first, about its definition; second, about its causes. Concerning the signs, two things must also be noted: first, about the signs that signal illness; second, about those that signal the thing provoking the illness. Concerning the cure, two things must be noted: first to be noted are certain ones for the body; second, certain ones for the spirit. Then we will also discuss certain helpful things for this disease.

Concerning the first. Note that *amor hereos* is an excitation of the thoughts about an individual or singular form and figure of human likeness, very similar to melancholic worry, aided by unfulfilled desire and concupiscence; for if they were fulfilled, *hereos* would be relieved. The disease and its form are noted in this definition. The cause of the disease is also noted. Also noted is the form of the disease's cure. The form of the disease is noted where it is said: *Excitation of the thoughts etc.* For in them [i.e., patients] the thoughts are excited by that which he calls *about an individual* etc. He accounts for this species or impress with respect to the efficient cause, as will be apparent in [the section on] causes. *Aided by desire and concupiscence.* For unless these were present, in no way would [the patient] suffer such madness. *Unfulfilled.* For if they were fulfilled, then the disease would cease. *Very similar to melancholy worry.* This is said on account of two things: on the one hand because these [i.e. patients of *amor hereos*] are similar to those [the melancholic] in essence, on the other because when they are not cured, they become melancholic or mad.

---

18 forma] fons R     *22 speciei*] species *corr. in* speciei R    species P            **25** *concu-*
*piscentia*] cetera R          pateretur] --entur P              **26** *Inexpletis*] in exemplis *corr. in* ex-
empletis P          **27** *persimilis*] similis P          **28** tum] tū R    tñ P          **29** tum] q
tū *ut videtur* P          non] *om.* P          **30** manici] maniaci P

Tunc nota de causis. Auctor ponit duas causas,
scilicet pulchritudinem mulieris et necessitatem expellendi
superfluitatem. Sed ego dico quod est tamen una causa
principalis, scilicet extrinsicum apprehensum quod putatur
35 conveniens et amicum,[4] sicut forma alicuius mulieris que
est ita fortiter apprehensa et ita firmiter a cogitatione
amplexata quod placet ipsi patienti super omnia. Dico autem
quod illa duo que ponit auctor sunt coadiuvantia, scilicet
pulchritudo mulieris et necessitas expellendi superflui-
40 tates. Hoc autem quod ego dico est causa principalis. Hoc
enim est quod movet fantasiam vel intellectum.[5] Ista autem
movent rationem et obvolvunt[6] ita quod non discernit sed
ducitur tamen super cogitationem quasi iam habeat determina-
tum iudicium ad unam partem. Istud autem contingit in qua[7]
45 ex illa principali causa quam dixi, coadiuvantibus tamen
pulchritudine mulieris et necessitate expellendi
superfluitates.

Tunc nota de signis et primo de signis que signant
egritudinem. Horum autem signorum quedam sumuntur a forma
50 corporis, quedam vero ab operationibus moralibus, quedam
vero ab operationibus virtutis spiritualis sicut sunt pulsus
et hanelitus. Signa que sumuntur a forma corporis illa
tangit auctor satis.[8] Oculi enim eorum concavantur,
exsiccantur, et contrahuntur, nec fiunt lacrimosi nec humidi
55 nisi fiat eis memoria de divortio sive separatione a
dilecta; in aliis casibus non lacrimantur. Facies istorum
est similis faciei ridentis et quasi illius qui vult esse
iocundus. Sompni eorum sunt parvi, non profundi. Palpebre
eorum sunt tumide propter vigilias. Corporis eorum fit
60 arefactio. Item querunt solitudinem[9] et quando sunt soli tunc
flent aut cantant; etiam in sompno accidit eis aliquando
cantus aliquando fletus. Hec igitur sunt signa a forma
corporis et ab operationibus moralibus.

Tunc nota a parte operationum virtutis spiritualis cuiusmodi
65 operationes sunt hanelitus sive <pulsus. Quando audiunt que
displicent>,[10] retardant; quando vero audiunt que placent
tunc fit hanelitus eorum quasi habens estuantis. Item

---

31 Tunc] Item P      33 quod est] *om.* P      44 in qua] *om.* P      45 ta-
men] cum P      48 Tunc] Item P      49 sumuntur] ponuntur P      forma] parte
P      50 vero ab operationibus moralibus] a parte anime P      51 vero] *om.* P

Then note concerning the causes: The author gives two causes, namely the beauty of a woman and the necessity to expel superfluity. But I say that there is, however, one principal cause, namely an extrinsic apprehension that is thought fitting and congenial, such as the form of any woman that is so strongly apprehended and so firmly embraced by the thought that it pleases the patient above everything. I say, moreover, that those two [causes] that the author gives, namely the beauty of a woman and the necessity of expelling superfluities, are coadjuvant causes. That, however, which I say is the principal cause, for this is what moves the fantasy and the intellect. These moreover move and obscure the reason such that it does not distinguish, but is rather led upon that thought as though it already had a settled judgment on one side [i.e., that the object is desirable]. Moreover, this occurs in the subject on account of that principal cause that I have said, aided, however, by the beauty of the woman and the necessity of expelling superfluities.

Then take note concerning the signs, and first of those that signal illness. Some of these signs are taken from the appearance of the body, some indeed from behavior, some indeed from the functions of the spiritual faculty, like pulse and breathing. The author deals sufficiently with signs that are taken from the appearance of the body. Their eyes grow hollow, dry out, and contract, nor are they tearful or moist unless they are reminded of parting or separation from the beloved; in other cases they do not cry. Their faces are similar to the face of someone laughing and, as it were, to that of someone who wishes to be merry. Their sleeps are light, not deep. Their eyelids are swollen because of sleeplessness. Their bodies dry out. They also seek solitude, and when they are alone, then they weep or sing; sometimes also in sleep song or weeping befalls them. These are the symptoms from bodily appearance and from behavior.

Then note concerning the functions of the spiritual faculty, whose functions are breathing and <pulse. Breathing and pulse> slow down <when patients hear what is displeasing>; when indeed they hear what is pleasing,

53 enim] *om.* P        56 dilecta] re d. P        56 casibus] talibus P        64 a parte operationum] ab operationibus P        cuiusmodi] eius P        65–66 <pulsus . . . displicent>] *om.* RP *suppl.*        66 placent] placeant P        67 habens] *om.* P

frequenter hanelant cum suspirio. Item pulsus eorum est
parvus, diversus, habens intersectionem.

70    Tunc nota signa super re amata. Aliquando enim ipsi
celant et nullo modo volunt manifestare rem quam amant. Sed
si sciretur hoc esset magna pars cure. Propter hoc necessaria
sunt ista signa. Sic autem scies que sit res amata. Tene
pulsum pacientis et narra ei de muliere aliqua quam credis
75    ipsum amare.[11] Illam multum lauda et multum extollas de
pulcritudine de honestate et huiusmodi et ita fac successive
de pluribus et diversis mulieribus inter quas credis illam
esse quam amat. Si igitur veneris in sermone tuo ad illam
que est amata, tunc pulsus eius mutatur et fit latior et
80    maior et velocior quam prius. Postea iterum redeas vel fac
ut alius redeat super easdem mulieres quas tu prius
laudaveras; fac quod alius vituperet illas successive unam
post aliam et dicat multa turpia et multa vilia de eis. Si
igitur venerit ad illam que est amata, tunc impossibile est
85    quin mutetur pulsus eius et sic optime invenies signum super
re amata. Quando enim gaudet tunc fit hanelitus latus et
pulsus maior; quando vero tristatur propter turpia et vilia
que narrantur de sua dilecta tunc retardat hanelitum et fit
pulsus minor et fit intersectus et suspenditur hanelitus ac
90    si non posset liberum hanelitum habere. Item bonum est quod
puella quam amat ducatur ante eum et ducantur successive
multe ante ipsum inter quas creditur illam esse quam amat.
Tunc optime per ista signa scies que sit illa quam amat.

    Tunc nota de cura. Cura autem consistit in duobus: uno
95    modo ex parte corporis, alio modo ex parte anime. Item ex
parte corporis consistit duobus: quedam enim reducunt corpus
gratia compositionis, quedam gratia humorum. Si igitur de
humoribus aliud est adustum quod cognoscitur per adustionem
et siccitatem oris et lingue[12] et per amaritudinem gutturis
100    quasi comedisset pruna novella immatura, tunc debes evacuare.[13] Hoc autem optime fit cum .iiii. herbis que sunt
iste: capud monachi, lactucella abbatis, radix volubilis
maioris, et basilicon.[14] Accipe de istis ana; fiat decoctio;
deinde in fine decoctionis adde de epithimo[15] quantum est
105    medietas unius predictorum et fac bullire. Et nota quod

---

**68** hanelant] *om.* R    **70** Tunc] Item P    **73** scies] scietur P    **74** pulsum]
pl *scrib. et* -sus *add. sup. lin.* P    **76** de] et P    fac] fiat P    **81** super] *om.* R
**82** laudaveras] laudaveris P    **84** venerit] veneris P    **85** signum] ipm̄ *exp. ante* s. P

then their breathing becomes feverish, as it were. Also they frequently breathe with sighs. Their pulse is also small, uneven, and intermittent.

Then note the signs concerning the beloved, for sometimes these [patients] conceal the thing they love and in no way wish to reveal it. But if it were known, this would be a great part of the cure. Hence these signs are necessary. In this way, then, you will know who the beloved is. Hold the patient's pulse and speak to him about a certain woman whom you believe he loves. Praise her greatly, and highly extol her beauty, honor, and such, and do this successively with many different women among whom you believe is the one he loves. If therefore in your talk you come upon the one who is loved, then his pulse will change, and become broader and greater and faster than before. Afterwards, go back over or make another go back over the same women whom you had previously praised. Make someone else scorn them successively, one after the other, and let him say many disgusting and vile things about them. If he comes to the one who is loved, then it is impossible for his pulse not to change, and thus you will best find the sign about the beloved. For when he rejoices, then his breathing becomes deep and his pulse greater; when indeed he grows sad on account of the disgusting and vile things that are related concerning his beloved, then his breathing slows down and his pulse is less and is intermittent, and his breathing is interrupted as though he could not draw a free breath. It is also good that the girl whom he loves be led before him, and that many be led before him successively, among whom is believed to be the one he loves. Thus by these signs you will best know which may be the one he loves.

Then note concerning the cure. The cure consists in two things, one for the body, another for the mind. The bodily cure also consists of two parts, for some restore the body on account of its composition, others on account of humors. If, therefore, humors [are involved], one sort is burnt, which is recognized by burning and dryness of the mouth and tongue and by bitterness in the throat, as though he had eaten new, unripe plums; then you ought to purge. Now this is best done with four herbs which are these: dandelion, larger wild endive, root of larger honeysuckle, and basil. Take equal parts of these and make a decoction; at the end of its cooking add dodder—half the amount of the previous herbs—and bring it to a boil.

---

89 minor] etiam m. P    90 est] *om.* P    92 illam] illa P    93 per ista signa]
*om.* P    94 Tunc] Item P    100 debes] debet *corr. in* debes P    101 iiii] quatuor P

ultimo debes apponere epithimum ita quod non transeat super
ipsum nisi una bullitio vel due secundum quod bullire
solent ova.

Item si causa fuerit magnificata et morbus[16] tunc evacua
110 cum ieris sicut cum iera pigra, iera logodion, iera memphitum.[17]
Ego autem aliquando dedi electuarium de suco rosarum.[18] Si
vero non sit processus tantus, tunc sufficit mel violaceum
et cassia fistula[19] sed tamarindi nullo modo in hoc casu
competunt. Sed supra in casu ubi est colera naturalis, alie
115 due predicte cum predicta decoctione distemperentur. Post
evacuationem duc eum ad balneum et reducas eum cum bona
dieta.[20]

Et nota quod illud quod in hac cura respicit corpus, hoc
est balneum, quies, et sompnus; et nota quod sompnus est magnum
120 bonum in ista egritudine. Et nota quod auctor prohibet
ebrietatem, tamen sciendum est quod modica ebrietas multum
valet quia inducit sompnum.[21]

Tunc veniamus ad ea que sunt ex parte anime. Nota igitur
quod isti homines qui patiuntur hanc egritudinem aut sunt
125 homines quibus est aliqua discretio et qui sunt corrigibiles
aut homines quibus nulla est discretio et qui sunt incorrigibiles. Tunc faciendum circa eos sicut fit circa pueros
quos sine verberibus sed cum omni mansuetudine docemus
primo a.b.c., quibus promittimus nuces, poma, et alia.
130 Taliter cum omni cautela est procedendum circa istos. Debemus eis promittere aliqua et iungere eos cum sociis et cum
paribus suis et promittamus eis honores et beneficia si
sint scolares et si in hoc delectentur. Per hunc modum
aliquando recedunt a sua insania, et aliquando non rece-
135 dunt sed magis insaniunt. Unde ista non sunt documenta
universalia sed particularia, et etiam ea que ponit auctor
non sunt universalia.[22] Dicit enim quod cantilene et
soni instrumentorum musicorum conferunt. Hoc autem non est
universale. Et propter hoc medicus de sua industria adminis-
140 tret illa que viderit valere ad curam. Verumtamen hoc est
optimum quod <coeat> cum aliis mulieribus et etiam cum
diversis. Si vero paciens aliquo modo sit corrigibilis, tunc
debemus narrare rem cum feditatibus et turpitudinibus suis et

**107** bullitio] bibitio R   **109** magnificata] manifestata P   **111** aliquando] *om.* P
**113** Sed] et *exp. et* sed *add. sup. lin.* R   **116** balneum] balnea P   **123** sunt] *add. sup.*
*lin.* P   **124** aut] autem P   **127** Tunc] primo modo t. P   **128** quos] quod P

Note that you should add dodder last so that it comes to the boil only once or twice, as long as eggs are usually boiled.

If the cause is aggravated and [becomes?] a disease, then evacuate with *hieras*, such as *hiera pigra, hiera logodion*, and *hiera memphitum*. I have sometimes given an electuary of rose juice. If indeed it has not progressed so far, then violet honey and purging cassia suffice, but tamarinds in no way help in this case. But above, in the case where there is natural choler, the two aforesaid with the aforesaid decoction will be imbalanced. After purging, lead him to the bath and restore him with a good diet.

And note that which cóncerns the body in this cure, that is bathing, rest, and sleep; and note that sleep is a great good in this illness. And note that the author forbids drunkenness, but it must be known that moderate drunkenness is very helpful because it brings on sleep.

Then we come to those things that concern the mind. Note therefore that these people who suffer this illness are either people who have some discretion and are corrigible, or people who have no discretion and are incorrigible. Then they are to be treated as we do boys whom we first teach the ABCs without blows but with all gentleness, and whom we promise nuts, apples, and other things. In such a fashion with all caution we should proceed with them. We ought to promise them something, and join them with companions and with their equals, and promise them honors and benefices if they are scholars and if they delight in this. In this way sometimes they desist from their madness; sometimes they do not, but grow madder. Whence these are not universal recommendations but particular, and also those which the author suggests are not universal, for he says that songs and the sounds of instrumental music are beneficial. This, however, is not universal. And because of this let the physician by his efforts administer those things that he sees will be useful for the cure. Indeed, this is best, that he have intercourse with other women, and also with different ones. If indeed the patient is in any way corrigible, then we ought to discuss the [beloved] object with its filthy and loathsome qualities, and relate all the

---

**129** poma] prunas P      alia] talia P      **132** paribus] *corr. ex* partibus P      promittamus] promittemus R      **139** de] in *exp.* de *add. sup. lin.* P      **140** illa] ea P
**141** <coeat>] ·comedat *corr. in* cohiret R      comedat *in marg.* vel coeat P      **142** paciens]
*om.* P      **143** rem] *om.* P      cum] *add. s.l.* P      feditatibus] fetiditatibus P
turpitudinibus] turpidinibus P

narrare omnia vicia que possumus de re amata. Item pacienti
145  debemus proponere dampna et odium amicorum suorum que
proveniunt ex tali insania. Item cavere debemus ei animo
moderato quia per hoc stimulatur. Sed ista non sunt
universalia.

Sed nunc nota documenta universalia: primum igitur est
150  mutatio regionis[23]; secundum est occupatio in litigiosis
contentionibus; aliud est in necessariis occupationibus;
quartum est in coitu cum aliis mulieribus.

Mutatio igitur regionis est valde bona et hoc vidi prodesse,
unde feci quod quidam de consilio et consensu parentum
155  suorum fuit <accusatus?>[24] homicidii et compulsus fuit
exulare a patria et sanatus est. Item bonum est facere eum
impeditum in occupationibus necessariis ut inducatur ad hoc
quod sollicitus sit de victu et vestitu et quod
depauperetur et quod dicatur ei: "Quid modo comedes? Quid
160  bibes? Quid expendes? Unde vives? Omnia bona tua pereunt et
sic tu miser eris."[25] Item bonum est quod super eum veniant
occupationes de litigiosis contentionibus. Hoc enim expertus
sum prodesse. Ista facienda sunt si paciens non posset
habere illam quam amat. Verumtamen si posset eam habere tunc
165  est summa et optima cura quod associentur. Sed si non potest
eam habere vel si posset et cum periculo vel cum peccato
tunc bonum est quod ipse conversetur cum honestis et maturis
et quos vereatur et qui dicant et suadeant ei de virtutibus
et moribus.

170  *Basilicon.*[26] Siccus in .ii. gradu. Sed a parte
qualitatum activarum est vicinum temperamento. Et hoc scio
experimento, quia si cum aqua rosacea irroretur, infrigidat; si
vero cum vino irroretur, calefacit. Unde aliquando feci emplastrum
super caput ad infrigidandum de basilicone asperso cum aqua
175  rosacea. Item incorporetur cum oleo rosato optime valet
contra ustionem et excoriationem factam ex igne.[27] Item aperit
opilationem cerebri odoratum et naribus instillatum.[28] Item
sucus eius cum oleo violaceo[29] instillatus naribus optimum
caputpurgium[30] est, vel cum oleo camomillino[31] sed non fui
180  usus eo cum oleo camomillino.

---

**144** vicia] vilia P      **145** proponere] promittere P      odium] *om.* R      **146** pro-
veniunt] p. ex P      **147** moderato] temperato P      stimulatur] stilantur R
**149** nunc] vero P      est] *om.* R      **150** regionis] *corr. ex* religionis P      **151** aliud]
alius P      **154** quidam] cuidam R      **155** fuit[1]] *om.* P      <accusatus?>] *om. cum*
*spat. 5–6 verb.* R      *om.* P; *suppl.*      **156** exulare] exire P      est] fuit P      **157** in-

vicious things that we can concerning the beloved object. Then we ought to describe to the patient the rejection and hate of his friends that will result from such madness. Also we ought to caution him with a moderate spirit, because he will be upset by this. But these are not universal.

But now note universal recommendations: first is change of locale; second is entanglement in lawsuits; third is necessary business; fourth is intercourse with other women.

Change of locale is very good and I have seen it work, whence I caused someone <to be accused of> homicide with the advice and consent of his relatives, and he was forced to flee the district and was healed. It is also good to burden him with necessary business, so that he is persuaded to be worried about food and clothing, and that he might become impoverished and that it be said to him: "How will you eat? What will you drink? What will you spend? How will you live? All your goods will perish and thus you will be wretched." It is also good that entanglement in lawsuits befall him. I know by experience that this works. These things are to be done if the patient cannot have her whom he loves. But if he can have her, then it is the greatest and best cure that they join together. But if he is not able to have her, or if he is, but with danger or with sin, then it is good that he converse with honest and mature people whom he respects, and who will speak to him and persuade him concerning virtue and morals.

*Basil.* [It is] dry in the second degree. But the active qualities are nearly temperate. And this I know by experience, for if it is sprinkled with rose water, it cools; if indeed it is sprinkled with wine, it heats. Therefore sometimes I have made a plaster for cooling the head with basil sprinkled with rose water. Also let it be mixed with rose oil; it is most useful against burning and peeling caused by fire. It also opens blockage of the brain when smelled and instilled in the nostrils. Also its juice with violet oil or chamomile oil instilled in the nostrils is an excellent head purge, but I have not used it with chamomile oil.

---

ducatur] dicatur P    **158** quod¹] ut P    vestitu] de v. P    **159** quod dicatur
ei] dicetur P    **165** associentur] associetur R    **167–8** honestis . . . quos] bonis
et maturis et honestis et eos P    **168** ei] *om.* R    **171** vicinum] in P    **176** us-
tionem] ultionem P    **177** et] *ante* odoratum R    Item] sicut P    **180** eo] et P

Item nota optimum experimentum[32] contra fluxum ventris
qui est sine excoriatione et qui est antiquatus,[33] ita quod
est ex debilitate membrorum plus quam ex vicio humorum—expertus
sum. Sed si esset cum excoriatione non bonum esset; sed in
185    fluxu qui est sine excoriatione expertus sum. Accipe semen
basiliconis frixa in patella cum oleo rosato et da bibere
vel da comedere qualitercumque paciens sumere posset.
Mirabiliter prodest. Nos fecimus de amigdalis et de isto
tortellas et dedimus comedere. Item potest dari ad
190    comedendum cum pullis ita quod pulli de eo farciantur vel
potest dari cum ovis frixatis vel alio modo.[34] Optimum est.

---

**184** cum] *add. s. l.* P     **185** expertus] expertū P     **187** da] *om.* P     **189** tor-
tellas] -os P     **190** pullis] *corr. ex* puellis P     **191** frixatis] fractis P

Also note an excellent remedy for diarrhea that is without peeling and that is persistent, such that it is from weakness of the members rather than from a fault of the humors—I have tried it. But if it were with peeling, it would not be good, but in a flux which is without excoriation I have had experience. Take basil seed fried in a pan with rose oil, and give it to be drunk or eaten however the patient is able to take it. It works wonderfully. We made tortillas from this and almonds, and gave them to be eaten. It can also be eaten with chicken, such that the chickens are stuffed with it, or it can be given with fried eggs, or in other ways; it is excellent.

# NOTES

## Abbreviations

Arnald, *Tractatus*  Arnald of Villanova, *Tractatus de amore heroico*, ed. Michael R. McVaugh (Barcelona: Seminarium historiae medicae cantabricense, 1985).

Avicenna, *De anima*  *Liber de anima seu sextus de naturalibus*, ed. Simone van Riet, 2 vols. (Leiden: E. J. Brill, 1968–72).

CMG  *Corpus medicorum graecorum* (Leipzig: Teubner, 1908—).

DSB  *Dictionary of Scientific Biography*, ed. Charles C. Gillispie (New York: Scribner, 1970–80).

EI²  *The Encyclopedia of Islam*, 2nd ed., ed. H. A. R. Gibb (Leiden: E. J. Brill, 1954–79).

PL  *Patrologiae cursus completus, series latina*, ed. J. P. Migne, 221 vols. (Paris, 1844–64).

PSQ  *The Prose Salernitan Questions*, ed. Brian Lawn (Oxford: Clarendon, 1979).

QDA  Peter of Spain, *Questiones super De animalibus*, Madrid, Biblioteca Nacional, MS 1877.

SLA  Peter of Spain, *Scientia libri de anima*, ed. Manuel Alonso, 2nd ed. (Barcelona: Juan Flors, 1961).

TK²  Lynn Thorndike and Pearl Kibre, *Incipits of Mediaeval Scientific Writings in Latin*, rev. and aug. ed. (Cambridge, Mass.: Mediaeval Academy of America, 1963).

## Introduction

1. The phrase is from the *Knight's Tale*, lines 1373–74. All quotations of Chaucer will be taken from the edition of Benson 1987. "Hereos" is a corruption of "eros," discussed in the introduction to Constantine's *Viaticum* in Part 2. Modern inquiry into medieval lovesickness was launched (in Anglo-American scholarship, at least; cf. Chrohns 1905) by Lowes' discovery (1913) that Chaucer's text referred to the medical tradition of *amor hereos*.

2. For the symptoms of depression I have consulted Maxmen 1986. Tennov 1979 proposes the concept of "limerance," an "involuntary reaction . . . mediated by physiological mechanisms" (256). It is characterized by, among other things, intrusive thinking about the object ("cognitive prepossession"), acute longing for reciprocation, aching of the "heart," buoyancy, and a general intensity of feeling. The other types of love are all discussed in Sternberg and Barnes 1988.

3. Liebowitz 1983.

4. Rubin in Sternberg and Barnes 1988, ix.

5. On the relations between culture and symptoms see MacDonald 1983, 72; Zola 1983 [1966]; Douglas 1982 [1973], "The Two Bodies" as well as the works of Foucault listed in the bibliography.

6. Herzlich and Pierret 1987, xi.

7. Previous works that touch on these issues from other perspectives include: Couliano 1987, 13–23, Karnein 1985, Schnell 1985, Jacquart and Thomasset 1985a, Schadewaldt 1985,

Boase 1977, Agamben 1977, and Ciavolella 1976; Lowes 1913 is still valuable. In its earliest stages my work was conceived as a challenge to the assertions of Robertson 1962 about the relationship of the medical tradition of *amor hereos* to theological condemnations of cupidinous love. My work differs from the other studies listed above in proposing a functional relationship between lovesickness and the conventionalized love variously called "amare per amores," "paramours," or "noble love" in the context of late medieval gender and social relations. Kelly 1987 reminds us of the dangers of using the multivalent term "courtly love" without specifying its content, as did Donaldson 1970 [1965] in his essay on "The Myth of Courtly Love." I introduce the term here in quotation marks to signify that it is problematic; having done so, I do not retain them throughout.

8. The quotation is from Greenblatt 1988, 75. Jacquart and Thomasset 1985b discuss medieval medicine's contribution to both a *scientia sexualis* as well as an *ars erotica*.

9. Geertz 1973, 10.

10. Demaitre 1980, 84 notes that Bernard of Gordon composed a commentary on the *Viaticum* that has not survived. Medieval medical sources containing discussions of lovesickness consist of translations from Arabic medical texts (e.g., *Viaticum*, Avicenna's *Canon*, al-Rāzī's *Liber ad almansorem*); commentaries on those texts by university masters; Western handbooks of medicine (e.g., Bernard of Gordon's *Lilium medicinae*); and independent treatises on love (e.g., Arnald of Villanova's *Tractatus de amore heroico*, Gerard of Solo's *Determinatio de amore hereos*). Häring 1982 offers a general introduction to medieval commentary literature.

11. Cf. Jacquart and Thomasset 1985b, 9.

12. Cadden 1986 outlines the complexity of medieval medical discourse on sexuality. See, too, Jacquart and Thomasset 1985b.

13. A good sense of the handbooks can be gained from the reproductions in Cogliati Arano 1979. A facsimile edition of the Vienna *Tacuinum sanitatis* was published in 1967.

## Chapter One: Pathology and Passion

1. Kristeva 1987, 4–5.

2. Ed. Vollmer 1914. For a recent discussion of authorship, themes, and structure, see Bright 1987, 222–44. On the bronze statuette in fig. 1.1, see Chamoux 1962.

3. On lovesickness in antiquity, see Ciavolella 1970, 1976; Schadewaldt 1985; Giedke 1983; Rohde 1914; and Chrohns 1905. I encountered the stimulating work of Winkler 1989 late in the writing of this book. Though we are working with the problem of eros in two different cultures (ancient Greece and medieval Christian Europe), our interpretations converge in a number of respects.

4. *Mutatis mutandis*, Greenblatt 1988, 75 (on Renaissance medical treatises) articulates the significance of such an innovation. By stimulating and organizing medieval medical discourse on lovesickness and sexuality at an early stage, the *Viaticum* contributed to the "culture's sexual discourse [that] plays an important role in the shaping of identity. It does so by helping to implant in each person a system of dispositions and orientations that governs individual improvisations."

5. Beecher's and Ciavolella's forthcoming (1989) extensive introduction to Jacques Ferrand's *Treatise on Lovesickness* will survey the history of lovesickness from the ancients to the seventeenth century, but its focus, as far as I know, will be on the history of ideas.

6. Quoted in Biesterfeldt and Gutas 1984, 53.

7. The writings preserved in the Hippocratic Corpus do not deal explicitly with morbid love, though the doctrines on melancholy are pertinent antecedents to medical teaching on lovesickness. *Aphorism* 6.23, for example, is a useful reminder of the correlation between emotional state and bodily condition that marks the medical tradition on love: "Fear or depresssion that is prolonged means melancholia"—that is, a condition of black bile. This most pernicious of bodily substances lends its name to the psychological condition accompanying its pathological presence: loss of appetite, sleeplessness, excitation and depression. Klibansky et al. 1964, Flashar 1966, and Pigeaud 1981 provide detailed treatment of melancholy in antiquity. For a modern assessment of the *typus melancholicus*, see Tellenbach 1980; for sleep disturbances, *ibid.* 21–23, 102.

Roman medicine was just as taciturn about lovesickness as early Greek medicine. Celsus (fl. ca. 25 C.E.), whose medical handbook for laymen had a limited transmission in the Middle

Ages (Reynolds 1983), connects black bile with one form of insanity he terms frenzy or *phrenesis*, whose cures are similar to those later developed for lovesickness. Since the body must be rid of the offending substance, Celsus recommends purgation by vomiting, bloodletting, and exercise. Sorrow, too, has its own therapy: the healer should allay the patient's fears and offer good hope. The patient's works should be praised and he should seek out pleasure in stories and games. His groundless sorrow should be gently admonished.

8. *Knight's Tale*, lines 1373–75.

9. Pigeaud 1981, 1987.

10. The problem of boundaries is particularly evident with questions of sexuality. For individual studies in this area see Jacquart and Thomasset 1985b; Green 1985, 1989b (forthcoming); Lemay 1981, 1982; Cadden 1986. Karnein 1985 analyzes the interrelation of imaginative literature, didactic literature, and theology on the subject of passionate love in the twelfth and thirteenth centuries.

11. For a brief introduction to his life and works, see DSB 5:227–37. On the circulation of Galen's works in the Middle Ages, see Beccaria 1959 and Baader 1981.

12. Ed. Heeg 1915, 206–07 (= CMG V 9,2).

13. Translated from the Arabic version into German by Pfaff 1940 (= CMG V 10,2,2), 494–95; I have rendered his version into English.

14. Galen wrote, for example, a treatise entitled *Quod animi mores corporis temperamenta sequuntur* (*That the disposition of the soul follows the temperament of the body*), ed. Marquardt et al. 1964 [1821–33], 2:32–79; trans. Hauke 1937.

15. Nutton 1979 (= CMG V 8,1), 94–95 and 100–103. Though Galen's works on prognostics were not known in the West until the fourteenth century, they considerably influenced the Arabic medical treatises latinized in the eleventh and twelfth centuries, for which see Nutton 1979 and Baader 1981.

16. Gourevitch 1984, 73–77.

17. On Galen's social standing and that of his clientele, see Kudlien 1986, 84–88 and Scarborough 1969, 115–21. On the social status of mimes and pantomimes, see Treggiari 1969, 138 ff., and on the scandal of upperclass women's affairs with them, see Balsdon 1974, 280–81. *Tituli Ulpiani* 13.2 proscribed marriage between freeborn men and actresses; The *Digest of Justinian* 23.2.44 pr. prohibited marriage between, on the one hand, the daughter of a senator or granddaughter by a son or great-granddaughter by a son and grandson, and a freedman or a man who himself or whose father or mother practices or has practiced the stage profession. I would like to thank my colleague Susan Treggiari for her help with the legal and social questions involved.

18. A brief biography and further bibliography may be found in DSB 10:230–31. For an edition of the Greek text, see Raeder 1964 [1926], VIII:8, 249–50; for the Latin, Bussemaker and Daremberg 1876, 6:215. The edition by Mørland 1940 contains only the first two books; apparently it was never completed. Vazquez Bujan 1984 challenges Mørland's localization of the Oribasius translations in Ravenna and proposes southern Italy as their source. Ciavolella 1976, 51–53 discusses both Oribasius' and Paul of Aegina's contributions to the history of the lover's malady.

19. The Latin and Greek versions differ here. According to the Greek (Raeder 1964 [1926], 250), their eyes are filled with pleasure (*hedones*); the Latin MSS (Bussemaker and Daremberg 1876, 6:215) contain *liborem* and *laborem*.

20. Beccaria 1956; Mørland 1932.

21. Beccaria 1956, no. 8; Newton 1976. The point is of interest because Lowes 1913, 523 suggested that the term *amor hereos*, found in many *Viaticum* manuscripts, was not Constantine's doing, but rather must be sought "in some such early Latin translation of a Greek medical text as that which has given us, in the Laon MS of Oribasius, *ton heroton*." For discussion of the problem, see the introduction to the edition of the *Viaticum* in Part 2.

22. From al-Rāzī's *Divisiones* (Lyons, 1510), cap. xi "de amore." For Rufus of Ephesus' treatise on melancholy see Klibansky et al. 1964; Flashar 1966; and Garbers 1977, which contains both Isḥāq ibn ʿImrān's Arabic treatise on melancholy derived from Rufus', and Constantine the African's Latin rendering of the Arabic.

23. Ibn al-Jazzār's work is briefly discussed in chapter 2.

24. Text and translation in Drabkin 1950. Hereafter page numbers from this edition will be given parenthetically in the text. On Cassiodorus' citation and its implications, see Vazquez Bujan, 1984, 661–80. For medieval transmission of the text, see Reynolds 1983, 32–35; for the

translation of Soranus, DSB 12:538–42. Pigeaud 1987, 129–41 contains a full discussion of Caelius Aurelianus on mania.

25. For extensive discussion of Caelius Aurelianus' remedies for mania, see Pigeaud 1987, 145–219.

26. Foucault 1986 discusses the ascetic strains in late Roman medicine and philosophy that surface here in Caelius' work. Brundage 1987 traces the Church's rulings on sexuality, while Cadden 1986 and Jacquart and Thomasset 1985b, 121–32 outline some of the discrepancies between medicine and theology on sexual topics.

27. See Tellenbach 1980, 60 on Abraham's theory that hate, paralyzing the capacity for love, is at the root of manic-melancholic illness. See also Pigeaud 1981, 259–64.

28. Ed. Hett 1937, 30.1. Biesterfeldt and Gutas 1984, 22 point out that "Both the influence of Hippocratic humoral pathology, as standardized by Galen, on the systematic description of mental diseases, and the impact of the *Problemata Physica* [assembled in Alexandria ca. 4–7th c. C.E.] on the form of scientific discussion can be observed in a peripheral part of the field of mental diseases, the malady of love." They further note concerning the *Problemata Physica* that "the subject of love was touched upon by way of explaining the physical manifestations of human affects. These discussions, which made use of humoral reasoning but operated on a more popular level, provided evidence for the psychogenic interpretation of somatic processes." Biesterfeldt and Gutas offer an edition and translation of an Arabic work, surviving in a number of versions, that draws upon the tradition of the *Problemata Physica* to describe the malady of love. Walzer 1962 (1939) erroneously claimed that it represented part of a lost Aristotelian dialogue; as Biesterfeldt and Gutas show, the work is medieval.

29. Kurdziałek 1963, 3–4.

30. Reynolds 1983, 32–35.

31. Talbot 1978, 393.

32. As in, for example, Karlsruhe, Landesbibliothek 120 (Beccaria 1956 no. 56.3). Drabkin 1950, xv discusses Isidore's use of Caelius Aurelianus. For a discussion of melancholy and other mental diseases in Isidore, see Pigeaud 1984.

33. Ed. Lindsay 1911: "Alii Graeca etymologia feminam ab ignea vi dictam putant, quia vehementer concupiscit: Libidinosiores enim viris feminas esse tam in mulieribus quam in animalibus. Vnde nimius amor apud antiquos femineus vocabatur." I would like to thank Monica Green for drawing my attention to this passage.

34. Ed. Heiberg 1912. For the Greek text see Heiberg 1921, and for translations and commentaries Rice 1980, 146–91. Biographical information may be found in DSB 10:417–19. Sharpe 1974 discusses mental disease in the *Epitome*. On the Montecassino MS in Beneventan script, see Beccaria 1956, no. 97.

35. In *Sacerdos ad altare* (Haskins 1924, 372). The medieval reception of Ovid's poetry is a vast topic. In the present context, see Hexter 1986 and Offermans 1970. For a review of literature and discussion of Ovid's importance to twelfth-century clerics who wrote love poetry see Moser 1987. On Ovid in medieval Iceland see Kalinke 1984. For Ovid in twelfth-century monastic culture, see Leclercq 1979, 62–85. More specialized studies include Pellegrin 1957 and Viarre 1966. Schnell 1975 outlines Ovid's influence on "höfische Minnetheorie."

36. A convenient translation of Longinus with commentary is found in Arieti and Crossett, 1985. See also Plutarch's citation of her in his story of lovesickness in the life of Demetrios, 38.1, ed. Flacelière 1977.

37. Oxford, Corpus Christi College MS 189, fol. 14 verso: "Ovidius de remedio amoris dat huiusmodi morbi curam cum dicit sunt fora sunt leges quod tuearis amore."

38. Cf. Jacquart 1984, 98.

39. Blonquist 1987, 1 and 5. The Old French text is edited by Roy 1974.

40. Blonquist 1987, 106.

41. Mesk 1913 offers a thorough analysis of the story in ancient literature; Stechow 1945 traces the motif in art. See Ciavolella 1976, 21 for medieval versions of the story.

42. In addition to the bibliography in n. 2 and the preceding note, see Bright 1987, 234–36, who offers parallels from Seneca's *Controversies* (VI.7), pseudo-Quintilian's *Declamations* (291), and Calpurnius' *Declamations* (46).

43. Ed. Ogle and Schullian 1933.

44. On the manuscript history of Valerius Maximus and his medieval commentators see Reynolds 1983.

45. Dionigi da Borgo San Sepulcro 1470, 5.7 (no foliation). David Anderson kindly brought this commentary to my attention.

46. Fulgentius, ed. Helm 1898, III.2. The passages in Vatican Mythographer I (227) and II (153) may be found in Kulcsár 1987. Vatican Mythographer III (7.3) is printed in Bode 1968 (1834).

47. Leclercq 1982, 75–76. Ciavolella 1976, 31–40 surveys what Church Fathers have to say about morbid love.

48. The story was frequently illustrated. Examples may be found in Laborde 1911, 1:pl. 155 and Robertson 1962, plates 93–95. I would like to thank R. E. Kaske for sharing his research on Amnon and Thamar with me.

49. The Old French translator of Ovid's *Ars amatoria* remarks a number of times on the duplicitous use of lovesickness to win a woman: "One should pretend that one is distressed because of the love for the lady and that one is close to death because of her. Because of this, amorous young men sing and say: 'You who will see her, for God's sake, say to her: / I will die if she does not have mercy on me.'" (Blonquist 1987, 38). See also pp. 67–69 on acquiring a convincing pallor and other symptoms of lovesickness.

50. Laborde 1911, 1:pl. 155: "Hoc significat divites luxuriosos qui omnem voluntatem suam et desiderium volunt facere, et cum non possunt habere quod desiderant, dono vel simulatione verborum illud acquirunt." In addition to the sources in n. 26 above, see Kristeva 1987, 209–33 on "love-hatred in the couple" and the quotation from Hildegard of Bingen in chapter eight, note 1.

51. Freud 1957 (1914), on which Kristeva 1987 is a lengthy meditation.

52. PL 204:539–46.

53. Leclercq 1982, 84–86; Leclercq 1979, 27–61; Ohly 1958.

54. Newton 1976, 41. On Gregory as the "doctor of desire" see Leclercq 1982, 25–34.

55. "Amor languor est et infirmi animi passio." PL 204:53–59.

56. Briefly covered by Pollman 1966, 54–59, and in greater detail by Dronke 1979 and Hunt 1981.

57. Origen's homilies on Canticles are printed in PG 13:35–58; his commentary on Canticles, translated into Latin by Rufinus, appears in PG 13:59–198. Lawson 1957 contains an English translation. On the influence of Origen's exegesis of the Song, see Ohly 1958, 13–27; de Lubac 1959, 1:221–38; and Leclercq 1982, 94–97. On the problem of ambiguity in medieval love language and literature, see Patterson 1987 [1979], 115–53 and Schnell 1985.

58. Lawson 1957, 29. Further quotations (all from Bk. 3 of Origen's commentary on the Song) will be noted parenthetically in the text.

59. PL 15:2030–31. Glorieux 1952 attributes the work to an unknown twelfth-century author (pseudo-Ambrose).

60. Dumeige 1955. See chapter 7 for further discussion of this fascinating treatise.

61. *De anima* 33 in *Opera omnia* 2.192.

62. *Summa aurea* fol. ccc verso.

63. Hendrix 1980a and 1980b. For further discussion, see chapters 3 and 8.

64. A comparison of an early medieval commentary on the Song such as Gregory's with twelfth-century expositions by Gilbert of Hoyland, Baldwin of Canterbury, pseudo-Ambrose (= anonymous twelfth-century author), and Guillaume of St. Thierry shows the influence of a medicalized language of love on religious discourse. For a general discussion of the penetration of secular medicine into religious discourse, see Agrimi and Crisciani 1978, 36–55.

65. John of Fécamp as quoted in the important article of Dinzelbacher 1981, 194. Cf. Brundage 1987, plate 15.

66. Nichols 1983, 110–47.

67. PL 168:1601. On this passage, see Dinzelbacher 1981, 197.

68. Dinzelbacher 1981 and Bynum 1987, 246–59 point out the increase in such experiences from the twelfth century on. Büttner 1983 reproduces a number of medieval paintings depicting such experiences of union with the crucified Christ.

69. Miles 1985, 63–93 analyzes viewers' relations to fourteenth-century Tuscan painting; her discussion of Mary Magdalen is on pp. 80–81. Giotto's Crucifixion in the Scrovegni Chapel, Padua (reproduced in Miles), parallels the work by Niccolò da Bologna reproduced here. Nichols 1983, 120 comments on the Virgin Mary's performing of "the responses the audience is meant to have" in the Clermond-Ferrand *Passion*. "Mary shows us the importance of the human mediating figure in these representations of the Passion. Standing between Christ and the audience, linked to each, she enables the text to generate emotional correlates."

70. Miles 1985, 81.

71. The example of the Dominican is found in the *Vitae fratrum* 4.3.3, ed. Reichert 1897,

158; Leclercq 1982, 52 reports on Julian. See Agrimi and Crisciani 1978, 1–24 for the medieval understanding of the *infirmus* as an *imitator Christi*; Nichols 1983, 117–26 for eleventh-century understandings of *imitatio Christi* and Bynum 1987, 249 and 256–57 on late medieval notions of *imitatio*. Büttner 1983 studies iconographical traditions of *imitatio pietatis*.

72. Quoted from Hatto 1967.

73. Woolf 1962, 12.

74. Guibert's parents' unconsummated marriage was attributed to bewitchment and broken by magic (I.12, Benton 1970, 63–68). Christina of Markyate, a twelfth-century recluse, refused marriage; her mother attempted to break her resolve through love potions (Talbot 1959, 72–75). Blöcker 1982 is a richly-documented study of women and magic, with an emphasis on love magic in the early Middle Ages. Müller 1984 surveys love potions and love magic in medieval literature, while Birchler 1975 examines the connection between love magic and lovesickness in the Renaissance. Canonical and penitential sources are discussed in Peters 1978 and are collected in Lea 1939, 1 and Hansen 1901.

75. E.g., Hansen 1901, 41 (from Burchard of Worms, ca. 1025): "Credidisti aut particeps fuisti illius incredulitatis, ut aliqua femina sit, quae per quaedam maleficia et incantationes mentes hominum permutare possit, id est aut de hodium in amorem aut de amore in hodium."

76. Ed. Dillon 1953; trans. Dillon 1951. Michie 1937 argues that a native tradition of faery love-madness or lovesickness was fused with the medical tradition of lovesickness in the early romances, and that such a fusion is evident in the story of Cú Chulainn's wasting sickness. If the earlier of the two manuscripts containing the story dates to the twelfth century, then Constantine's *Viaticum* or possibly Avicenna's *Canon* are the only likely sources for medical influence. The Irish adaptation of Bernard de Gordon's chapter on *amor hereos* (lovesickness) from the *Lilium medicinae* that Wulff 1932 prints and translates is from a sixteenth-century manuscript; other Irish MSS of the *Lilium* date from the fourteenth and fifteenth centuries. The Middle Welsh story of Math, son of Mathonwy, one of the branches of the *Mabinogi*, opens with an episode of lovesickness. The story is preserved in fourteenth-century manuscripts, but the tale itself is older. See Ford 1977, 1–2 and 91–92.

77. In an important article on women in Celtic society, Ford 1988, 419 explains that he has chosen to call Celtic women "'the opposing sex' because such a designation seems to suggest more clearly a kind of independence and equality with Celtic men, and because it also points to the aggressive and martial natures associated with them; it also suggests quite rightly that sex was the principal instrument of such opposition." Cú Chulainn's visionary experience of victimization and his "unmanning" in sickness (cf. Emer's lament: "A month and a season and a year without sleeping in wedlock") are intelligible as reactions to his initial slighting of his wife in a social context where women are perceived as hostile, powerful (thus able to enact hostility), and sexually threatening.

78. Paraphrased from Blöcker 1982, 14–15.

79. Love magic and lovesickness are surveyed in penitentials, sermons, and texts on magic in Wack 1989; see, too, Blöcker 1982. To the sources in these articles may be added an example from *L'Art d'amours* (Blonquist 1987, 78–79): "[women] think that these herbs move men to love, but they make them mad." Men's fears of being victimized by women's love-magic pervade the surrounding passage. The translator of Ovid enjoins his readers under no circumstances to allow a woman to read his book; he who trusts a woman enough to let her read it "gives her the sword whereby she will do damage to him and to many another valiant man."

80. Ed. Broomfield 1968, 389–90.

81. On the "discovery of love" in the twelfth century, see Dinzelbacher 1981 and Leclercq 1979. Winkler 1989 ("The Constraints of Eros") discusses medical and magical approaches to eros in ancient Greece as forms of control.

## *Chapter Two: Constantine's* Viaticum

1. Walzer 1962 [1939], 50.

2. See, for example, the studies of Gregory 1966, Chenu 1968, and Courtenay 1984.

3. Lawn 1963; Wetherbee 1972.

4. Nemesius is edited by Burkhard 1917. The quotation of the Archpoet is from "Estuans intrinsecus" (Langosch 1975, 258). On elements in twelfth-century medical and philosophical thought, see also McKeon 1961 and Silverstein 1954.

5. On Qustā ibn Lūqā's treatise, see Bono 1984, esp. 92–97, and Thorndike 1923, 1:657–61.

6. Stock 1983, 1984/5, and 1985.

7. See, for example, Benton 1982 and Leclercq 1979.

8. Duby 1988, 143–44.

9. The most recent summaries of Constantine's life are Green 1989b and Bloch 1986, 1:98–110, with references to earlier literature. Bloch prints parallel texts from *De viris illustris* and the *Chronicle* with annotations on 127–34. See also McVaugh 1970; D'Alverny 1982, 421–25; and von Falkenhausen 1984. For Constantine's contributions to intellectual life in the West, see Sudhoff 1932; Schipperges 1964; Baader 1978; Kristeller 1956 (reprinted with additions 1986); and Silverstein 1978.

10. Bloch 1986, 1:99 gives the details of the Salernitan legend; for the Montpellier tradition, see Singer 1917.

11. Singer 1917.

12. On the relations between Constantine and Alphanus, see Kristeller 1986, 27–38 and Bloch 1986, 1:93–98, with references to earlier literature.

13. D'Alverny 1982, 423 questions the common assumption—shared by Bloch 1986—that Constantine was a Muslim.

14. See Cowdrey 1983, Bloch 1972 and 1986, Newton 1976, Creutz 1930 and 1932.

15. Bloch 1986, 1:104 and 135–36 reviews the biographical evidence for Atto in *De viris illustris* and points out that "Romana lingua," which has generally been understood to mean French, can also refer to Latin. For the older view, see Creutz 1932, 428–33.

16. Jacquart and Troupeau 1980, 85–88; Creutz 1930; Lehmann 1930.

17. Wack 1987.

18. There is no edition of the Arabic text. Manuscripts are listed in Ullmann 1970, 147 n. 6 and in Sezgin 1970, 3:305. For biographical information, see Dols 1984, 67–69. Daremberg 1853 translates a number of chapters into French. Bürgel 1978 surveys the general context of medieval Islamic medicine.

Despite the impressive list of Constantine's linguistic accomplishments in the Montecassino chronicle, there is no evidence from his surviving corpus that he worked with any languages other than Arabic and Latin. Earlier scholars, including Lowes 1913/14, 515–16 and 521–34 thought that Constantine either worked from or even created the Greek version of Ibn al-Jazzār's *Zād al-musāfir* known as the *Ephodes*. Recent scholars follow Daremberg 1853, 78 in rejecting a connection between Constantine and the Greek version. See McVaugh 1985, 14–15. The Greek translation of the chapter on lovesickness is printed in the works of Rufus of Ephesus, ed. Daremberg and Ruelle 1879, 582–84; it was also translated into Hebrew in 1259 by Moses ibn Tibbon as *Zedat ha-derachim*. Constantine's Latin version was turned into Hebrew in 1124 (Ullman 1970, 148 and Schipperges 1964, 42).

19. Dugat 1853 translates the chapter on love into French.

20. Noted by Ciavolella 1976, 61. Indeed, a contemporary of Ibn al-Jazzār's, the physician Abū l-Qāsim Ḥalaf ibn al-ʿAbbās al-Zahrāwī (Abulcasis or Alsaharavius, d. ca. 1009), compiled a handbook entitled *Kitāb at-Teṣrīf* that also contained a chapter on ʿishk similiar to Ibn al-Jazzār's (Ullmann 1970, 149–51; Sezgin 1970, 3:323–25; Sarton 1927, 1:651, 681; DSB 14:584–85; Ciavolella 1976, 63–64). The Latin text, translated by Gerard of Cremona, was printed under the title *Liber theoricae necnon practicae Alsaharavii* (Augsburg, 1519). The chapter on love is in the *Lib. pract.*, tract. 1, sect. 2, ca. xvii. The two chapters resemble each other more than they do any of the other discussions of love in Arabic treatises rendered into Latin during the Middle Ages. In the absence of any clear evidence for a connection between the works or their authors, we can only say that they embody one tradition in a flourishing body of Arabic medical thought concerning passionate love.

21. For parallels between *De melancholia* and *Viaticum* I.20, see the text and notes below, Part 2. Garbers 1977 prints both the Arabic and Latin versions of *De melancholia*. There are two important studies of Constantine's *De melancholia*: Creutz and Creutz 1932 and Schipperges 1967a. See also Klibansky et al. 1964, 82–86 and Flashar 1966.

22. Cf. McVaugh's statement (1985, 16–21 and 29) that Arnald of Villanova's focus on *amor hereos* "had the effect of cutting it free from *melancolia*."

23. EI² 4:118–19. See also Bell 1979, esp. 34–45 and 162–67.

24. EI² 4:119.

25. Quoted in Bell 1979, 162–67. On *adab* literature, see Arberry 1953, 11–13; 197–201

are an Arabic literary treatment of lovesickness. Other Arabic stories involving lovesickness found their way into European culture in Petrus Alphonsi's collection *Disciplina clericalis*.

26. Bell 1979, 107–19.

27. On the pseudo-Aristotelian *Problem* 30 (on melancholy), see Klibansky et al. 1964, 15–41.

28. EI² 4:119.

29. Couliano 1987, 16.

30. Couliano 1987, 21.

31. Menocal 1987, 91–113.

32. On Gerard's translations see D'Alverny 1982. For other Arabic treatments of the malady of love, see the important article of Biesterfeldt and Gutas 1984. Graham 1967, 48–50 briefly mentions the mid-eighth-century treatise on mental disorders by Najab ub din Unhammad, *Ashab wa Ullamut*. It contains a chapter on ʿishk, which "gets its name from the word ishka, a creeping plant which wraps around a tree and kills it slowly" (50). Meyerhof 1928 summarizes the section on love in an eleventh-century compendium of medico-philosophical definitions by Ibn Abî Usaibî'â, *Ar-rauda at-tibbiya* (*The Medical Garden*). See too Browne 1962 [1921], 84–88.

33. ". . . artem querentibus litteratoribus inquam et proueccioribus liber pantegni a nobis est propositus . . . Verum propter aliud ad proficuum scilicet questus festinantibus quia in illius magnitudine forsan tediosi uidentur esse, huiusmodi compaciens quoquo modo me exinaniui formam eorum suscipiens simplicitatis. qui tamen si huic libro studiose adquieuerunt, non male succedet eorum exercitus." Quoted from British Library, Egerton 2900, fol. 1.

34. Noted by Daremberg 1853, 81. As Baader 1967 and 1974 has shown, in his translations Constantine hammered out a language which, though not classically elegant, nonetheless contributed significantly to the development of Latin as a vehicle for technical writing. Although the canon of Constantine's works has not yet been fully established, nor their relative chronology worked out, current scholarship is beginning to penetrate the thicket of misattribution, doubtful works, and independently circulating excerpts of larger works. Though this type of research is beset by technical difficulties, beginning with unedited Arabic manuscript sources, continued effort promises to yield even more about Constantine's linguistic and intellectual contributions to the twelfth-century renaissance. Bloch 1986, 1:127–34, 3:1101–02 discusses his canon as contained in Peter the Deacon's list. Still useful are Steinschneider 1866 and Schipperges 1964. On Constantine's contributions to the *Articella*, see the recent work of Kristeller 1986, 144–51. New editions of some of Constantine's smaller works may be found in: Montero Cartelle 1983, Garbers 1977, Green 1987. These editions of various *opuscula* may prove rich sources for the study of Constantine's innovations.

35. On Richard de Bury, see Lowes 1913/14, 528–32; cf. John of Tornamira's (fl. last quarter of 14th century) claim that "proprie tamen amor hereos vertit se ad mulierem propter deliciam carnalem ultimate eis deliciosam habendam" (*ibid.*, 504).

36. My reasons for reading *eros* rather than *heros* or *hereos* are given in the introduction to the edition, Part 2 below.

37. Temkin 1973, 54–55. The location of lovesickness in the brain or the heart becomes controversial in the commentaries of Egidius and Peter of Spain, once medicine came to grips with Aristotelianism in the thirteenth century. For late summaries of the controversy, cf. chapter 9 of Ferrand in Beecher and Ciavolella 1989, and Burton (ed. Jackson 1977), part 3, pp. 57–58.

38. Couliano 1987, 11–12.

39. See the text printed in Part 2.

40. Temkin 1973, 83; a full discussion is on 82–92.

41. Ciavolella 1970 traces the interaction of ancient medicine and literature on the subject of lovesickness.

42. The discussion of love in the theoretical part of the treatise is brief, with no discussion of causality and a short list of symptoms. The chapter on love in the practical part of the *Pantegni* (Lyons 1515, II.99v = lib. 5 practice, cap. 21) is largely taken from the *Viaticum*; it does, however, contain a number of therapeutic medicines that do not appear in the *Viaticum's* chapter on love.

43. These are signalled in the notes to the edition in Part 2.

44. Ed. Daremberg and Ruelle 1876, 306, 320, 508–09. As one of the six "non-naturals" to be regulated for health, coitus was sometimes depicted in health handbooks. See Cogliati

Arano 1976. Klibansky et al. 1964, 86 say that therapeutic intercourse poses an insoluble contradiction between medical and theological or ethical psychopathology. Therapeutic intercourse was still current in the Renaissance. See Leibbrand and Wettley 1961, 160 and Shakespeare's and Fletcher's *Two Noble Kinsmen*, Act V scene ii.

45. The phrase is from Duby 1988, 145. Just as modern medicine until recently has taken the male body as its norm for many experimental studies, so ancient and medieval medicine may have assumed that discussion of the generically male patient obviated the need for discussion of women's lovesickness. Further discussion of women and lovesickness appears in chapters 6 and 8.

46. On the availability of prostitutes, see Otis 1985; Baldwin 1970, 1:133–37; and Bullough and Brundage 1982, 34–42, 176–86.

47. A passage from Avicenna's treatise on ʿishk (Fackenheim 1945) that explains the value of surrounding oneself with good-looking companions (twice enjoined by Constantine):

> For this reason one will never find the wise—those who belong to the noble and learned, and who do not follow the way of those who make greedy and avaricious demands—to be free from having their hearts occupied with a beautiful human form. . . . Therefore the prophet says: *Seek ye satisfaction of your needs in those of beautiful countenance,* the plain meaning of which is that beauty of form is to be found only where there is a good natural composition, and that this good harmony and composition serve to improve the internal disposition and to sweeten the character.

48. See the illustrations in Orofino and Casetti Brach 1984; the discussion in Schipperges 1985, 233–40, "das Badewesen"; and Grotzfeld 1970.

49. See Cosman 1978, 1–36 for recent bibliography, as well as Kümmel 1977.

50. Olson 1982 analyzes therapeutic justifications for literature in the Middle Ages.

51. For a fuller discussion of this text, see Wack 1987. Bloch's suggestion (1986, 1:136) that Atto may have merely polished and improved the style of Constantine's originals, rather than turned them into vernacular poetic versions, raises a possibility I did not sufficiently consider in my article, i.e., that Johannes and Atto collaborated on the *Liber de heros morbo.*

52. I have adapted the last phrase from Winkler's analysis (1982) of the "invention of romance" in Greek culture: "Just as we expect Aristophanic comedy to reverse the roles and violate the boundaries of daily life, and by that expression to reinforce our sense of them, so the emergence of romantic plots in a non-romantic culture is not entirely strange. What most interests me in this is the curious phenomenon that an artistic pattern may endure for a long time in a grey area of irrelevance to actual life and then much later take on new existence as a concrete social norm" (22).

53. The most recent contribution to this debate is Green 1989b. The sheer number of surviving manuscripts is telling: I have located 123 manuscripts of the *Viaticum* earlier than 1400, and I believe that a thorough search of European libraries would uncover more.

54. Kristeller 1986, 36–37.

55. Lawn 1963, 52–54; Sudhoff 1916, 348–56. St. Amand and Durham catalogues are listed in Becker 1885, 233, 243. I would like to thank Monica Green for this and other references to *Viaticum* manuscripts. Kristeller 1980, 9 notes in passing the early and wide diffusion of Salernitan texts.

56. In Seidler 1967, 44–54 and Powicke 1931, 84–85.

57. Schum 1887. The mss are Erfurt Amplonian F 266, Q 174, Q 180, Q 190 and Q 221. Kibre 1946, 257–97 notes that the *Viaticum* is among the medical titles most frequently encountered in late medieval libraries.

58. Cavanaugh 1980, 1:97–99; 1:289; 2:525, 535; 2:667–69; 2:753. See also James 1909, 2–96 for the bequest of John Erghome (75–76).

59. Haskins 1924, 374; *Chartularium universitatis parisiensis,* ed. Denifle and Chatelain 1889–97, 1:no. 453.

60. Bullough 1961, 600–12.

61. Bullough 1961, 604–05. See also Getz 1982.

62. Bullough 1962, and Robb-Smith 1971.

63. McVaugh 1985, 25. On the Montpellier physician Bernard of Gordon's familiarity with the *Viaticum,* see Demaitre 1980, 108–09.

64. MacKinney 1938, 240–68.

65. Sarton 1927, 2:1089–91; for biographical information, see Wickersheimer 1979 [1936], 476–78.

66. Pagel 1894, 14.

67. Wickersheimer 1979 [1936], 634 and Pagel 1894. Pierre's entry for *amor hereos* is found in Pagel 1896, 11.

68. Stock 1983, 12, 99ff., 244–52, and elsewhere (see index s.v. "culture").

69. For medicine as a social process, see Schipperges 1978a, 264 and 1978b, 447–89.

70. See chapter 8 below for examples.

# Chapter Three: Gerard of Berry

1. Hugh of St. Cher, *De doctrina cordis* (ca. 1235), in Hendrix 1980a.

2. On the transformation of medicine in the twelfth and early thirteenth centuries, see Crisciani 1983; Kibre and Siraisi 1982; Talbot 1978; and the articles of Kristeller on the School of Salerno (1976, 1980, 1986). Bullough 1966 traces the development of the medical profession.

3. Literature on Ovid in the Middle Ages is cited in chapter 1, note 38. For the *Liber de heros morbo* see Wack 1987.

4. I have found the investigations of Karnein 1985, who studies the *Wirkungsgeschichte* of *De amore*, useful for my assessment of Andreas. Jacquart 1984 places Gerard of Berry and Andreas in the same Parisian milieu, and asserts Gerard's familiarity with the *De amore* based on the similarities of their definitions of love.

5. Erfurt, Wissenschaftliche Allgemeinbibliothek, F 266, CA 174, CA 180, CA 190, CA 221. For descriptions see Schum 1887.

6. Gerard's commentary on the *Viaticum* and/or his chapter on love were used by Peter of Spain (see chapter 5), Arnald of Villanova (McVaugh 1985, 27), William of Brescia (Corvi) in the *Practica* (Venice 1508, fol. 23r), Bernard de Gordon (Demaitre 1980, 84; there are a number of borrowings from Gerard in Bernard's discussions of *amor hereos*), and John of Gaddesden (Littré 1847, 405). Jacquart and Thomasset 1985b, 120 note that "la passion 'héro-ïque' stimula la pensée médicale et l'aida à préciser les liens qui unissent états mentaux et mécanismes physiologiques." As far as surviving evidence allows us to judge, Gerard of Berry was the first to attempt this synthesis.

7. On the implications of the title *physicus* (rather than *medicus*) see Kristeller 1986, 43–48. Previous biographical notices of Gerard include: Littré 1847, 21:404–08; Pignol, 1889; Wickersheimer 1979 [1936], 1:203; Jacquart 1979, 92–93; De Renzi 1967 [1857], 402–09.

8. Basel D.III.6 is the earliest dated manuscript; for a description see the introduction to the edition, part 2 below. On the dating of Hugh of St. Cher's (pseudo-Gerard of Liège) *De doctrina cordis*, see Hendrix 1980a. Hugh's quotations from Gerard of Berry are given in note 61 below.

9. The text is in De Renzi 1859, 5:289: "Frater (sic) Salernitanorum sive Lumbardorum qui vocatur Arpia de quo Girardus sexto viatici capitulo de egressione secundine loquens de hoc dicit, argumentum huius rei talis est." Compare Gerard's statement in the *Glosule* (Basel D.III.6, fol. 64v): "De egressione secundine. *Postquam ergo peperit.* capitulum illud est de egressione secundine. eggresso enim fetu a matrice secundina retinetur aliquando uero per se solam, aliquando uero cum plurimo sanguine menstruoso non educto quam educi oportet, aliquando cum peccude, que peccus apud lombardos dicitur arpia. peccus enim ista apud quasdam gentes generatur in matrice et nutritur cum embrione sicut apud illos qui fructibus, radicibus, et herbis nutriuntur, ut sunt lombardi. est autem peccus ista similis bufoni et appellatur talis fetus frater lombardorum."

10. De Renzi 1858, 329, followed by Pifferi 1962, 5.

11. De Renzi 1852, 1:282–86; 1853, 2:779–80; 1857, 402–09.

12. See Lawn 1963, 67–72 on Parisian medicine at this time.

13. See D'Alverny 1957 and 1982, and Van Riet 1972, 95*.

14. The texts are given in the notes in Lawn 1979, 285–87. For the dating of the Salernitan masters, see Kristeller 1980. Though these authors discuss the same phenomenon of the *arpia* or *frater lombardorum* there are not enough verbal echoes with Gerard's passage to make the direction of borrowing or influence clear.

15. Lawn 1979, 285–87. Gilles de Corbeil refers to the "fratrem Salernum" in *De compositis medicamentis* 4.664–719 (ed. Choulant 1826) and claims that the "gens Beneventana"

wrongly ascribed it to the Salernitans so that they might have companions in shame. Lawn dates Gilles' poem around 1194 (1963, 71).

16. Specific parallels to the works of Urso and Maurus are given below, nn. 22 and 27. On the commentary form at Salerno, see Kristeller 1976, 1980, 1986.

17. McVaugh 1985, 24–25.

18. D'Alverny 1957, 80; Demaitre 1975, 104–05. However, if Montpellier were the site of Gerard's encounter with Avicenna's works, it is odd that Avicenna's *Canon* does not appear in the earliest attested Montpellier discussion of lovesickness, Arnald of Villanova's *Liber de amore heroico* (ca. 1260–70); see McVaugh 1985, 24–25.

19. Vieillard 1909; Sudhoff 1928; Lawn 1963, 69–71.

20. "Licet autem auctor iste ualde plane et aperte in pluribus locis procedere uideatur, ita uidelicet ut nulla expositione penitus egeat in superficie intuenti, uerumptamen si quis exquisite perscrutari desiderat, difficultatem multam reperiet in causis, signis et curis passionum."

21. See Kristeller 1976, 1980 on the *accessus* among twelfth-century Salernitan physicians and commentators. Gerard's prologue survives in a shorter and longer form, called in some manuscripts *prologus maior* and *prologus minor*, a terminology I have adopted. Both prologues are printed in the Venice 1505 edition of Gerard of Solo's works. The shorter form abbreviates the initial theoretical overview and differs in its phrasing in a number of places, though the overall content is roughly the same.

22. "Cum omne elementum et ex elementis corpus generatum in materia communitatem habeant, satis est euidens quod per modum agendi et paciendi mutuo nata sunt sese adinuicem permutare. Corpus ergo humanum ex predictis motus et immutationes non effugit non solum secundum affectationes et dispositiones plurimas quas appetit materierum diuersitas, sed etiam secundum passiones illas ratione quarum medicinalis artifex corpus humanum considerat ut subiectum. Cum igitur predictus artifex speculetur omne sic immutans illud per quem illud habet sibi subiacere, ex necessitate consequitur quod omne elementum ex elementis corpus generatum ab eodem cognosci et considerari habeant quodam modo ut in quibus cause subiecti et passionum suarum repperit evidenter" (Basel D.III.6, fol. 1r). This passage appears to echo a number of Salernitan discussions of the elements, including Bartholomaeus, *Glossa in Johannitium* (Kristeller 1976, 85): "Tercia pars huius scientie medicina dicitur. hec quidem de actionibus et passionibus elementorum in commixtis corporibus pertractat. Licet enim gratia humani corporis inventa fuerit, nichilominus tamen de omnibus humanum corpus immutantibus agit et disserit . . ."; Maurus' commentary on Hippocrates' *Aphorisms* (De Renzi 1852–59, 4:34–35): "Cum omne corpus animatum vel inanimatum, sensibile vel insensibile a lunari globo contentum et ab elementis aliud ex quatuor elementorum conficiatur commixtionibus, tanta in uno-quoque eorum extitit quantitas, quanta sue compositionis modum extitit necessitas. . . ."; and Urso, *Glosulae* 25, 37 (Creutz 1936).

23. On glossing as a form of textual commentary see Kenny and Pinborg 1982, and on medical glosses at Salerno, Kristeller 1976, 1980.

24. See the discussion of "selective will" and "hermeneutic filters" in Couliano 1987, 11–12.

25. Noted by Wack 1982 and, more cautiously, by McVaugh 1985. Van Riet 1968, 1972 contains a modern critical edition of Avicenna's *De anima*. For detailed comparison of Gerard's text with its sources, see the edition below in part 2. For further discussion of the inner wits, see Harvey 1975 and Wolfson 1973.

26. McVaugh 1985, 23. In Avicenna's scheme, the *virtus imaginativa*, located in the second ventricle, is not to be confused with *imaginatio*, located in the first. In contrast Urso locates the *virtus fantastica* in the first ventricle in *Glosula* 41 (Creutz 1936).

27. Translated from Lawn 1979, 275–76. Compare the similar accounts in Urso's *Glosses on Aphorisms* (Creutz 1936), nos. 24, 84 and 85, and the case noted in PSQ P 95 (Lawn 1979, 242).

28. For a fuller account of the Salernitan theories and their probable use by Andreas Capellanus, see Wack 1986a.

29. All emphases are mine. In *De anima* I.5 Avicenna uses similar metaphorical terms. In discussing which faculties rule (*imperant*) others, and which serve (*famulantur*), he says, for example: Two faculties serve (*deserviunt*) the estimation; the appetitive faculty serves the imaginative faculty with obedience (*deservit cum oboedientia*); the estimative orders (*imperat*) others. Gerard's retention of this language of service and rule is significant; its implications will be argued below.

30. Bloch 1983, 17–18, 223–27. An important essay in this connection is Benton 1982.

31. Bloch 1983, 17.

32. See chapter 1 and note 60 below.

33. Jacquart and Thomasset 1985b, 15–28; Bloch 1983, 54–57.

34. The semantic development of *hereos* has been discussed by Lowes 1913; Ciavolella 1976; Agamben 1977; Jacquart and Thomasset 1985a.

35. Wack 1987.

36. Montero Cartelle 1983, 160.

37. Constantinus Africanus, *De melancholia* 1536, 283.

38. Kurdziałek 1963, 3–4. David of Dinant's "Aristotelian notebooks" (*Quaternuli*) were condemned in Paris in 1210 as heretical; all copies were to be burned. Though four manuscript fragments have survived, it is difficult to tell what kind of circulation the text had before the ban.

39. Rocha Pereira 1973 prints the text; cf. Wack 1989a for a brief discussion of this point.

40. I have used the text and translation in Walsh 1982, though I have occasionally modified the translation. Further references to this edition are given in the text. On Andreas' psychology of love, see Karnein 1985 and Wack 1986a. Jacquart and Thomasset 1985a, 1985b and Jacquart 1984 explore the intersections of medical and literary views of love and sexuality. Jacquart and Thomasset 1985b, 135–52 suggest that Andreas' text offers an important step in the mastery of sexuality in the Middle Ages by advocating the technique of *coitus interruptus*.

41. Wack 1986a.

42. Karnein 1985, 106–07, 262–66.

43. Leclercq 1979; Dinzelbacher 1982; Schnell 1985, 18–40.

44. The passage may be found in Ewart 1960, 13–14, lines 393–436. The translation is from Burgess and Busby 1986, 48–49.

45. Quoted from Blonquist 1987, 67; cf. 38 for another recommendation to feign love-sickness. The Old French may be found in Roy 1974, 152 and 114. Andreas Capellanus notes: "He who is troubled by the thought of love finds it harder to sleep and eat" and that the loss of sleep caused by love induces poor digestion and great physical weakness (3.57–58).

46. Speroni 1974, 272: ". . . quant il est devant vous simples, pensis, plains de souspirs, et face uns regars piteus et amoureus, et samble, quant il vous regarde, k'il doive plourer en riant: saciés que c'est une des plus beles et des plus vraies espreuves c'on puis trouver en son ami, s'il aime de cuer u non."

47. I have used the reprint edition (1964) of the *Canon medicine* originally published in Venice 1507. The relevant section is liber 3, fen 1, tract. 4, cap. 23 and 24.

48. McVaugh 1985, 24–30.

49. Because Gerard did not conflate Avicenna with Constantine uncritically, as his attempt at causal analysis shows, I am inclined to view his adoption of Avicennan symptoms as deliberate choices that can be interpreted as symptomatic of the social and intellectual energies shaping his interpretation of the *Viaticum*.

50. Hatto 1960, 42. The Middle High German text may be found in Marold and Schröder 1969, 2–3, lines 81–122.

51. Walsh 1982, 296–98 = 3.36–37. Origen's description of *amor languens* (*Commentary on the Song of Songs*, Bk. 3) is conveniently translated in Lawson 1957, 198: ". . . he yearns and longs for Him by day and night, can speak of nought but Him, would hear of nought but Him, can think of nothing else . . ."

52. These are handily collected in Karnein 1985, 288–301. Gerard's symptom corresponds to *Hec sunt duodecim signa* no. 2 ("Qui videre non potest eum vel eam, libenter audit loqui de eo vel ea"); *La Regle des Fins amans* no. 6 ("Li .vj. est oïr volentiers la parole de son ami").

53. The gender presumptions of medical discourse on lovesickness are treated more fully in chapter 6. Cf. Bona Fortuna's comment (below, part 2) that the physician ought to describe to the patient "the rejection and hate of his friends that will result from such madness."

54. Despars 1498, fol. Niii recto and following. For biographical information on Despars, see Jacquart 1980. Cf. Bona Fortuna's recommendation (below, part 2) that patients be treated "as we do boys whom we teach the ABCs without blows but with all gentleness, and whom we promise nuts, apples, and other things."

55. For stereotypes of women and the feminine in a context relevant to my analysis, see Bynum 1982, 110–69; Bynum 1987, 216–17, 266–73. Andreas Capellanus' Book 3 is a thesaurus of negative stereotypes about women.

56. Despars 1498, fol. Niii recto ff.; Andreas 303–13; for Boccaccio, see Branca 1964, 2:224.

57. On the metaphoric significance of symptoms see Sontag 1979; Kristeva 1985, 19–20 and 1987, 23; and Douglas 1975, 83: "The body communicates information for and from the social system in which it is a part. It should be seen as mediating the social system in at least three ways. It is itself the field in which a feedback interaction takes place. It is itself available to be given as the proper tender for some of the exchanges which constitute the social situation. And further, it mediates the social structure by itself becoming its image." Zola 1983 [1966] points out that the correspondence or divergence of signs and symptoms with a culture's major values accounts for the degree of attention they receive from patients and physicians; the West, in contrast to some other societies, is characterized by a high insistence on rationality and control. Thus to the extent that symptoms reveal a loss of rationality or control (traits of the feminine and/or infant in Western culture) they become worthy of medical notice.

58. Leube-Fey 1971, 138–46 and cf. Andreas in Walsh 1982, 44, 174, 198.

59. "Li premiers signes de vraie amour si est loiaus cuers, qui ne peut riens celer vers son ami" (Karnein 1985, 290). Cf. *Hec sunt duodecim signa* no. 11 ("Secretum servat nec denudat"); *La Rigle des Fins amans* no. 3 ("Li tiers est regehir et descourvrir souvent son cuer a son ami"); *Lez xij choses especialz qui apertient a amor* no. 9 ("Li nueuiesmes est couvrir lou secreit de son amin. Sallemons dist: qui descueure lou secreit de son amin, il pert foit").

60. Karnein 1985, 93–100.

61. Hendrix 1980a contains a modern edition of the text. Hugh's borrowings from Gerard may be clearly seen below:

| Hugh of St. Cher,<br>De doctrina cordis | Gerard of Berry,<br>Glosule super Viaticum |
| --- | --- |
| "De scissione cordis per amorem"<br>Sumitur alio modo amor extaticus pro amore mentem alienante secundum quod extasis dicit alienationem, qui scilicet amor apud medicos amor ereos appellatur. Est autem amor ereos magnum desiderium cum nimia concupiscentia et afflictione cogitationum. Ereos dicuntur viri nobiles qui propter mollitiem et delicias vite subiecti sunt huiusmodi passioni. | [Constantine, *Viaticum*]<br><br>heroes dicuntur uiri nobiles qui propter diuicias et mollitiem uite tali pocius laborant passione. (57–59) |
| Secundum signum amoris extatici est desiccatio membrorum. Amorosi etiam aresciunt in membris eo quod vehementi cordis applicatione circa rem dilectam multiplicantur spiritus ex quo interiorem desiccationem patiuntur. | Omnia membra eius arefiunt. (41; cf. 23–28) |
| Tertium signum amoris extatici est concavitas oculorum. Consueverunt enim amorosi habere oculos concavos seu profundos quia oculi secuntur spiritus sese retrahentes et concurrentes ad locum estimative. | profundatio oculorum, quia secuntur spiritus currentes ad locum estimatiue. (34–36) |
| Quartum signum amoris extatici est siccitas oculorum, carentia lacrimarum nisi fletus adveniat ex parte rei dilecte. | Item siccitas occulorum et priuatio lacrimarum nisi adueniat fletus ex parte rei desiderate. (36–37) |
| Sunt autem duo que lacrimas ab amantibus excutere consueverunt. Primum sunt cantilene amoris et musica instrumenta. Quando remoti sunt a re dilecta tunc enim coguntur rei amate recordari. | Sed tamen flet cum audit amoris cantilenas. (39–40) |
| Secundum quod excutit lacrimas ab amante est cum de separatione rei dilecte perterretur. | et precipue si fiat mentio de repudio et de separatione rerum dilectarum. (40–41) |
| Quintum signum amoris extatici est pulsus inordinatus. Omnis enim amorosus pulsus habet aut nimis tardum et rarum aut nimis frequenter | Pulsus eius inordinatus, quia aliquando frequens et velox dum res consimiles rei dilecte commemorantur. (42–43) |

et velocem secundum diversas apprehensiones quas habet de amato. Tardus est enim pulsus amantis dum desperat de dilecto habendo, velox dum sperat se a re amate vicem amores reportare.

| | |
|---|---|
| Sextum signum amoris extatici est profunda cogitatio et sollicitudo versa ad interiora, ita quod talis amorosus gerere videtur ymaginem dormientis qui evigilare non potest nisi cum de re amata fit ei mentio. Unde si cum amoroso loquaris de hiis que inter homines fiunt, que ad rem amatam non pertinent, vix intelligere potest. Si autem de re amata vel quod ad rem amatam aliquo modo pertineat statim intelligit et evigilantis gerit ymaginem eo quod tota intentio et cogitatio sua fixa est in re amata, adimata desiderio. | Ex parte anime sunt profunde cogitationes et sollicitudines, ut si quis de aliquo loquatur, vix intelliget, si autem de eodem, statim mouetur. (31–34)<br><br><br><br><br><br>tota intentio et cogitatio defixa est in pulchritudine alicuius forme uel figure desiderio coadiuuante. (3–5) |
| Septimum signum amoris extatici est quod animus tali amori subiectus cum videt rem rei amate similem quasi insanire videtur. | cum uidet consimilem rei desiderate magis mouetur et insanit. (68–69) |

If I am correct in my conjecture as to the identity of Egidius (see chapter 4), then Hugh's use of Gerard's commentary may have been facilitated by the Dominican studium in Paris ca. 1220–30. If Egidius is Giles of Portugal, a.k.a. Giles of Santarem, who studied and then taught medicine in Paris in the 1220s, then he may have been the one to alert Parisian Dominican circles to the importance of the *Viaticum* and Gerard's commentary. Egidius entered the order at about the same time as, and was closely connected with, Humbert of Romans, who in turn was a student and friend of Hugh of St. Cher.

62. Patterson 1987 (1979), 132.

63. Speroni 1974, 252: ". . . nepourquant, je me sui souvent aperceüs de le grant valour et de le grant douchour d'amours, que la ou je perdoie le boire et le mengier, le dormir et le reposer par destrece de bien amer, l'esperance de mon desirrier me confortoit, si que il me sambloit que ce ne me coustoit riens: ains, me plaisoit tant k'il me sambloit que il n'estoit autres paradis que d'amer par amours."

64. Otis 1985 and Brundage 1987, 203–07, 210–12, 308–11, 314–19 and *passim*. See also his plates 3, 4 and 8.

65. Despars 1498, fol. N iv recto and verso.

66. Jacquart and Thomasset 1985b situate *amor hereos* among a network of cultural problems including the relations between body and soul; the philosophy and theology of freedom and repression; and the physiology and psychology of pleasure. They argue that medicine both collaborated and conflicted with theology, and that within the space of medical discourse an *ars erotica* developed. See Figure 4.1 in Brundage 1987 for an amusing summary of the Church's restrictions on sexual activity.

67. E.g., that the lover distract himself with other women (*Remedia amoris* 441–44).

68. Cf. the illustrations of baths in Brundage 1987, plates 3 and 4.

69. *Lilium medicinae* (Lyons 1574), cap. 20; Lowes 1913/14, 497–502 prints most of the chapter, including the shock treatment alluded to here, in which a disgusting old crone thrusts a bloody menstrual cloth in the lover's face and says: "This is what your girlfriend is like!" See also Demaitre 1980, 26–27.

70. Bloch 1977, 231–58; 1983, 226.

71. Blonquist 1987, 18–19; Roy 1974, 88.

72. Speroni 1974, 265.

73. Speroni 1974, 269–71.

74. Speroni 1974, 275.

75. The point will be argued at length in chapter 8.

76. Freud's opinion (1957 [1914], 88) that men's sexual love entails overestimation of the desired object and hence an idealization of it is both a modern reformulation of this medieval

insight and its historical consequence. Kristeva 1987, 267 argues that "the amatory experience rests on *narcissism* and its aura of emptiness, seeming, and impossibility, which underlays any *idealization* equally and essentially inherent in love," and that the moral, religious, and psychological crisis of our time is related to the fact that "the social consensus gives *little* or *no* support" to the possibilities for idealization.

77. Hatto 1967, 42. In a study of humility in Old Provençal and early Italian poetry, Kittel 1973, 163 argues that the active humility of Christ and the receptive humility of the Virgin influenced the images of the ideal lady and her lover: the *lady* is heir to the "active, masculine virtues" while "the lover's devotion has some of the passive, receptive quality of the Virgin's humility."

78. Wack 1984.

79. Moi 1986, 19 is concerned with the political implications of courtliness when she argues that: "The whole point of the various courtly and chivalric exercises described in Andreas's and Chrétien's texts was to escape all comparison with villeins. Signalling their cultural superiority, the 'effeminisation' of the aristocracy paradoxically comes to signify their 'natural' right to power. It is precisely in its insistence on the 'natural' differences between rulers and ruled that courtly ideology achieved its legitimising function, a function which operates long after the feudal aristocracy has lost its central position in society."

## Chapter Four: Giles

1. The work is preserved in a unique manuscript: Gerona, Archivo Capitular, Codex (78 or 75) 20, e, 11, fols. 1–25. The microfilm I have used has two signature cards, one of which indicates that the old number was 78, the other 75.

2. Biographical information may be found in Reichert 1897, 154–56 (the thirteenth-century Dominican *Vitae fratrum*); *Scriptores ordinis praedicatorum* 1:241–44; *Acta sanctorum* Mai III (1680), 402–38; Kaeppeli 1970, 1:15–16.

3. *Acta sanctorum* Mai III (1680), 404 ff.

4. Reichert 1897, 154–55. If Egidius is Giles of Portugal, then he must have known his fellow Dominican Hugh of St. Cher; this may help to explain Hugh's knowledge of the *Viaticum* and Gerard of Berry's commentary on it.

5. Quoted from Schullian and Sommer 1948, 235.

6. For an account of the troubles, see Van Steenberghen 1955, 78–88. Since, according to De Rijk 1972, Peter of Spain studied in Paris in the 1220s and left for the north of Spain in 1229, as did Giles, he may have crossed paths with his fellow countryman either in Paris or en route to Spain.

7. Jacquart and Troupeau 1980.

8. Albertus Magnus can be used as a case in comparison. Though he drew upon Peter's *Questiones super de animalibus* for his own *Quaestiones* on that book, in some cases he also established clearer distinctions, defined ideas more sharply, and enlarged the problems (Goldstein-Préaud 1981, 69). When read side by side, one could not mistake the Madrid version of Peter's text (in Madrid, Biblioteca Nacional MS 1877) for the later of the two. So too with Egidius and Peter of Spain. In comparison with Peter's, Giles's questions seem, if not a step backwards, then at least quite simple. Given Bazàn's remark (1985, 141) that "la question disputée est un des instruments les plus importants qu'ils [les maîtres] se sont donnés pour affirmer cette liberté [intellectuelle] et cette conscience de soi, et pour chercher leur lieu propre dans l'histoire des idées," it is difficult to see why, if Giles is the later of the two, he did not crib more from Peter. Giles could only have benefited by using Peter's arguments as a point of departure. I take Bazàn's point (1985, 140) that prudence is called for when attributing texts, since "Dialogue et communication d'arguments et de formules établissaient dans un groupe universitaire une certaine communauté de style entre les maîtres." It is possible that the commentaries (especially in the section on *amor*) of Giles (whoever he was) and Peter of Spain are not directly related, but draw upon a common body of scholastic questions that has not survived in other sources.

9. The other Aristotelian text that I have been able to trace in the commentary is *De anima*. Giles' other authorities include: Galen (*Tegni, De simplicis medicinis*; *Super afforismos*); Isaac Judaeus ("in *Dietis*"); Haly ('Alī ibn al-'Abbās); Hippocrates (*Prognostics*; *Afforismos*); Avicenna; Rasy (al-Rāzī); and Alexander.

10. Though Thorndike 1965, 24 says that Michael Scot's translation of *De animalibus* was completed by 1220 at the latest, Wingate 1931, 72–78 fixes the date between 1200 and 1210, and claims that it "achieved a rapid diffusion in the schools." D'Alverny 1982, 437 notes that traces of Aristotelian works show up before the known versions of the thirteenth century (Michael Scot's and William of Moerbeke's). In what follows I have assumed the later dates for *De animalibus* (i.e., 1217–20), but whether earlier or later, Giles would have had no trouble quoting it in the 1220s.

11. Ferreiro Alemparte 1983, 205. He discusses Giles, "the Portuguese Faust," on 220–21. Despite his caution that "Es inútil pretender apurar más el núcleo histórico que sospechamos oculto en la leyenda," I have nonetheless ventured a plausible guess.

12. Note 7 above.

13. Though Wingate 1931, 72–78 notes a number of authors who used Michael Scot's translation before 1230, it became the subject of extensive interest after 1230 or 1235. Peter of Spain's *Questiones super de animalibus*, the earliest surviving commentary on that work, seems to have developed in two stages according to Goldstein-Préaud 1981: the Madrid version was apparently compiled in Paris (thus before 1245, according to Goldstein-Préaud, but if De Rijk's chronology is right, then before 1229), and the Florence version after 1248.

14. Bazàn 1985, 29.

15. Jacquart in Bazàn et al. 1985, 285–93.

16. *Ibid.*

17. In the first book Giles takes up, for example, the topics of PSQ P 31; N 17; B 231, 247; and B 188. More extensive study of the treatise may reveal more embedded Salernitan questions.

18. Bazàn 1985, 141.

19. The fact that Egidius, like Gerard of Berry, uses *heros* and *herosis* (*hereos* appears only once) suggests to me that his commentary is to be placed in the first half of the thirteenth century, antedating Peter of Spain's (ca. 1246–50), in which *amor hereos* consistently appears.

20. The unstated Aristotelian premise (from *Categories* 14a 15) of the question appears in Peter of Spain's Version A: "It is clearly the nature of contraries to belong to the same thing (the same either in species or genus)" (Barnes 1984). For a general discussion of the challenges to Galenic medicine posed by Aristotle's biology, see Siraisi 1981, 186–202. Elsewhere in the commentary Giles engages with Aristotelian biology. He takes up, for example, topics that occupied David of Dinant at length, that Peter of Spain addressed a number of times, and that attracted interest until the anatomical discoveries of the sixteenth and seventeenth centuries. Do women's sexual organs contain *testiculos* (gonads) analogous to men's? Do women contribute seed to conception? And what is the relation of their sexual pleasure to fertility? At one point he quotes Aristotle "in libro de animalibus" to the effect that since women do not have a seminal discharge, they do not have *testiculos*. In the chapters on sexual disorders Giles is concerned to establish that women do in fact have *testiculos* and to clarify what menstrual blood contributes to the embryo and fetus.

21. Van Steenberghen 1955, 66–77.

22. Kurdziałek 1963, 36–38: "Omnis autem affectus fit cum compassione cordis; nec sine cordis passione potest fieri affectus in anima. Dubitabile est autem, utrum propter passionem cordis fiat affectus in anima, aut propter affectum anime sit pasio in corde. . . . accidit quoque morbus aut etiam mors ex nimio timore aut amore aut quolibet alio affectu. Manifestum est igitur, quod licet passio cordis et affectus simul tempore fiant, passio tamen cordis causa est affectus, qui fit in anima. Dico, quod passio illa est immutatio diastoles et sistoles cordis . . . Rursus autem in amore fit velocior cordis dilatatio, tardior vero constrictio, tardior vero dilatatio pulsus arterie qui profundus sentitur."

23. See chapter 1 and Pigeaud 1981 and 1987. Cadden 1986, 165 notes that Bernard of Gordon raised this issue explicitly. In answer to the question "Should a physician *qua* physician take accidents of the soul into consideration?" Bernard "reiterates the position of Galen that, while properly the domain of philosophy, mental, emotional, and spiritual considerations affect health and are therefore appropriate subjects of a physician's practice."

24. The process is described in David of Dinant's Latin paraphrase of pseudo-Aristotle's *Problem* 30 on melancholy, ed. Kurdziałek 1963, 3–4.

25. This was a topic of the Salernitan questions: see Lawn 1963, Q 119 and note; Lawn 1979, P 21.

26. Note 1 above, fol. 1v.

27. "Aut nulla ebrietas / aut tanta sit, ut tibi curas / eripiat: si qua est inter utrumque, nocet."

## Chapter Five: Peter of Spain

1. Quoted from Favati 1957. "In that part where memory is [love] takes its place . . . Its essence is when desire is so great that it goes beyond the measure of nature; then it is no more adorned with repose. It moves, changing color, (from) laughing to weeping, and distorts the face with fear; it rests little. Moreover you will see that it is found most among people of worth" (trans. Bird 1940).

2. Bird's edition of Dino's commentary (1940, 1941), which contains extensive discussion of both the poem and the commentary, should be supplemented by Favati's corrections (1952). Fontaine 1985 surveys the commentaries on the poem. Nardi 1959 and Ciavolella 1970, 1976 discuss the commentary's relation to the tradition of lovesickness.

3. For biographical information on Peter of Spain, see notes 6–8. The two versions of his commentary are edited separately in Part 2 below. Suggestive parallels between Guido's poem and Peter's questions include:

| Cavalcanti | Peter of Spain |
|---|---|
| stanza I lines 2–3 | Version A lines 83–94 |
| II.15–16 | Version B 26–29, 168–69 |
| II.19–20 | A 83–94 |
| IV.43–50 | B 20–25, 34–45 |
| V.57–58 | A 215–31 |
| V.63–67 | A 30–54, B 170–78 |

My point is not to prove that Cavalcanti knew Peter's *Questions*, but rather to underscore their convergence on the common ground of a philosophical (specifically Aristotelian) analysis of love.

4. Peter's possible relation with Giles of Santarem (Aegidius Portugalensis) is treated in chapter 4, note 6. On his use of the Salernitan questions see Lawn 1963.

5. The quotation is from De Rijk 1972, XLI. Da Rocha Pereira 1973 contains an edition of the *Thesaurus pauperum*. *Amor hereos* does not appear among the diseases contained in the *Thesaurus*, though it does contain quasi-magical remedies for love, on which see Wack 1989a.

6. For Peter's place in scholasticism, see Ferreira 1960 and Grabmann 1979 [1936]; for a brief summary of opinions on Peter's philosophical achievements, see da Cruz Pontes 1968 and Craveiro da Silva 1977.

7. In my summary of Peter's life, I follow the chronology and conjectures of De Rijk 1972, IX–XLIII. Still useful is the monograph of Stapper 1898. Recent reviews of research on Peter of Spain include Craveiro da Silva 1977 and D'Alverny's review (1976) of da Cruz Pontes 1972. Older bio-bibliography appears in Sarton 1927, 2:889–92.

8. Though the chronology in Schipperges 1961a and 1973, 3:679–91 needs revision, his eloquent appreciation of Peter's achievements in medicine offer a valuable introduction to his *opera*.

9. Kibre and Siraisi 1978, 128.

10. The canon of Peter's writings is still uncertain. Alonso 1961 lists most of Peter's works in the introduction (pp. XI–XXII). The commentary on Isaac's *De febribus*, listed by Amplonius Ratinck as Peter's (Erfurt, Wissenschaftliche Allgemeinbibliothek Q 212, fols. 109–64) and listed in TK[2] 1421 as his, does not appear in Alonso's list. Alonso 1957 places Peter's commentary on the works of pseudo-Dionysius in this same period (1246–50).

11. For a general survey of the early reception of Aristotle, see Birkenmajer 1970 [1930], 73–87. For Peter's role in the process, see Grabmann 1979 [1929], 1:480–95 and Schipperges 1964, 177–85.

12. Grabmann 1979 [1929] 1:482.

13. Paravicini Bagliani 1981.

14. Da Cruz Pontes 1977, 1981 and Schipperges 1968 discuss the multiple versions of several of Peter's works.

15. There are not only two versions, A and B, but also two different forms of the B version. While the variations among the manuscripts of the B version (discussed in the introduction to the edition, part 2) may involve copyists' abridgements and expansions, no such explanation accounts for the differences between A and B. Though "A" and "B" imply a chronological relationship, the priority of either version will not be argued here, since the chapter on *amor hereos* alone is insufficient evidence from which to determine the priority of one version with certainty. In my limited study of the manuscripts' contents, I have found no cross references from one version to the other, though perhaps study of other chapters will reveal something of this sort. Further research into the manuscript tradition of Peter's medical works is needed to settle the question.

16. On the various types of questions and disputations in medieval universities, see Bazàn et al. 1985.

17. E.g. Oxford, Corpus Christi College 189 (s. 12[2]), fol. 4v: "ait quidam philosoffus amor est mentis insania . que vagum animum ducit per inania . sitit leticias et bibit tristicia crebris doloribus permiscit gaudia." The annotation is in a late twelfth- or early thirteenth-century hand. The poem also occurs in Bethesda, National Library of Medicine, MS 12, fol. 17r.

18. Moser 1986 and Speroni 1974, 250 and notes (on Richard of Fournival's *Consaus d'amours*) discuss this poem's sources and variants.

19. Lyons, 1574, p. 219: "Ultimo intelligendum, quod ista passio pulcherrimo modo potest describi sic: Amor est mentis insania, quia animus vagatur per *maniam cerebri*, doloribus permiscens pauca gaudia [emphasis mine]." Comparison with Peter's version suggests that the sixteenth-century editor of Bernard may have printed a garbled version of the poem: "Amor est mentis insania qua vagatur animus per *inania crebris* doloribus permiscens gaudia" (Version B, lines 11–12).

20. *Recepte super prima tertii Canonis Avicennae*, New York Academy of Medicine Library, MS (apparently unnumbered; cf. de Ricci 1937, 1312 no. 9), fol. 61r: "De hermete et est species melancholie qua vehemente quis contrahat cum tuetur circa pulcherrimas formas et figuras. . . . Eadem videtur esse cura amoris qui herios dicitur, scilicet cum statione et colloquio sapientum virorum et cum pulcherrimis mulieribus et pueris et coeat multum cum eis. . . ." Kibre 1939 and 1971 briefly surveys Domenico's career and writings.

21. *Practica* (Venice, 1508), cap. 24, fol. 23v.

22. On the subject of love and the material determinism associated with medicine see the brief discussions in Wack 1984 and 1986c.

23. The standard work on the internal senses is Wolfson 1935; Harvey 1975 provides a lucid summary of the vast material covered by Wolfson. Steneck 1974 is also helpful. On Peter's psychology in general, see Schipperges 1961b and 1969.

24. Alonso 1961, 259–62.

25. *Ibid.*, 263–64. The complicated relations between imagination and fantasy are traced in Bundy 1927.

26. For a more detailed analysis of this development see Wack 1989a.

27. The determination is preserved in Erfurt, Wissenschaftliche Allgemeinbibliothek F 270, fols. 77v–78v. McVaugh 1985, 34–37 gives a résumé of the work's contents. An edition will appear in Wack 1989b. The most recent study of Gerard of Solo is by Guénoun 1982, a work I have not been able to obtain.

28. Alonso 1961, xxxviii.

29. De Rijk 1972. Of interest on this point are Pires 1969 and Schipperges 1982.

30. Aristotle's comment on the equivocal meaning of "love" in *Topics* 106b clarifies the logic of the debate and offers another rationale for scrutinizing both the physical and emotional sides of love: "To love also, used of the frame of mind, has to hate as its contrary, while as used of the physical activity it has none; clearly, therefore, to love is homonymous" (Barnes 1984). Well aware of both this passage and the ambiguities of *amor*, Peter elsewhere (QDA fol. 265r) explores the problem of contraries in connection with physical love and "love according to the soul," concluding with the Philosopher that while physical love has no contrary, hate is the opposite of love as a frame of mind. For a summary of Aristotle's psychophysiology of love, see Ciavolella 1976, 20–22.

31. On the "non-naturals," see Demaitre 1975, esp. 106 note 9. Cf. Peter's definition of health in the *Liber de conservanda sanitate* (da Rocha Pereira 1959, 171).

32. SLA, 283–84. Cf. da Rocha Pereira 1959, 191: "Cor . . . terminus omnium operationum anime rationalis, testante Galeno. Operationes anime in cerebro incipiunt et suscipientur cordis complementum"; and the statement of William of Corvi (or Brescia, b. 1250) in his *Practica* (Venice, 1508), cap. 24 "de amore," fol. 23r: "Inchoat enim amor ab imaginatione et in corde perficitur, deinde manifestatur in cerebro; est ergo passio cordis et cerebri diversimode tamen." Tennov 1979, 64 cites modern research on two-way communication between the heart and the brain.

33. Da Rocha Pereira 1959, 181.

34. Walsh 1982, 198–205 (Bk. I, dialogue H).

35. The relevant passage is printed in da Cruz Pontes 1964, 265: "Et nota quod quidam est calor infixus in membris, radicatus in humido spermatico, et iste non fluit et refluit sed est radicalis et durat in corpore durante vita. Alius autem est calor qui generatur in corde et epate et iste calor est fluens; fluit enim et refluit quia generatur ex materia nutrimenti." Cf. also Peter's *Expositio de longitudine vite* (Alonso 1944, 425–26 and 461).

36. Cf. Wack 1986c and 1989b.

37. *Super Isagogen Iohannitii*, quoted from Lawn 1979, 230: "Desiderium est operatio composita ex virtute animali, sensibili, et appetitiva naturali, iuxta illud quod dicitur: stomachus sentiens suam inanitionem appetit. Et viget in ore stomachi, in collo matricis, et in virga." This idea also appears in Raoul de Longchamp's commentary on the *Anticlaudianus*. On Peter's familiarity with the Salernitan questions, see Lawn 1963, 76–78.

38. The questions on heat and cold in the commentary on Aristotle are in Madrid, Biblioteca Nacional 1877, fol. 264r and following; their reappearance in the *Viaticum* commentary is on fol. 159r–v.

39. PSQ P 95.

40. I have not been able to locate Avicenna's remark about a corrupted imagination as the cause of lovesickness, quoted by Peter in Version A (note 20), in editions available to me. Since Peter is usually careful in his citations of authorities, perhaps a student or copyist inserted Avicenna's name before statements possibly taken from Gerard of Berry. Or it is possible that Peter had a manuscript of the *Canon* containing passages not surviving in the printed editions that I have consulted. In any event, Avicenna's statements on the "corrupted" imagination reappear in Gerard of Solo's *Determinatio de amore hereos* in a similar context, suggesting that Gerard knew Peter's argumentation fairly closely. On the role of imagination in love see Wack 1986a.

41. McVaugh 1985, 14 and 53. On development of the melancholic character type, see Klibansky et al. 1964.

42. Gerard of Solo 1505, fol. 34; John of Gaddesden: Lowes 1913/14, 502–03; John of Tornamira 1490, fol. xxv ᵛ; Jacques Despars 1498, fol. N iii ʳ.

43. Da Rocha Pereira 1959, 185.

44. See chapter 3, note 56 and Couliano 1987, 21.

45. Da Rocha Pereira 1959, 183. Cf. Tennov 1979, 18–19: "The eyes . . . are so important in limerance that they, not the genitals or even the heart, may be called the organs of love."

46. *Anatomy of Melancholy* (Jackson 1977, 198).

47. *Summa conservationis et curationis* (Venice, 1502), cap. 18: "De melancholia ex amore vel ex desiderio repatriandi et vocatur ylischi." Cf. Savonarola, who calls love for a woman *amor haereos*, and love for one's country *ilisci* (Giedke 1983, 52).

48. *Divisiones* (1510, fol. 6v): "Cura eius [sc. amoris] est assiduatio coytus et ieiunium et deambulatio et ebrietas plurima assidue."

49. Da Rocha Pereira 1959, 211: "Nota quod balnea quodam modo sunt genus deliciarum."

50. Carley and Coughlan 1981 print a list of books that Walter de Monington (abbot 1342–75) acquired for Glastonbury Abbey. Item 75 in the catalogue reads: "Item vnum quarternum de nouem sexternis continentem questiones magistri Petri hyspanici super viaticum asaac. secundo folio incipiente *calor*." Amplonius' notation for Erfurt, CA 212 in his catalogue of his library reads: "Item glose et questiones optime Petro Hispani super libro Viatici Constantini" (Schum 1887).

51. For further comparison between Peter and Gerard, see Wack 1986c. Though Gerard may be drawing upon a common pool of scholastic questions to which Peter contributed, his duplication of Peter's arguments and authorities suggests closer contact.

52. McVaugh 1985, 34–37 summarizes both works.

53. 1574, 216.
54. See nn. 17–19 above.
55. McVaugh 1985, 24–25.
56. *Ibid.*, 45.
57. *Ibid.*, 46, 47. Since the relation of love to hope was debated in the schools around this time (e.g., Alexander of Hales, *Glossa in quatuor libros sententiarum*, Bibliotheca Franciscana Scholastica Medii Aevi, 12 [Quaracchi: Collegium S. Bonaventurae, 1951],pp. 9–10, dist. 1.6), both Peter and Arnald may be incorporating concerns from other faculties into their medical works.

## Chapter Six: The Measure of Pleasure

1. Blonquist 1987, 30. This chapter is a revised version of Wack 1986b, with updated and streamlined notes.
2. McWilliam 1972, 769. On Boccaccio's use of the medical tradition of lovesickness, see Ciavolella 1970.
3. Diepgen 1963, 162–63; Birchler 1975, 312.
4. For Gerard see chapter 3 above. Bernard of Gordon's discussion of *amor hereos* is found in the *Lilium medicinae* (1574) Particula 2, chapter 20 and is partially reprinted in Lowes 1913/14, 499.
5. Murdoch 1974, 62.
6. Trans. Richards 1982, part 2, chapters 55–60. Christine is not talking about lovesickness as such, but about women so faithful to their lovers that they sickened or died by sometimes violent means. She ultimately condemns such excessive love. *L'Art d'amours*, Book 1 gives a number of examples of women maddened by love: Byblis loved her brother "so much that she almost died of it"; "Myrrha was a woman who loved her father so much that she died for her love"; Pasiphae, Io, Europa, and Medea all suffered "deranged" or "frenzied" love (Blonquist 1987, 31–35). Duby 1988, 123–24 cites a story from Ordericus Vitalis of a woman who died of love.
7. Blonquist 1987, 2. Henderson 1979 includes an illuminating discussion of the backgrounds of Ovidian lovesickness. On the survival of Ovid in the Middle Ages, see Viarre 1966 and Hexter 1986. Auerbach 1965, 210–16 and Offermans 1970 discuss his influence on vernacular poetry. In Marie de France's *Guigemar*, Venus is depicted in a mural throwing "Le livre Ovide, ou il enseine / Coment chascun s'amur estreine" (ll. 239–40) into a fire.
8. Faral 1913, 63–157 catalogues examples from the *Roman d'Eneas* and the *Roman de Thèbes*.
9. Ed. Micha 1970, 2:92–94, lines 3023–85. Lejeune 1977 discusses the related theme of "la mort par amour" among medieval heroines.
10. See chapter 1 above. Wright 1966, 76–77, 99, 105, 142, 156 *et passim* notes the similarity of Ovidian and Christian vocabularies for "symptoms of affect." Hunt 1981, 196 prints an Old French translation of *Cant.* 2.5 amplified by borrowings from vernacular poetry.
11. Mentioned by Dronke 1979.
12. Könsgen 1974, 16.
13. Leclercq 1979, 52.
14. On Hildegard of Bingen, see D'Alverny 1977, 123; Cadden 1984; Dronke 1984. Women's excessive lust was of course a standard topic of clerical antifeminism, as in, e.g., Bk. III of Andreas Capellanus' *De amore* (Walsh 1982).
15. *De proprietatibus rerum* 6.6 (Seymour 1975, 1:302); *De proprietatibus rerum* 18.49 (Seymour 1975, 2:1200).
16. "Delectatio in coitu maior est in mulieribus quam in masculis, quia masculi delectantur tantum in expulsione superfluitatis. Mulieres dupliciter delectantur, et in suo spermate expellendo, et masculi recipiendo ex vulve ardentis desiderio"; *Pantegni* VI.17 in *Opera omnia Ysaac* (Lyons, 1515).
17. Jacquart and Thomasset 1985b, 113–16. Lawn 1979, 4 adduces parallels from the Pseudo-Aristotelian *Problems*, Adelard of Bath's *Quaestiones Naturales*, and the *Anatomia Nicolai*.
18. Blonquist 1987, 40.
19. Lawn 1979, 242: "Quare quedam puella dum amasiam expectasset facta est maniaca?"

20. De Renzi 1859, 5:299–300 (noted by Lowes 1913/14, 507).

21. Blonquist 1987, 2.

22. Andreas equates *morum probitas* and *nobilitas* in I.VI (Walsh 1982, 44). The rhetoric of languor and remedy tends to cluster in the nobleman's dialogues (I.E, I.G, I.H) and also appears in Andreas' own statements to Walter (II.VI, Walsh 1982, 242, 244). On Andreas' relation to the medical tradition of *amor hereos*, see Karnein 1985 and Wack 1986a.

23. Guillaume de Lorris associates love-suffering with nobility, wealth, leisure and masculinity in the *Roman de la Rose* (1230–45). The lover encounters Leisure (Oiseuse, a descendant of Ovidian *otium*) guarding the entrance to the Garden of Love and sees Wealth (Richece) dancing in the company of the God of Love. Poverty and Baseness are among the personages barred from entry. The God of Love instructs the young man, when he falls in love with the Rose, about the *mal . . . angoisseus* and the *doulors d'amors* with its panoply of symptoms.

24. *De anima* 33 in *Opera omnia* 1963 [1674] 2:192.

25. *Summa aurea* 1964 [1500], fol. ccc$^v$. De Rijk 1972, xxxiii cautiously surmises that William of Auxerre and William of Auvergne may have been among Peter's teachers of theology.

26. For information on the manuscripts and versions, see the editions in Part 2.

27. Lines 141–44 in Version A. The passage from Aristotle's *De animalibus* that Peter refers to became a commonplace in Renaissance medical writings on female psychology. See Maclean 1980, 41–43. Three centuries after Peter of Spain, the physician Francois Valleriola (1504–80) claimed that "hopeless love" is the cause of lovesickness (Giedke 1983, 61).

28. *History of Animals* IX, 608b 7–12 (Barnes 1984, 1:949).

29. Goldstein-Préaud 1981, 64 suggests that the commentary on *De animalibus* precedes Peter's medical commentaries, and may stem from his Parisian period in the 1220s. Schipperges 1968/9 dates the MS (Madrid, Biblioteca Nacional, 1877) to around 1255. See Grabmann 1979 [1928], 1:480–96 and Wingate 1931, 79–81 for general discussions of the commentary. On Peter's views of human sexuality in general, see Schipperges 1969.

30. Madrid, Bibl. Nac., 1877, fol. 284v: "Secunda causa est quia femina est humida. Humidum autem nullius est impressionis cum humidum sit male terminabile termino proprio, sicut dicit Philosophus. Mas autem, quia siccus, recipit impressione[m] et est bene terminabile siccum. Et ideo de promisso sibi aliquo diffidit femina ubi confidit mas."

31. "Ad aliud dicendum quod femina desperat et difidit tunc quia causa defectus in se portat. Generatur enim ex virtute debili et ex defectu virtutis et quia habet et sentit istud malum in[vi?]dit bonum alienum et inde consequitur invidiam. . . . Sed invidit propter causam iam predictam aut quia maxime est intenta circa filios suos, vel quia circa multa negocia est intenta, et ideo capit a multis ut ab ipsis possit extorquere et ex hoc causatur invidia et ideo invidia est."

32. Version A, lines 145–50.

33. Version A, lines 151–59.

34. Version B, lines 195–202.

35. Version B, lines 203–12.

36. Version B, lines 213–21.

37. Version B, lines 237–47.

38. Madrid, Bibl. Nac., 1877, fol. 263v: "Dicit Philosophus in libro physicorum quod materia appetit formas sicut turpe bonum sive pulchrum et femina masculum." Allen 1985 discusses this passage and its influence in the Middle Ages. The analogy was frequently cited in Renaissance medical works: see Maclean 1980, 40–41.

39. On the quantification of qualities and the intension and remission of forms, see Maier 1968, 10–11, 25–27, and McVaugh 1975, 89 ff.

40. Madrid, Bibl. Nac., 1877, fol. 284v: "Ad aliud dicendum quod in opere generationis maxime est verecundia. Una causa est quia mulier in opere coitus se ipsam agnoscat in recipiendo, vir autem se evacuat et liberat et ideo etc. Secunda causa est quia femina tenet locum materie, mas autem locum forme in quo gloriatur homo; mulier se in hoc vilipendit."

41. Madrid, Bibl. Nac., 1877, fol. 263v: "Constantinus dicit in pa[n]tegni quod femina delectat in duo, scilicet emittendo et recipiendo, masculus autem solum in emittendo. Ergo maior delectatio in femina quam in masculo. . . . Sicut scribitur in libro de coitu: calida complexio stimulat ad coitum. Ergo cum masculi sint calidiores feminis, maior est delectatio in masculis quam in feminis, quod concedo. Ad primum in contrarium dico quod masculus sicut agens et plus habet de calore et spiritibus quam femina. Iterum sperma in masculis est magis

digestum et propter hoc maior est delectatio in masculo quam in femina. . . . Licet in pluribus delectentur femine quam masculi, tamen magis intenditur maior delectatio in masculo quam in femina."

42. Peter of Spain's psychological works have been edited by Alonso 1944, 1952, 1961.

43. Arnald's text is found in McVaugh 1985, 47; that of Gerard of Solo in *Commentum super nono almansoris* 1505, fol. 34: "Causa finalis est delectatio coitus: et quamvis non habeant operationem tamen intentionem: et hoc sufficit: quia non oportet quod semper habeant operationem."

44. *Clarificatorium super nono almansoris* 1490, fol. xxv$^v$: "Nam hereos grece est multum delectabile latine: et licet talis amor excedens seu cum insania mentis se extendat apud plures homines ad plures res . . . proprie tamen amor hereos vertit se ad mulierem propter deliciam carnalem ultimate eis deliciosam habendam."

45. Murdoch 1975.

46. McVaugh 1975, 100–02.

47. Lawn 1963, 85–86. According to De Rijk 1972, xxxii Albert could not have been Peter's teacher at the University of Paris, as is sometimes supposed. Goldstein-Préaud 1981 briefly examines Albert's questions on *De animalibus*, and Jacquart and Thomasset 1981 outline his teachings on human sexuality.

48. Ed. Filthaut 1955, 155.

49. *Ibid.*: "Ad secundum rationem dicendum, quod quantitative maior est delectatio in muliere, verumtamen intensive maior est in viro."

50. Pierre de St.-Flour in Pagel 1896, 29. For the commentary on *De secretis mulierum*, see Lemay 1981, 172–73.

51. 1521, fol. 51: "Dicendum ad unum quod extensive plus delectatur mulier: perdurat enim voluptas in ea diutius . . . vir vero intensive voluptuatur peramplius: in modica enim hora qua delectatur plus ipsius intenditur voluptas."

52. 1574, cap. 20: "Quinto notandum, quod ista passio frequentius advenit viris quam mulieribus, pro tanto, quia viri sunt calidiores, & universaliter foemine frigidiores: & hoc patet in masculis brutorum, qui cum furia & impetu moventur ad coitum implendum. Nunc quia viri calidiores, ideo in coitu intensius delectantur, mulieres autem extensive plus, quia in semine viri, & in semine proprio." On Bernard's life and works, see Demaitre 1980. Manuscripts of Peter of Spain's *Questiones super Viaticum* were copied at Montpellier or in southern France during Bernard's time (Vatican, pal. lat. 1166). Erfurt, CA 212 (Version A) was written in Montpellier at the beginning of the 14th c., according to Schum 1887, 468; he gives Erfurt CA 221 a southern French origin and notes that the 2 hands of Peter's *Questiones* are "des frühsten 14. Jh" (477–78). Krakow, RBJ 781, copied in 1334, might also be from Montpellier.

53. For biographical information, see Wickersheimer 1979 [1936],1 : 185–86 and Jacquart 1979, 85–86.

54. Erfurt, Wissenschaftliche Allgemeinbibliothek, CA 270 fol. 78r. An edition of this text will appear in Wack 1989b (forthcoming).

55. 1505, fol. 34.

56. "Vir delectatur intensius quam mulier: quia calidior est: sed plus mulier extensive delectatur: quia in pluribus delectatur quam vir."

57. "Quarto delectatur in fricatione membri viri circa collum matricis: et propter hoc multe mulieres tam pauperes quam divites efficiuntur meretrices: quia quanto magis coeunt tanto plus appetunt."

58. Masters and Johnson 1966.

59. Castle 1987.

60. "Et dicitur hereos vel hereosus is insanus amor quia plus accidit viris nobilibus et viris heroicis quam viris simplicibus de communi plebe" (1498, fol. Niii$^r$).

61. Beecher and Ciavolella 1989. There is a reprint (1978) of the edition of 1623.

62. Lockwood 1951, 238–322 and Siraisi 1981, 276–78. For a passage suggesting that Bona Fortuna saw women patients in his practice, see chapter 7, note 21. Green 1989a surveys women's health care in the Middle Ages.

63. On the role of dialectic method in Peter's work in general see Schipperges 1969, 47–48.

64. Hendrix 1980a.

65. See Birchler 1975, 313–14 and notes, and Giedke 1983, 55–105, in which Gesner, Forestus, Platter, de Baillou, and Backhauss are all cited as referring to women's susceptibility

to lovesickness. Ciavolella 1988, 14 argues that "Le seule façon de réconcilier la froideur des femmes avec leur évidente extrême sensibilité et leur propension à l'*erotomania* consistait à associer la maladie avec le refoulement des sens et l'hystérie."

66. For a study of analogies between the body and society in Henri de Mondeville's work, see Pouchelle 1983, 180–205 and, more generally, Douglas 1982 [1973] and 1975, 83–89.

67. Peter debates whether the brain or the *testiculi* is the locus of *amor hereos* (Version A, lines 55–107; Version B, lines 61–98). McVaugh 1985, 32, 34 notes that in Arnald of Villanova's later explanation of *amor hereos* in *De parte operativa* (incomplete when he died in 1311) cerebral localization of causality seems not to interest him as much as does the complexion of the generative members. Arnald wrote *De parte operativa* after he had returned to teaching at Montpellier in the 1290s, hence at a time when Peter of Spain's commentary was being copied there.

68. Beecher 1988 discusses the theories of erotic melancholy in the Renaissance; a fuller treatment appears in Beecher and Ciavolella 1989.

69. McVaugh 1985, 49–50.

## Chapter Seven: Bona Fortuna

1. See the edition (below, Part 2) for a description of the manuscripts. On the library of the Sorbonne at this period, see Rouse 1967.

2. Quotations from Bona Fortuna's text are taken from: P = Paris, BN lat. 15373; R = Rouen, Bibl. mun., A 176. "Dico modo quod in alie die dixi" (P 5v); "Ideo volo aliquid loqui extra intentionum istius capituli" (P 12v); "de hoc etiam dixi alia die" (P 56r).

3. E.g.: "Unde statim in principio flebotomare, si potes . . . Si autem non confidis virtuti, nec audes flebotomare, tunc infrigida" (R 64v); "et nota quod antequam ponas huiusmodi fortia debet prius unguis remolliri cum emplastris remollitivis" (R 72v).

4. On the *reportatio*, see Hunt 1950, 3–6 and Smalley 1964, 201–08. The manuscript appears to preserve several moments of classroom dialogue, which suggests that the treatise in the form we have it comes from a student's hand rather than from the master's. Thus: "Ego dabo tibi exemplum ut non possis errare quamvis etiam nulla febris precessit. Ponatur igitur quod febris quasi [?] incipiat in aliquo flegmatico habente venas strictas qui multum et diversa comederat prius et multum laboraverat et intemperat in eo in primo autumpni et antecessit eam oscitatio multa et gravitas sompni. Tunc quid dices de isto? Certe. Quantum ad eius complexionem . . ." (R 64v). A sentence or two further he again asks someone in the class what he would say in response to a problem: "Si vero incepisset in medio autumpni tunc quantum ad hoc debent esse ex humore melancolico naturali. Quid igitur dices de isto?" (R 64v).

5. "Et nota quod cutis habet tres intersticia sive pelliculas quod potest videri in pergameno" (P 2v).

6. P 102v; R 68r.

7. "Hoc facto intinge pannum sicut faciunt illi qui faciunt pannos curatos ad libros et isto curatorio utere" (R 71v).

8. In the early fourteenth century Henri de Mondeville (Wickersheimer 1979 [1936]), 1:282) and Barthelemy de Bruges (*ibid.* 1:60) were associated with both universities, as Gerard of Berry possibly was several generations earlier. The manuscript of Bona Fortuna's *Tractatus*, located at the Sorbonne after 1338, contains the works of the Montpellier masters Bernard of Gordon and Arnald of Villanova. Once Bona Fortuna refers to his own teacher without giving a name: "et nota quod de tertiana non vidi aliquem mori sed magister meus vidit unum mori" (R 62v). He also mentions a Master William who suffered a certain type of pain: "Et talem dolorem habuit magister Wilhelmus spasmatus" (R 68r). Neither reference offers much clue to the author's locale.

9. See the introduction to the edition, part 2 below.

10. Jacquart 1981, 200–02.

11. Private communication. On Bernard of Bona Hora, see Wickersheimer 1979 [1936] 1:72 and the *Cartulaire* of Montpellier (1890, 1 nos. 30 and 39). The identification of Bernard de Bona Hora with the Beneto documented at Llerida in 1311 made by Cardoner i Planas 1973, 81, and followed by Jacquart 1981, 42 seems unlikely to me. Cardoner i Planas cites Rubió Y Lluch 1921, 2:lxv as his source, who, however, mentions only Beneto and not Bernard de

Bona Hora. Rubió Y Lluch in turn refers to Denifle 1888, 252, who reports that in April of 1311 the king offered a teaching position in medicine to a master P. Gaveto, who refused it. In October of the same year, "magister Beneto" was invited to lecture in medicine. I have not been able to examine the archival document (ACA, Reg. 208, fol. 20v) in question, and so have not been able to ascertain whether Beneto is identified there with Bernard de Bona Hora.

12. *Cartulaire* (1890, 249–50, no. 39): "Bernardus de Bonaora, clericus conjugatus, et Jordanus de Turre, laicus, magistri in medicina in Studio Universitatis predicte . . . temere veniente, dicto Cancellario et ejus locumtenenti obedire non curant, dicentes publice quod, nec pro Cancellario et locumtenente predictis, quantum pro uno ansere facerent. Preterea dictus Bernardus, predictis nequaquam contentus, unum magistrum in medicine de Universitate predicta verbis vituperavit et facto, percutiendo eundem."

13. McVaugh 1976 discusses surviving collections of Montpellier *experimenta*.

14. On the subject of scholasticism in treatises like Bona Fortuna's, see Demaitre 1976.

15. Among the authors Bona Fortuna refers to are: Aristotle; Hippocrates, *Epidemiarum, Aphorisms, De regimine acutarum, De humana natura*; Galen, Commentaries on the *Aphorisms, Prognostics,* and *Liber Epidemiarum; Liber interiorum, Liber de virtutibus naturalibus*; Rufus; Johannes Alexandrinus, Commentary on the *Epidemiarum*; Johannes Damascenus, *Antidotaria;* Johannitius; Dioscorides; Serapion; Avicenna; Averroes, Commentary on *De somno et vigilia* (fol. 8v); Haly; al-Rāzī; *Tractatus de flebotomia.* To take just one example of many in which Bona Fortuna disagrees with the *auctores:* " *Tunc nota ut non oriantur pili:* auctores ponunt multa, sed nullum est ita efficax sicut est istud. Recipe arsenicum in aqua sublimatum . . ." (P 1v).

16. E.g.: "Item Ypocras dicit quod in principio egritudinis cronice non est adhibenda fortis medicina. Constat autem quod huiusmodi egritudo est cronica, ergo etc. Ergo male dicit auctor (= Constantine) quod incipiendum est a forti medicina" (R 59v); "Quidem autem excusant auctorem, et dicunt quod ipse commiscuit ista propter intentionem laxandi ut videlicet isti faciant perturbationem in stomacho et intestinis propter quam sequatur postea laxatio. Sed hoc non accepto ego, sed dico quod non debent simul permixti dari" (R 65r).

17. "Ita semper procedendum est rationabiliter. Et si vides te non proficere in una medicina tunc transferre ad aliam quantum valeat ad propositum. Et si una non videtur prodesse coniunge duas et postea tres et sic deinceps. Deinde tamen non facias ut administres aliquid impertinens vel sine ratione. Ista cautela generalis est in omni cura. . . . Sed si non vides iuvamentum tunc muta de una in aliam, sed non recede a via rationali sicut dictum est prius" (P 25v).

18. "Hoc debes tu considerare secundum industriam tuam prout vidis expedire" (P 24r). He repeats this elsewhere, e.g., R 69r.

19. On the influence of the late medieval debate on universals and particulars upon medical thought, see Laín Entralgo 1961, 58–81. For Bernard's opinions on reason and experience, see Demaitre 1980, 117–35, and for an example of Arnald's adjustment of theory and practice, see Jacquart and Thomasset 1985b, 204–05.

20. "Unde vidi quod de uno domo omnes tam mulieres quam viri fuerunt depilati propter mures qui ceciderant in oleum et putrescant in eo" (R 67r). "Vidi enim quemdam de cuius corpore quasi in centum locis exivit sanguis propter morsus et corrosiones pediculorum . . . Tunc nota quod vidi quemdam qui a corpore cuiusdam eduxit plenam scutellam de pediculis" (P 3r). Physicians at Montpellier around 1300 were among those who attempted to reconcile these two worlds of theory and practice—perhaps another clue to our author's place of activity.

21. Such statements as: "Unde *nuper* [emphasis mine] vidi quandam mulierem qui fuit disposita ad lepram cuius menstrua retinebatur et ipsa tota calebat quia sanguis ille menstruas adurebatur" (R 69v) suggest that Bona Fortuna was engaged in practice during his professorship. On the relation of theory to practice at Montpellier, see Demaitre 1975.

22. "Tunc nota de cura istarum passionum. Si igitur sit propter habundantia spermatis et cum hoc sit etas adolescencie vel iuventutis et sint alia particularia convenientia et virtus fortis, tunc quantum est de consilio medicine, quicquid etiam sit de consilio theologie, non est tutum rumpere virtutem talium. Unde nota quod generatio spermatis est una de bonis rebus. Tunc enim letificatur anima et est virtus fortis. Unde ego quantum est de consilio medicine non resisterem sed aliud facerem" (R 55r). On the relations between medical discourse on sexuality and theology see Jacquart and Thomasset 1985b.

23. For an explanation of the disease and its treatment by a writer in the second half of the thirteenth century, see Lemay 1981, esp. 177–78. For norms of propriety in medieval scientific and medical views of sexuality, see Cadden 1986.

24. "Si autem materia sit spermatica, tunc non flebotoma quamvis etiam sit venenosa, sed

fac quod spermatizet. Inunguat igitur obstetrix digitum in aliquo oleo odorifero et immittat vulve et fricet et moveat quousque spermatizet. Et ultimum consilium est quod ipsa nubat viro bene potenti coire. Hec enim passio utplurimum fit ex spermate frigido retento; propter hoc mulier indiget forti subagitatore qui bene possit eam calefacere et sperma provocare. Tales autem viri sunt qui habent corpora bruna, pectora lata, venas amplas" (R 57v).

25. McVaugh 1985, 46; Favati 1952, 90, 91, and *passim*. Although Gerard of Solo still locates the cause of *amor hereos* in the object (as does Dino del Garbo), he nonetheless discusses the role of *species* in his two works on lovesickness, the *Commentum super nono almansoris* 1505, fol. 34: "[Causa] principalis est obiectum delectabile imprimens suam speciem in virtute yma-ginativa et estimativa, et virtus estimativa mediante specie impressa"; and the *Determinatio de amore hereos* (Erfurt Ampl. F 270, fol. 78r). For the term *species*, see Michaud-Quantin 1970, 113–50 and the thorough account of Tachau 1988.

26. Roger Bacon also uses the terms *species* and *passio* interchangeably; see Lindberg 1976, 114 and Tachau 1988, 8 n.14.

27. McVaugh 1985, 48. The *Epistolae duorum amantium* (Könsgen 1974) are an early ex-ample of the rhetoric of individuality in medieval love literature. See the index *s.v.* singularis, unicus.

28. See note 19 above.

29. Jean de St. Amand (Pagel 1894, 299); del Garbo in Favati 1952, 101. For later thir-teenth-century thinking on similitude as the cause of love, see Aquinas, *Summa Theologiae* Ia IIae 26–30.

30. Alonso 1952, 367: "Dicitur igitur quod intellectus ille practicus est qui ratiocinatur propter aliquid, idest, qui apprehendit rem per suam speciem non in quantum ens est sed in quantum bona vel mala, ut consequenter moveat ad imitandum vel fugiendum illud."

31. *Ibid.*, 366–67: "Dicit igitur in parte prima quod hec duo, scilicet, intellectus practicus et appetitus sunt moventia. Et hoc si nomine intellectus comprehendimus intellectum et ima-ginationem. Et si non dicamus tantum duo esse moventia, sic comprehendentes duo sub uno nomine, erunt tria moventia, scilicet, intellectus, appetitus et imaginatio sive phantasia. . . . Et, hoc habito, resumit quod prius posuit, scilicet, quod utraque, videlicet, appetitus et intel-lectus, sunt motiva secundum locum et sub intellectu comprehendit imaginationem."

32. In his chapter on *amor hereos* (1508, fol. 23r) William not only states that similarity is the cause of love ("[Amor] dicitur delectatio quia delectatio est apprehensio convenientis et coniunctio convenientis cum convenienti sive similis cum simili, quia simile appetit simile et cum eo delectatur"), but also claims that the *causa primitiva* is the *aspectus rei* having the form of a beautiful woman. This sight kindles the heart just as the sun ignites straw through a lens. For Gerard of Solo, see note 25 above.

33. On the problems surrounding *species in medio* see Tachau 1988.

34. Wack 1989a.

35. Seidler 1967, 90.

36. 1508, fol. 23v.

37. For discussions of the pulse test see Ciavolella 1970, 496–517 and 1976, 23–27, as well as Mesulam and Perry 1972.

38. On the adoption of the *Canon* into medical curricula see Siraisi 1984, 47 and 69 n.2. Nutton 1979, 23–26 discusses the authorship of the Latin version of Galen's *De praecognitione*.

39. See chapter 1.

40. The story is translated into German in Giedke 1983, 64–65.

41. Laín Entralgo 1961, 81.

42. *Summa pulsuum* in Grant 1974, 745.

43. In their analysis of sexuality in medieval medical writings Jacquart and Thomasset 1985b suggest modifications of Foucault's notion that medicine represents a normalizing, re-pressive discourse. Although parts of Bona Fortuna's chapter appear to support Robertson's contention (1962, 459) that "the physician of the Middle Ages had no more respect for the passionate lover than had the theologian," the treatise as a whole by no means condemns or attempts to repress sexuality (cf. notes 22–24 above). Cadden 1986 rightly stresses that medi-eval physicians show a range of attitudes toward sexuality, from "explicit treatment of sexu-ality unadorned by ethical trappings" to reticence or disapproval for particular sexual or medical practices. Patterson 1987, 26–39 trenchantly analyzes the unifying and harmonizing vision (i.e., doctors and theologians think alike, and think like Augustine) of Robertsonian "Exegetics."

44. See Sutton 1984, plates 81, 124 and catalogue nos. 105 and 80 for a brief introduction

to the genre. See also Holländer 1913. Schama 1979, 1980 argues that seventeenth-century Dutch painting encodes the tensions of a culture at once hedonistic and puritanical; this may help to explain the popularity of the "doctor's visit/lovesick maiden" genre. For Renaissance accounts of lovesickness, see Giedke 1983, 55–105.

45. The following section has been adapted from Wack 1986b. McVaugh 1976 provides evidence for the practical activities of physicians as they have been documented in surviving *experimenta*.

46. Unfortunately, the passage is corrupt in the manuscripts; see the note *ad loc.*

47. 1978 [1623], 177. Beecher and Ciavolella 1989 have completed a comprehensive edition and translation of Ferrand's treatise.

48. In addition to the "adustio humoris" noted by Gerard of Berry and Peter of Spain (A version), cf. Avicenna, *Canon*, lib. 1, fen 1, doctr. 4, cap. 1.

49. For a caveat on using medical texts as evidence for the realities of practice, see Siraisi 1982, esp. 233 n.4.

## Chapter Eight: Recreating a Context

1. Hildegard of Bingen, *Causae et curae*, Bk. 2 (Kaiser 1903, 75–76).

2. Keen 1986, 79–80. In his study of William Marshall's career, Duby 1984 touches a number of times on the question of "courtly" love.

3. See Blonquist 1987, 18–19 for the *Art*. Christine's counsels in the *Treasure of the City of Ladies* have been translated by Lawson 1985, 102–05. The wife's speech is edited by Wright 1906, 175–76.

4. Arnoul 1940, 21–22: "Quant n'ose parler a ascune qe jeo quide q'elle serroit dangerouse, jeo envoieroi ascune makerel a qi jeo parleroie mult piteousement et dirroi: 'Jeo ne su qe mort, si vous ne me eidetz.'"

5. Benson 1984, 249. Régnier-Bohler 1988, 361–63 points out that hair was an important element of self-image in the Middle Ages.

6. Monica Green, private communication, 3 July 1988. Before the advent of case histories in the Renaissance, there is little documentation for the patients of lovesickness. The published collections of *consilia* (individualized therapeutic recommendations) have so far revealed no treatments for the lover's malady. The academic physicians do argue that the patients of lovesickness are, variously, men, the young, those with hot temperaments, the nobility, knights, and women. Yet what seem to be reflections of medical practice and social reality may in fact be no more than the rustle of parchments in dialogue. Medieval academics tended to achieve new insights by studying authoritative texts in new contexts rather than by observing the world. The new theorizing about lovesickness found in these commentaries, for example, grew in large part from reading Avicenna and Aristotle and applying the fruits of that reading to medical doctrine. One could plausibly argue that the "patients" in these texts were called into being by theory and method rather than by the realities of medical practice.

7. See, for example, Steadman 1968, esp. 20–26; Robertson 1962, 47, 457–60; and Benton 1961.

8. Sabra 1987 argues the case for Islam's creative appropriation of Greek science.

9. See the seminal if flawed work of Foucault 1973 and 1978–86; Sontag 1979; Ingleby 1982; MacDonald 1983, 70–75, and Herzlich and Pierret 1987. For studies of culturally-shaped views of the body and of sexuality in the Middle Ages, see Pouchelle 1983 and Jacquart and Thomasset 1985b. Silverman 1983, 140, 149–93 usefully discusses the cultural construction of madness and sexuality. My focus in this chapter is deliberately limited in time, social class, and gender. Since the "meaning" of lovesickness resides in a complex negotiation between individual psychology and social context, that meaning must be reinterpreted in different periods, cultures, social classes, and genders. Winkler 1982 and 1989 has offered interesting suggestions about the interplay of psyche and society in the erotic life of antiquity. Nearly thirty years ago D. W. Robertson (1962, 108–10; 457–60) offered a powerful model for the cultural context of the lover's malady, viewing the medical tradition as an echo and a reinforcement of the theological condemnation of cupidinous love. Since then, significant work in the history of medicine has shown the relative independence of medieval medicine—especially in sexual matters—from ecclesiastical strictures (e.g. Lemay 1982, Jacquart and Thomasset 1985b, Cadden 1986). My approach therefore differs from Robertson's in not privileging ecclesiastical moral

views on passionate love. Although I do use written and visual religious sources, I elucidate them from a psychological and social, rather than theological, point of view.

10. Despars 1498, fol. Niii recto.

11. Translated from Lowes 1913/14, 509–10.

12. Despars 1498, fol. Niii recto.

13. For Arnald see McVaugh 1985, 50–51. William of Brescia (Corvi), *Practica* (Venice, 1508), fol. 23r connects "herois id est dominis" with German *Heer*, "dominus," as does Valescus of Taranta (Lowes 1913/14, 505).

14. Douglas 1982 [1973], 70.

15. Goldin 1967.

16. 1508, fol. 23r. Other physicians who remark on this idealization are Bernard of Gordon, Arnald of Villanova, and John of Tornamira. Cf. Freud's remarks on idealization, 1957 [1914], 14:88.

17. Bird 1940, 1941.

18. McVaugh 1985, 50–51.

19. Bynum 1987. Freud 1957 [1917], 14:249–50 notes: "We have elsewhere shown that identification is a preliminary stage of object choice, that it is the first way—and one that is expressed in ambivalent fashion—in which the ego picks out an object. The ego wants to incorporate this object into itself, and, in accordance with the oral or cannibalistic phase of libidinal development in which it is, it wants to do so by devouring it. Abraham is undoubtedly right in attributing to this connection the refusal of nourishment met with in severe forms of melancholia."

20. On the metaphoric significance of symptoms, see Sontag 1979, Kristeva 1987, 23 and 1985, 19–20. The correspondence of signs and symptoms with a society's major values accounts for the degree of attention they receive from patients and physicians; the West, in contrast to some other societies, is characterized by a high insistence on rationality and control. Thus to the extent that symptoms reveal a loss of rationality or control (traits of the feminine and the infantile in Western culture) they become worthy of medical notice. See Zola 1983 [1966] for the relation between culture and symptoms.

21. Ed. Dumeige 1955.

22. Robertson 1962, esp. 104–10, offers a moral-theological rather than psychological answer to the problem: "It is significant that the lover's malady as it is envisaged in the late Middle Ages is an extreme form of the pattern of action typical of the abuse of beauty."

23. Bynum 1982, 110–69 and 1987, 266–73.

24. Furnivall 1866, 156. Wimsatt 1978 explicates the poem in the context of exegesis on the Song of Songs; Stouck 1987 stresses its relation to currents of affective mysticism.

25. Kristeva 1985, 36–37 understands mystical experience as "un mouvement d'identification qu'il faut bien appeler primaire, avec une instance aimante et protectrice." She notes that Augustine compares the faith of a Christian in his God to the relations a baby has with its mother and suggests that mystical rapture is sustained by "processus psychiques infra- ou trans-langagiers qui obéissent à la logique des processus primaires et gratifient l'individue dans son noyau narcissique."

26. See previous note; Kristeva 1987, 234–63; and Jacoff 1984.

27. Ed. Roy 1891, 2.6, lines 168–78.

28. Koenigsberg 1967, 42. A similar psychoanalytical interpretation of courtly love was made by Moller 1960. He sees it, however, as a reflection of preoedipal object relations, whereas Koenigsberg argues that oedipal conflicts lie at the root of courtly love.

29. On incest in medieval stories and legends, see Rank 1926, 312–36.

30. Filgueira Valverde 1985, 43–55.

31. Brereton and Ferrier 1981, 100–01.

32. Furnivall 1868, 1. On the significance of the Virgin's bare breast in art see Miles 1986.

33. Rousselot 1908, 65–80; Manzaneda 1984.

34. Boase 1977, 134–37.

35. Foster and Boyd 1967, 207.

36. Bowlby 1969, 361–78 reviews psychoanalytical theories on the child's tie to the mother. Chodorow 1978 stresses the differential role gender plays in the nature of the attachment. Readers familiar either with critiques of Freud or with controversies over childhood in the Middle Ages may question whether "mother" in the sense that I am using it here is anachronistic. Medieval sources suggest otherwise, and to them one can add a large body of recent

scholarship on medieval childhood and family life that shows that families were characterized by close affective ties; parents loved their children and children their parents. According to Herlihy (1978, 1983), social and psychological investments in children were growing substantially from approximately the eleventh and twelfth centuries through to the end of the Middle Ages. Ideally, a mother nourished her own infant, yet even if a child was put out to a wetnurse, it was still "mothered" by a woman (cf. Demaitre 1977). To my knowledge, there is no medieval evidence that fathers or men played a significant role in nurturing and caring for infants—that was the domain of women. At one end of the Middle Ages, we find Augustine who writes of the "comfort of woman's milk" he received from the breasts of his mother and nurses and who speaks of himself to God as "a creature suckled on your milk and feeding on yourself" (*Confessions* 1.6 and 4.1). At the other end we find the Menagier of Paris, who describes children's love for women who feed and clothe them and give them affection when their own parents or stepparents neglect them. "These children love the company of strangers who take care of them more than that of their relatives who don't care about them." What was important then as now was nurturing and affection, not biological motherhood; the former, not the latter, shaped psychological development.

37. Walsh 1982, 306–21.

38. Bowlby 1973, 9–10, 12–13, 21, 245–57. Gold 1985, a study of images of and attitudes toward women in twelfth-century France, emphasizes patterns of ambivalence surrounding them.

39. Benton 1970, 41, 74.

40. See Klapisch-Zuber 1985, 117–31 on the "cruel mother" in Florence in the fourteenth and fifteenth centuries. Though she focuses on economic motives for abandoned children's recriminations, her evidence also attests to their emotional distress.

41. The quotations are from Bowlby 1973, 256. Bowlby 1980, 23–43 reviews psychoanalytic literature on the place of loss in mourning. Cf. Freud, "Instincts and their Vicissitudes," *SE* 14:133–40 and "Mourning and Melancholia," *SE* 14:251: "The melancholic's erotic cathexis in regard to his object has thus undergone a double vicissitude: part of it has regressed to identification, but the other part, under the influence of the conflict due to ambivalence, has been carried back to the stage of sadism which is nearer to that conflict." See also Chodorow 1978, 57–76.

42. Bowlby 1980, 310. Summarizing earlier studies, he explains how it may do so on p. 258: "The experience of loss can contribute causally to depressive disorders in any of three ways: (a) as a *provoking* agent which increases risk of disorder developing and determines the time at which it does so . . . (b) as a *vulnerability* factor which increases an individual's sensitivity to such events . . . (c) as a factor that influences both the *severity* and the *form* of any depressive disorder that may develop."

43. Hemorrhage, infection, and anemia were but a few of the complications. Abnormalities of presentation and maternal anatomy threatened death for mother and child. The harrowing story of Guibert's birth (Benton 1970, 41–42) gives some idea of the dangers. They are briefly discussed in Alexandre-Bidon and Closson 1985, 38–45 and in the excellent study of medieval children by McLaughlin 1974, 111. Herlihy 1975 discusses medieval women's life expectancies.

44. Klapisch-Zuber 1985, 132–64 describes the system of wetnursing in Florence, 1300–1530. See also McLaughlin 1974, 115; Shahar 1983, 183–89; and de La Roncière 1988, 220, 275. I am indebted to Hester Gelber for suggesting this line of argument and for alerting me to the implications of Bowlby's work for the Middle Ages.

45. McLaughlin 1974, 111.

46. Klapisch-Zuber 1985, 117–31.

47. Duby 1983a, 223–24. McLaughlin 1974, 129 and n. 175 discusses the separation of young boys from their families. Plates 13–25 in Bynum 1987 testify to the psychological importance of mothering in the Middle Ages, concerning which McLaughlin 1974, Herlihy 1978, 1983, and Arnold 1980 offer ample documentation.

48. Bowlby 1980, 234–37 comments on the role of idealization in mourning and depression. Though above I have concentrated on instances of maternal loss, a young child's loss of the father may also play a role in rendering him vulnerable to a depressive condition like lovesickness, by raising the levels of idealization and anxiety in his attachments. McLaughlin 1974, 128 notes that fathers were frequently absent from a child's early life in a military and expansionist society.

49. *SE* 14:50–51: "The loss of a love-object is an excellent opportunity for the ambivalence in love-relationships to make itself effective and come into the open. . . . In melancholia, the occasions which give rise to the illness extend for the most part beyond the clear case of loss by death, and include all those situations of being slighted, neglected, or disappointed, which can import opposed feelings of love and hate into the relationship or reinforce an already existing ambivalence. . . . If the love for the object—a love which cannot be given up though the object itself is given up—takes refuge in narcissistic identification, then the hate comes into operation on this substitutive object, abusing it, debasing it, making it suffer . . . the patients usually still succeed, by the circuitous path of self-punishment, in taking revenge on the original object and in tormenting their loved one through their illness, having resorted to it in order to avoid the need to express their hostility to him openly." Bowlby 1980, 145–46 offers supporting evidence.

50. *Art*, Bk. 3, 4734, ed. Roy 1974, 263. Dante's poem is from Foster and Boyd 1967, 1:no. 41.

51. Hildegard of Bingen, in Kaiser 1903, 73–74. Cadden 1984 and Dronke 1984, 144–201 discuss her attitudes toward sexuality.

52. Crane 1890, 105, CCL. On the popularity of the tale, known in Middle English as *Dame Sirith*, see McKnight 1913, xxi–xliii.

53. A translation of the story into modern French may be found in Paris 1868, 1:246–63. According to Sommer 1909, 1:xi, the revenge portion of the story is a later addition to *L'Estoire*. See also Spargo 1934, 204–05 for the story of Hippocrates and 136–206 for Vergil.

54. *Decameron*, third day, tenth story, of Alibech and Rustico.

55. For its analysis of magically caused lovesickness, the *Malleus* draws on Johan Nider's (c. 1380–1438) *Formicarius* (Lyons 1569, 326–27). Though the *Malleus* was published during the transition from the late Middle Ages to the early modern period, its attitudes toward women and love reach back into the fourteenth century, if not earlier. It also articulates in extreme form feelings characteristic of medieval culture in less exaggerated garb. In this regard, Duby's outline (1988, 77–82) of aristocratic men's fear of women is telling: "Women were held to be the principal, and insidious, source of domestic danger. They administered poison, cast spells, sowed discord, and caused weakness, disease, and death. . . . The first duty of the head of household was to watch over, punish, and if necessary kill his wife, sisters, and daughters, as well as the widows and orphans of his brothers, cousins, and vassals. Since females were dangerous, patriarchal power over them was reinforced." Blöcker 1982, 29 sums up the impetus behind accusations of love magic in the *Malleus*: "Dass heftige Aggressionen, besonders gegen Frauen, dabei abreagiert worden sind, erkennt jeder, der einen Blick in den Hexenhammer wirft." See Russell 1972, 273–86 on men's fears of women's sexuality as an impetus to the witchcraft craze and Monter 1977 on courtly love and witchcraft. Boase 1977, 78–79 notes that Gervais of Tilbury sent a young girl to the stake for resisting his erotic advances.

56. I have used the edition of Frankfurt, 1582. Magically-caused *amor hereos* is discussed in part 2, question 2, ch. 3 and in part 1, q. 6 and 7.

57. Trans. Summers 1971 [1928], 45 (= part 1, q. 6) and 97–98 (= part 2, q. 1, ch. 1).

58. In his study of erotic magic in ancient Greece, Winkler 1989 concludes that men dealt with threats of *eros* by fictitious denial and transfer: whereas men are the agents seeking love in magical papyri and tablets, in literature the lovesick clients are usually female. Magical rites supported pretensions of male control, and patterns of gender-transfer hid men's vulnerability and erotic agency.

59. The text is printed in Hansen 1901, 109–12. See also Wack 1989a.

60. Kelly 1977 and 1984, 1–18. See the response of Herlihy 1985b, 1–22 and the important study of Howell 1986. Herlihy 1985a, 100–101 notes that in the central and late Middle Ages women lost some of their functions in economic production and administration, and that as a result the contributions they made to their families through service or skill diminished.

61. Wright 1906, *passim*; Williamson 1985, 393–408. Christine's handbook, the *Treasure of the City of Ladies*, is translated by Lawson 1985 and discussed by Willard 1975.

62. Shahar 1984, 89–90.

63. Walsh 1982, 291.

64. Wolf 1864, 140. The text of *De vero amore* may be found in Karnein 1985, 298–301. Burns 1984/5 argues that woman in troubadour lyric is a projection of male desire and fear; that love feminizes the lover; that the poet desires to bring the woman under control; and that service is a fiction concealing his power. See, too, Gravdal 1985 and Bloch 1987.

65. Ed. Tarbé 1849, 59.
66. Walsh 1982, 308–09; 314–15; 318–21. See also Duby 1983a, 87–106, 144, 211–19, and 280–81.
67. Speroni 1974, 269–71; see also R. F. Green 1988 on erotic duplicity in the later Middle Ages.
68. On the development of courtliness, see Jaeger 1985 and Duby 1983b, 15–16. Duby summarizes his interpretation of courtly love (1988, 76): "What we know about those rituals [of courtly love] and their development from the middle of the twelfth century on suggests that the lord used his wife as bait, as a sort of decoy, offering her as the prize in a game whose rules, increasingly sophisticated as time went by, obliged participants—the unmarried knights and clerics of the households—to control their instincts ever more firmly." Kelly 1987 rightly critiques some of the less plausible elements in Duby's view. On the value of bodily integrity, see the question raised in Andreas Capellanus (Walsh 1982, 262–65) about a lover who lost an eye or some other part when fighting and was rejected by his partner.
69. Woolf 1962 describes the tradition in which Christ is figured as a knight and lover. I disagree with her assumption (1968, 44–63) that the lyrics employing the theme of Christ the lover-knight must have been written for and read by women. The twelfth-century allegorizations of the Bride of Canticles as the human soul shows that in a devotional context medieval men could view themselves through a female persona. See, too, Auerbach's studies of the semantic development of *passio* (1941, 1965).
70. For a general introduction to the institutional context of medicine, see Kibre and Siraisi 1978. By "clerical culture" I mean the intellectual culture of the universities (characterized in Middle English as "clergye") which was heir to, among other things, classical and patristic misogyny. In this respect a "secular" university like Bologna was no better than a "clerical" one like Paris.
71. Courtenay 1987, 24–27 discusses the reasons for the relative youthfulness of English universities in the fourteenth century, when it would have been "rare in any faculty to find a master over the age of forty." Most students would have ranged in age from fourteen to thirty. Geremek 1987 [1971], 148 ff. comments on the consequences of the youthfulness of the Parisian students.
72. Le Goff 1980, 135–49; Baldwin 1970, 133–49.
73. Bynum 1987, 157 and 161 notes instances of mystical love-languor, as does Leclercq 1979, 52. See chapter 6 above, a revised version of Wack 1986b. Duby 1983b, 11 argues that women's voluntary love, love that carried them out of themselves, was theoretically to be directed toward God alone, with the result for married love that: "Leur devoir est non point de partager leur amour, mais de se partager elles-mêmes. Dissociation, dédoublement de la personne: d'un côte (du cô du terrestre, du charnel, de l'inférieur) l'obéissance passive; de l'autre, l'élan vers le haut, l'ardeur, bref, l'amour. Dédoublement dans le mariage, mais de la personne féminine seule." If Duby is correct in this analysis, then perhaps this dissociated sensibility worked against the experience of lovesickness for an earthly object.
74. See Giedke 1983, 55–105; Birchler 1975; and now Ciavolella 1988.
75. Summarized in Giedke 1983, 64–65.
76. See note 44 to chapter 7 above.
77. Birchler 1975; Giedke 1983, 77; and Maclean 1980, 41.
78. Green 1985, 1989a, and forthcoming.

# Constantine

## Manuscripts

1. A handlist of *Viaticum* manuscripts is in preparation. The limit of 1400 has its source in an earlier study; there is a significant number of fifteenth-century *Viaticum* manuscripts. I would like to thank Monica Green for generously providing me with a transcription of Oxford, Bodleian Library, MS Bodl. 489.
2. The mss are: Bern, Burgerbibliothek A 94 (10), 11/12th c.; from the twelfth century: Cambridge, Gonville and Caius 411/415; Cambridge, Trinity O.1.40; London, British Library, Egerton 2900; New Haven, Yale Medical Library 16; Oxford, Bodleian Library, MS

Bodl. 489; Oxford, Corpus Christi College 189; Oxford, Bodleian Library, MS Laud misc. 567; Paris, Bibliothèque Nationale, lat. 6951; Vatican, Biblioteca Apostolica, Pal. lat. 1158; Vatican, Biblioteca Apostolica, Pal. lat. 1163. From the thirteenth century: Baltimore, Johns Hopkins Medical Library, Lat. 13.1; Bethesda, National Library of Medicine, MS 12; Cambridge, Gonville and Caius, 97; Cambridge, St. John's D.24; Durham, Dean and Chapter Library, MS C.IV.4; London, British Library, Harley 3140; London, British Library, Royal 12.D.IX; London, British Library, Sloane 371; London, British Library, Sloane 1610; Munich, Bayerische Staatsbibliothek, Cod. lat. mon. 452; Oxford, Bodleian Library, MS Laud lat. 106; Vatican, Biblioteca Apostolica, Pal. lat. 1161; Vatican, Biblioteca Apostolica, Pal. lat. 1162; Vatican, Biblioteca Apostolica, Pal. lat. 1165. Fourteenth century: Cambridge, Trinity R.14.35; Erfurt, Wissenschaftliche Allgemeinbibliothek, F 266; London, British Library, Arundel 215; Munich, Bayerische Staatsbibliothek, Cod. lat. mon. 13086; Paris, Bibliothèque Nationale, lat. 6890; Paris, Bibliothèque Nationale, lat. 14390; Philadelphia, Library of the College of Physicians, MS 8; Vatican, Biblioteca Apostolica, lat. 4425; Vatican, Biblioteca Apostolica, Pal. lat. 1149; Vatican, Biblioteca Apostolica, Pal. lat. 1164; Vatican, Biblioteca Apostolica, reg. lat. 1305. I have not seen Edinburgh, Advocates Library, 18.6.8 (s. 12/13) or Erfurt, Wissenschaftliche Allgemeinbibliothek, CA 190 (s. 12$^2$, Italy). Because I have worked with a number of these mss on microfilm, it is possible that errors involving show-through, erasures, very faint marks, etc. that are not perceptible as such on microfilm or prints from microfilm have crept in.

3. Newton 1976, 41–45 remarks on the surprising absence of Constantine's works in the list of books copied at Desiderius' behest.

4. Schipperges 1964, 54 notes that the twelfth-century manuscripts are most trustworthy. However, New Haven, Yale Medical Library 16 and Vatican, Biblioteca Apostolica, Pal. lat. 1158 have been excluded because they do not offer any readings not found in the other early mss. Vat. pal. lat. 1158 offers a unique text that is heavily altered, probably as a result of teaching needs.

5. Used by Garbers 1977 for the edition of *De melancholia*.

6. Given the siglum P in Wack 1987.

7. The *Pantegni* may, therefore, provide some clues to the mystery of the origins of *hereos*. However, the only *Pantegni* manuscript that I have been able to consult (Cambridge, Trinity College R.14.34 (906), s. 12), contains *amor* in the text (*Theorica*, Bk. 9, cap. 7, fol. 102v) and both *amor* and *eros* in the list of chapter headings (fol. 96v). Whether the chapter headings are Constantine's or a scribe's is unclear.

8. Baader 1967 and 1974.

9. Daremberg 1853, 87; Jacquart and Thomasset 1985a, 151.

10. Some of the early manuscripts have been corrected by later hands that changed *eros* to *hereos*. The earliest manuscript known to me containing *hereos* in the text without signs of correction is Oxford, Corpus Christi College 189, which Richard Rouse suggests (private communication) belongs to the second half of the twelfth century. Lowes 1913, 523 asserted that "the first use of the term *hereos* is to be sought, I am convinced, in some such early Latin translation of a Greek medical text as that which has given us, in the Laon MS of Oribasius, *ton heroton*." While this possibility cannot be excluded, the testimony of the *Viaticum* manuscripts I have checked does not support Lowes' hypothesis. As he points out, initial *h* was freely added and subtracted in medieval Latin. Its addition to *eros* in the Oribasius manuscript is independent, I believe, of its addition in the *Viaticum* manuscripts. As far as I have been able to determine, medical discussions of love before the 11th c. were so rare that Constantine is unlikely to have pressed an early medieval *hereos* (if there was such a term) into service.

11. Vat. pal. lat. 1161, Trinity R.14.35 (907), and Nat. Lib. Med. 12 read *eriosos*; Vat. pal. lat. 1162 reads *erios*; and British Library, Sloane 371 reads *heriosos*.

12. Goetz 1888–1901, 2:15–16, 314–15, 552 and 3:4, 137, 334. Alfanus, Constantine's first patron, translated the *Premnon physicon* of Nemesius from Greek. On Greek and Greeks at Montecassino, see Newton 1976, 52–53 and Bloch 1986, 1:1–98.

13. Noted by Saffron 1972, 11; Baader 1967, 38–39, and 1974, 112.

14. E.g., Goetz 1888–1901, 5:25, 73. It is remotely possible that school commentaries on Ovid's *Heroides* played some role in the genesis of the term. An accessus to the text notes: "Unde quidam intitulant eum 'O(uidius) heroum' idest matronarum uel 'liber heroydos'. 'heros, herois' grecum est masculinum et significat grecas mulieres nobiles" (Hexter 1986, 160).

15. The manuscript forms of the nominative are: Amor qui *eros* dicitur (Bern A 94): *et eros* Vat. pal. lat. 1163, Cambridge, Gonville and Caius 411/415, Paris, Bibliothèque Nationale, MS lat. 6951; *et . .os* Yale 16 (damaged); *et heros* Vat. pal. lat. 1158, British Library Egerton 2900, Cambridge, Trinity 0.1.40; *heros* Oxford, Bodleian Library, MS Bodl. 489; *et hereos* Oxford, Corpus Christi College 189; *zeros* Oxford, Laud misc. 567.

*Heros* est nomen maxime delectationis: Bern A 94, Vat. pal. lat. 1158, British Library Egerton 2900, Oxford, Bodleian Library, MS Bodl. 489, Cambridge, Trinity 0.1.40; *Eros* Vat. pal. lat. 1163, Paris, BN lat. 6951, Oxford, Corpus Christi College 189; *Eroi* Yale 16 (damaged); *heres* Cambridge, Gonville and Caius 411/415; *zeros* Oxford, Laud misc. 567. The peculiar reading *zeros* may support an original reading of *eros* if we see in it a misreading of a tironian *et* sign: 7eros (for "et eros").

16. *Expositio in tertium canonis Avicennae* (Madrid, Biblioteca Nacional, Inc. 1743), fol. 113r. I would like to thank Joseph Gwara for sending me a transcription of the passage from this extremely rare edition.

## Edition

1. See the introduction for a discussion of *eros/heros/hereos*.

2. *Contiguus* is puzzling as an expression for "in the brain"; the variant *continuus* in later mss indicates that it baffled medieval scribes as well. Although the lemma in Gerard of Berry's gloss is *contiguus*, the meaning assigned, *assiduus*, shows that it was understood as *continuus*. The *Thesaurus Linguae Latinae* notes that *contiguus* "transit in notionem *continuus*" and cites Boethius, *Top.* 4.2: "quod continuatur contiguum est." Dugat's translation (1853) of the Arabic does not clarify Constantine's word choice: "L'amour ('ichq') est une des maladies qui prennent naissance dans le cerveau."

3. Baader 1974, 109 points out that *extremitas* is one of Constantine's contributions to the development of medical Latin. On love as excess in Arabic thinking (ultimately from Aristotle, *Nic. Eth.* viii.6 1158a), see Bell 1979, 162.

4. The early mss agree on this reading; the variant *causa*, frequent in later mss, seems to be a gloss that has slipped in to replace the *lectio difficilior*.

5. Rufus of Ephesus (1–2nd c. C. E.), whose treatise on melancholy is preserved only in quotations and extracts from other writers. These are gathered in Daremberg and Ruelle 1879. See also Flashar 1966, 84–104 and Klibansky et al. 1964, 48–55. Rufus' pronouncements on the advantages of intercourse influenced therapeutic practice until the Renaissance. They were incorporated into the works of the great Byzantine compilers Oribasius (326–403), Aetius of Amida (fl. ca. 527–67), and Paul of Aegina (625–90), from which the Arabs drew heavily. Cf. *Constantini liber de coitu*, ch. 10 (ed. Montero Cartelle 1983, 126–28) "de utilitate coitus": "Rufus vero ait quod coitus solvit malum habitum corporis et furorem mitigat, prodest melancolicis et amentes revocat ad noticiam et solvit amorem concupiscencie, licet concumbat cum alia quam concupivit"; and *De melancholia* (ed. Garbers 1977, 185): "Coitus etiam adiuvat, *Rufo* testante. Coitus, inquit, pacificat, anteriorem superbiam refrenat, melancolicos adiuvat. Nonne enim vides, cum bruta irascuntur animalia, qualiter post coitum fiant mitia" (added by Constantine to his Arabic source).

6. Lawrence Berman kindly checked the Arabic text and reported that the Arabic word rendered by *herois* (B) is a genitive meaning "of love" or "of the lover." Hence *erous, erois, erroris*, etc. must be seen as attempts at the genitive of *eros*.

7. Although sense and syntax demand a genitive, I have left the mss reading because the mss are surprisingly consistent in preserving an uninflected form. Several explanations are possible. Constantine may have given up on the declension of *eros* after the previous sentence, and settled for an uninflected form. Or, since he is compressing his Arabic source at this point, which appears to contain a nominative form ("Quelquefois l'amour est le désir ardent de l'âme . . ."), he may have shifted constructions mid-sentence. It may also be a hopelessly corrupt passage. Cf. the *Liber de heros morbo* (Wack 1987): "Huius autem herois causa aliquando est . . ."

8. The Platonic theory of beauty as the cause of love clearly underlies this passage, a view that was widespread in Arabic philosophical and mystical treatises. The Arabs stressed the connaturality of the lover and beloved. See Bell 1979, 34–37, 107 ff.

9. In the Arabic and Greek texts, and the *Liber de heros morbo*, sleeplessness causes the

motion of bile (*coler*) which in turn causes swelling and jaundice of the eyelids. The variants *caloris/calore* and *motu/motus* reveal uncertainty about the proper object of *ex* and hence about the relation among heat, motion, and yellowish eyelids. An early scribal mistake of *calor* for *coler* may have caused the confusion.

10. Mesulam and Perry 1972 and Ciavolella 1970 comment on the "lover's pulse" from different perspectives.

11. That the soul is affected by the state of the body was a commonplace of medieval medicine. The allusion is to Galen's *Quod animi mores corporis temperamenta sequuntur* (Müller 1891, 2:32–79, trans. Hauke 1937). The notion is particularly emphasized in discussions of melancholy (e.g., 2:49), including Constantine's *De melancholia* (Garbers 1977, 103): "Corpus enim animam sequitur in suis actionibus, anima vero corpus in suis accidentibus."

12. Cf. *De melancholia* (Garbers 1977, 104): "Sicut dixit Hippocrates in epidimiarum libris, sexta particula: Animae, inquit, labor est cogitatio. Sicut autem corporis labor pessimos generat morbos, utpote laborem, itidem labor animae in melancholiam facit cadere, quod autem dicendum est de eis qui amata sua perdiderunt."

13. Cf. *De melancholia*, Bk. 1 (Basel, 1536) p. 289: "Letatur enim anima de complexione sua temperata, utpote a vino humectata"; Bk. 2 (290): "Cum ergo passio melancholica anime habeat accidentia timenda et periculosa . . . tollendo que in anima sunt plantata, cum diversa musica, et vino odorifero claro et subtilissimo."

14. According to ancient consolation literature (Kassel 1958), the most powerful drug against sorrow is the word.

15. See Olson 1982.

16. Bell 1979, 23 cites a treatise which attributes the following to the Prophet: "Three things clarify the vision: looking at greenery, looking at water, and looking at beautiful faces." Cf. *De melancholia*, Bk. 2 (Basel, 1536) pp. 394, 395: "Laudabilia sunt exercitia pedum temperata"; "Melancholici ergo assuescant ad pedum exercitia aliquantulum, apparente aurora, per loca spatiosa, ac plana, arenosa, et saporosa." *Pantegni*, pars practica, Bk. 5, cap. 21 (Lyons, 1515) 2:99v: "Hanc passionem [amor] cum vino odorifero et gratis verbis et diversis musicorum generibus curabis colloquiis cum dilectissimis; somnis; fructiferos videre hortos et odoriferos et lucidos; et aquam currentem videre et claram; spaciari cum pluribus mulieribus seu maribus. hec omnia tristiciam et timorem auferunt."

17. Cf. Rufus in Oribasius (ed. Bussemaker and Daremberg 1851–76, 5:7): "the remedy for sorrow is wine" and al-Rāzī, *Continens*, tr. IX (Daremberg and Ruelle 1879, 454–59): "et qui potest sustinere potum vini non indiget alia cura, quia eo solo sunt omnia quae sunt necessaria in cura hujus passionis." *Pantegni*, pars practica, 5.25 (1515): "Rufus inquit: vinum est fortis medicina tristibus timidis curiosis et hereosis; similiter balneum. Unde fit cum quidam balneum intrant ad cantandum excitantur vel animantur." Cf. Pigeaud 1981, 497–503.

18. The Arabic, Greek, and *Liber de heros morbo* all attribute the saying to Galen, but I have been unable to find anything resembling it among his works. Something similar is attributed to Orpheus in *De melancholia* (ed. Garbers 1977, 184): "Idem *Orpheus*: Sapientissimus, inquit, fuit, qui succum extraxit uvae in torculari, cum & tristem animam laetificet, immo laetitiam generet."

19. Zeno is quoted in Diogenes Laertius, 7.1.22 (Hicks 1937) and Galen, *Quod animi mores* (Müller 1891, 39–40).

20. In *De melancholia* and *Liber de heros morbo* these words are also attributed to Orpheus (Garbers 1977, 152–55): "Orpheus enim dixit, qui tonos adinvenit: Imperatores me ad convivia invitant, ut de me se delectent & gaudeant, sed ego de ipsis delector animos immutando, de ira in pacem, de tristicia in laetitiam, de gravitate in levitatem, de timore in audaciam." The Arabic and Greek texts name al-Kindi as the source for this quotation, but a search of his works available to me in translation failed to unearth the saying. Compare Macrobius, *Commentary on the Dream of Scipio*, trans. William Harris Stahl (New York: Columbia University Press, 1952), p. 195.

21. *Pantegni*, pars practica, 5.21 (1515): "Galie[nus]: colloqui inquit cum amantibus laborem eijcit et gaudium elicit a membris interioribus. Similiter cibaria letificantia sicut borago, basilicon, crocus, vinum odoriferum, ambra, ligna aloes, ciperum sericum crudum, ustum, aurum, muscus, electuarium quod leticia vocatur, et antidoton helmiferatum ut muscata malorum et omnia animam letificant."

22. Cited in PSQ N 6 (Lawn 1979, 280). A gloss in Bethesda, National Library of Medicine, 12 notes: "minus grauatur quod a duobus portatur."

# Gerard of Berry

## Manuscripts

1. A handlist of manuscripts is in preparation. I owe warmest thanks to Monica Green, who checked manuscripts in London, Paris, Munich, and Rome, and to Patricia Stirnemann, who checked prologues of Gerard's commentary and confirmed the dates of manuscripts in Paris. The marginal glosses to the *Viaticum* in Cambridge, St. John's College D.24 (99) are not from Peter of Spain's commentary, as noted in TK² (257), but from Gerard's *Glosule*.

2. Examples of additions:

| | | |
|---|---|---|
| actores grecos | *for* | auctores |
| forte credit | | credit |
| uitio uel adustio | | adustio |
| curatur secundum Avicenna | | curatur |
| diuersentur siue diuertantur | | diuertantur |
| ludorum multum prosunt | | ludorum |
| hereos siue heriosi | | heroes |
| dilecte uel desiderata | | desiderata |
| calidam colericam | | colericam |
| communi uicti uel usu | | conuictu |
| graui amore | | amore |
| moderate sumptum | | moderatum |

3. The following preliminary list of the greater and lesser prologues may be of use to future editors of Gerard's work: *Prologus minor*: Inc.: "Cum omnia ex .iiij. elementis generata a medicis sint quodammodo cognoscenda . . ."

Found in: Cambridge, Gonville and Caius 117/186 (no biographical information); Bethesda, National Library of Medicine 11 (no biographical information); Admont 386 [sold in 1934]; Oxford, Exeter 35; London, British Library, Sloane 3096; Cambridge, University Library 938; Vatican, Biblioteca Apostolica, reg. lat. 1304; Prague, Biblioteka Jagiellonska 2349; Paris, Bibliothèque Nationale, lat. 6889, 6890, 16181; edition of Gerard of Berry's text in Gerardus de Solo, *Opera omnia*, Venice, 1505.

*Prologus maior*: Inc.: "Cum omne elementum et ex elementis corpus generatum in materia communitatem habeant . . ."

Found in: Baltimore, Johns Hopkins Medical School, MS lat. 13.1; Basel D.III.6; Cambridge, Trinity R.14.35; Erfurt, Wissenschaftliche Allgemeinbibliothek F 266 and CA 221; Vatican, Biblioteca Apostolica, lat. 2453, 2454, and 4432; Vatican, Pal. lat. 1149, 1161, and 1165; Munich, Bayerische Staatsbibliothek 3512; Cues 303, 307; Paris, Bibliothèque Nationale, lat. 6888, 6892, 15115, 15116, and 16182; and the Venice 1505 edition of Gerard of Solo's works.

## Edition

1. On the variants *auctores-actores grecos* see Chenu 1927, 81–86. T and its relatives, recognizing the following paraphrase, substitute *Avicenna*. The definition is from Avicenna's *Canon medicinae*, lib. 3, fen 1, tract. 4, cap. 24 (Venice, 1507): "Hec egritudo est sollicitudo melancolica similis melancolie, in quo homo sibi iam induxit incitationem cogitationis sue super pulchritudine quarundam formarum et figurarum que insunt ei. Deinde adiuvat ipsum ad illud desiderium eius et non consequitur."

2. On the technical rather than moral sense of "error" here see Demaitre 1985, 339. As far as surviving sources allow us to judge, Gerard is responsible for introducing impairment of the estimative power into the etiology of the disease. Impaired judgment had been associated with melancholy since ancient times, and was reaffirmed by Avicenna, *Canon*, lib. 3, fen 1, tract. 4, cap. 19: "dicitur melancolia mutatio extimationum et cogitationum a cursu naturali ad corruptionem et ad timorem et ad malitiam."

3. "Sensed intentions" is a technical term in medieval faculty psychology. *Intentiones* are, roughly speaking, intentions, though the creature harboring them need not be human or possess volition in the usual sense. In the standard medieval illustration of this concept, as well as

of the functioning of the estimative faculty, a sheep will instinctively perceive the hostile "intention" of a wolf toward it. "Intentions" involve judgments of the object's desirability or lack of it. "Accidents" inhere in or befall substance; they are sensible and contingent qualities, such as coloring, hair color, height, etc. Gerard is saying, therefore, that once an object has been judged exceedingly desirable, the mind will perceive physical qualities that may not be there. Cf. David of Dinant (Kurdziałek 1963, 6): "Deinceps autem sciendum, quod facile decipimur circa sensum propter passiones quibus dispositi sumus, ut timidus in timore et amans in amore" (cf. Aristotle, *On Dreams*, 460b1–5).

4. While the idealization of the beloved may be distantly related to strategies for advantageous marriages (cf. Isidore, *Etymologies* 9.7.29 on desirable qualities in a prospective wife), Gerard's formulation corresponds more directly to lyric descriptions of the *domna* (e.g. Bernart de Ventadorn, "Non es maravelh s'eu chan"). On the lover's delusion that the woman is more noble than she is in reality, compare the class-consciousness in Andreas Capellanus, *De amore* I.D.181 (Walsh 1982, 90): "Amor enim personam saepe degenerem et deformem tanquam nobilem et formosam repraesentat amanti, et facit eam plus quam omnes alias nobilem atque pulcherrimam deputari."

5. Avicenna, *De anima* 2.2.18 (1972, 119): "Ergo aestimatio apprehendit res materiatas et abstrahit eas a materia, sicut apprehendit etiam intentiones non sensibiles, quamvis sunt materiatae." On the internal senses in general, see Wolfson 1935, 86–113 and Harvey 1975. Gerard applies to an inward sense a phenomenon discussed by Aristotle and Avicenna with respect to the outer senses, namely, that "the greater stimulus tends to expell the less" (*De sensu*, c. 7, 447a; Aristotle, *De anima* III 429a; Avicenna, *De anima* 5.2.12–25 [1968, 97]). An exceedingly pleasurable stimulus eclipses subsequent, less pleasurable stimuli, with the result that the original stimulus is the only one available for the inner senses to operate upon—hence balanced judgment, which involves comparison, becomes impossible.

6. Avicenna, *De anima* 4.3.96 (1968, 35): "Dicemus ergo quia aestimatio excellentior iudex est in animalibus."

7. The hierarchy of faculties by which the estimation governs desire and ultimately motion is described in Avicenna, *De anima*, 1.5.93ff. (1968, 100): "Deinde virtuti imaginativae deserviunt duae virtutes diversarum actionum: virtus enim appetitiva deservit ei cum oboedientia, quia aestimativa imperat ei moveri aliquo modo praeceptionis; virtus autem imaginativa servit aestimativae, per hoc quod ostendit ei formas retentas in ea quae sunt aptae ad recipiendum compositionem et divisionem. Deinde hae dominantur aliis: virtuti autem imaginativae servit fantasia; fantasiae vero serviunt quinque sensus; virtuti autem appetitivae serviunt concupiscibilis et irascibilis, sed concupiscibili et irascibili servit virtus movens quae est in lacertis."

8. On *spiritus* see Bono 1984. The role of *spiritus* as a medium between intention and operation was discussed by the Salernitan Urso of Calabria in his *Aphorisms* and *Glosule*, ed. Creutz 1936. Gerard in effect describes a process also outlined by Urso while using the set of mental faculties, including the estimation, named by Avicenna. Cf. Urso's Glosula 24 (Creutz 1936, 51): "Aliquotiens per sensum concupiscendo ad ymaginanda sensibilia incitamur, utpote cum aliquae delectabilia sensu percipiamus, intentione mentis ad haec deflexa, spiritu recurrente ad fantasiae instrumentum et incitante virtutem fantasticam, statim ad concipiendos effectus delectabiles rei sensae et cum sitienti appetitu per ymaginationem movemur et ymaginatione completa animae intentione duce spiritus ad illa membra trahitur, quae membra utpote instrumenta ad tales effectus perficiendos sunt deputata, ut membrorum natura per spiritum mota hos conceptos effectus percipiat."

9. McVaugh 1985, 23 points out that Gerard's location of the *virtus imaginativa* in the first ventricle does not follow Avicenna's scheme of cerebral localization of mental faculties. Perhaps Gerard derives his explanation from Salernitan teaching as exemplified by Urso's analysis of illicit passionate love in Glosula 85 (Creutz 1936, 119): "Similiter omnis vis imaginaria, quae virtus animae est appetitiva, per spiritum ad aliquid detestabile imaginandum movetur, cum videat quae concupiscuntur haberi nequeat, ut desiderium compleatur ad movendum spiritum amplius incitatur, quo motu intercluso sic spiritus calefit et subtiliatur, ut suae motionis impetu occulta substantia aduratur vel substantialis humiditas penitus aduratur et propter hoc exsiccatione cerebri non modica illiciti amantes sequuntur mente desiderata volentes; cum ea habere nequeant, sollicita et sedula cogitatione maniaci vel melancolici seu ethici efficiuntur, qua causa nitituri in vetitum cupimus semper quae negata." Cf. also PSQ, N 1.

10. In the thirteenth century this becomes a widely-repeated sign of love. It is found in

Bk. 3 of Andreas Capellanus' *De amore* (ed. Walsh 1982, 296): "nec, si aliquis ei de quocunque facto loquatur, ipsius dictis intentas adhibet aures, nec precantis solet ad plenum verba percipere, nisi aliquid de suo referendo loquatur amore. Tunc etenim si continuo secum uno mense loquatur non unum iota de omni fabulatione dimitteret." Hugh of St. Cher, who borrows extensively from Gerard's semeiology of love (see chapter 3), lists this among his *signa amoris.* See Hendrix 1980a, 127: "Sextum signum amoris extatici est profunda cogitatio et sollicitudo versa ad interiora, ita quod talis amorosus gerere videtur ymaginem dormientis qui evigilari non potest nisi cum de re amata fit ei mentio. Unde si cum amoroso loquaris de hiis que inter homines fiunt, que ad rem amatam non pertinent, vix intelligere potest. Si autem de re amata vel quod ad rem amatam aliquo modo pertineat statim intelligit et evigilantis gerit ymaginem eo quod tota intentio et cogitatio sua fixa est in re amata." Cf. Karnein 1985, 288, *Hec sunt duodecim signa*: "Qui videre non potest eum vel eam, libenter audit loqui de eo vel ea."

11. Avicenna, *Canon* III fen 1 tract..4, cap. 24: "Et signa quidem sunt profunditas oculorum et siccitas ipsorum et privatio lachrymarum nisi cum fletus adest: et motus continuus palpebrarum risibilis quasi aspiciat aliquid pulchrum delectabile aut audiat rumorem iocundantem aut letificetur."

12. Cf. Hugh of St. Cher, *De doctrina cordis* (Hendrix 1980a, 121): "Secundum signum amoris extatici est desiccatio membrorum. Amorosi etiam aresciunt in membris eo quod vehementi cordis applicatione circa rem dilectam multiplicantur spiritus ex quo interiorem desiccationem patiuntur."

13. Avicenna, *Canon* III fen 1 tract. 4, cap. 24: "Amplius cum non invenitur cura nisi regimen coniunctionis inter eos secundum modum permissionis fidei et legis fiat."

14. Nearly verbatim from Avicenna, *ibid.* cap. 25: "Considera an eius dispositio pervenerit ad adustionem humoris per signa que nosti et evacua. Deinde administra eis somnum et humectationem et nutrimentum ipsorum cum laudabilibus, et fac ipsos balneari secundum conditionem humectationis notam."

15. Condensed from Avicenna, cap. 25: "Et vetule ad eum incitentur ut vituperent illud quod diligunt ipsi et rememorentur eius dispositiones . . . narrent iste vetule formas eius quod diligunt cum similitudibus fetidis."

16. Avicenna, *ibid.*: "Et ex occupationis predictis est corruptio (Venice, 1595: emptio) puellarum et plurimus concubitus ipsarum et renovatio ipsarum et delectatio cum ipsis."

17. The underlined phrases indicate the portions of Constantine's text that are being glossed. For *heros* = "lord," "noble" see Wack 1987, 336 ff. On the connection between leisure and erotic desire, see Constantine the African, *De coitu* (ed. Montero Cartelle 1983, 160): "adaugent libidinem, ut cor ociosum et cotidiana leticia, secundum quod ait Filumenus." Cf. Hugh of St. Cher, *De doctrina cordis* (Hendrix 1980a, 119–20): "[amor exstaticus in malo] est autem amor ereos magnum desiderium cum nimia concupiscentia et afflictione cogitationum [Constantine, *Viaticum* 20.1]. Ereos dicuntur viri nobiles qui propter mollitiem et delicias vite subiecti sunt huiusmodi passione."

18. On the subjects of loyalty and secrecy the vocabulary of spiritual friendship and of vernacular passionate love intermingle. On the mutual obligations *celar-retener* between poet/lover and lady, see Leube-Fey 1971, 138–46 and Andreas Capellanus, *De amore* I.6, I.H (Walsh 1982, 44, 174, 198). On secrecy as one of the key elements in friendship, see Hendrix 1980a, 120 n. 35: the sixth *signum amoris* is "secretorum revelatio." See also Karnein 1985, 288: "Secretum servat nec denudat" [from *Hec sunt duodecim signa*]. Compare the French translation (Karnein 1985, 290): "Li premiers signes de vraie amour si est loiaus cuers, qui ne puet riens celer vers son ami."

19. Cf. Richard de Fournival, *Consaus d'amours* (Speroni 1974, 264): "Ja soit ce que maladies vienent a homme par destemprance d'aucunes des humeurs ki soustient le vie del homme, les maladies d'amours ne vienent pas par destemperation ne par corruption, ne li mal d'amer ne sont mie mal comme autre, ains sont grant desirrier ki carcent le cuer. Et, tout aussi conme on a veü aucune fois par grant joie le gent perdre le boire et le mengier et morir, tout en tel maniere li desirriers envoie ces manieres de maladies d'amours."

20. Cf. Aristotle, *De anima* II.4.415b 18: "All natural bodies are organs of the soul" and *Summa pulsuum* in Grant 1974, 746: "The soul thus moves the pulse, like an artificer; and in the same way, with the artificer absent, his instruments are stilled."

21. The closest parallel that I have been able to find is Guillaume de Conches, *Dragmaticon*, Stanford University Library, Dept. of Special Collections, fol. 85v (Philosophus speaks): "Corpora vero humana ex quatuor elementis proportionaliter et concorditer coniunctis sunt

constituta. Sed proportio et concordia animam allicit et corpori coniunxit et in corpore reti-
net. . . . Unde ea que illam proportionem conservant appetit; et que illam destruant fugit. Sed
ex quo incipiunt elementa discordare abhorret anima corpus et ab eo separatur."
     22. Cf. Urso of Calabria, *Glosula* 41 (Creutz 1936, 74): "Ex natura complexionis sic
variantur animae passiones, quare si quis habuerit cor calidum et siccum debet esse animosus,
furiosus, iracundus. . . . Ex longa vero consuetudine, utpote ex altera natura, prima natura
convincitur." Ultimately from Galen, *Microtegni seu ars parva* in *Articella* (Venice, 1498, 167r).

## Giles

     1. Cf. the similar arguments in Peter of Spain's *Questiones super Viaticum*, Version A,
lines 55–97 and Aristotle, *Categoriae* 14a15 (Minuo-Paluello 1961, 37): "Manifestum est autem
quoniam circa idem vel specie vel genera nata sunt fieri contraria; aegritudo namque et sanitas
circa corpus animalis."
     2. Cf. Peter of Spain, *Questiones super Viaticum*, Version A, lines 85–90.
     3. Cf. *De melancholia* (Basel, 1536) p. 393: "Tamen reprehendant nos quidam obijciendo.
Vinum et mentem percutit, et mala sua uitia ostendit."
     4. *De dietis universalibus et particularibus* (Basel, 1570) 2.5, p. 574: "uinum uetustissimum
auget calorem naturalem ultra temperamentum, nocetque membraneis cerebri, et mentem percutit." See Peter of Spain, *Questions on the Viaticum*, Version A, lines 232–48, and Version B,
lines 266–81.
     5. *Remedia amoris*, lines 809–10: "aut nulla ebrietas, aut tanta sit, ut tibi curas / eripiat:
si qua est inter utrumque, nocet." Cf. Peter of Spain, *Questions on the Viaticum*, lines 268–70.
     6. Walther 1963, 28237a; see also 4034 and 6416.

## Peter of Spain, Version A

### Manuscripts

1. Da Cruz Pontes 1964, 253.

### Edition

     1. The manuscripts list four questions on sneezing, the subject of the chapter after *amor*
in the *Viaticum*, together with the questions on love. I have omitted questions 11–14 on sneezing as irrelevant to the topic of lovesickness.
     2. *Isagoge* III.1 (Gracia and Vidal 1974–75, 337): "Morbus est qui principaliter corpori
nocet nullo mediatore qui eum adiuvet." Cf. *Pantegni*, IV.20 theorice: "Infirmitas ergo est quod
sensuali actioni nocet"; Peter of Spain, *Glosae super introitum sciencie tegni Galieni*, Madrid, BN
1877, fol. 50v: "Morbus enim est mala dispositio infi' nocumentum operationibus naturalibus
immediate."
     3. See *Viaticum* above, lines 1–2. On the cogitative power, see SLA, 263: "dicitur [fan-
tasya] autem cogitativa eo quod considerationi et speculationi circa formas sensibiles deputa-
tur. . . . cum autem intellectus imperium [sequitur], cogitativa vocatur."
     4. *De anima* 1.5.48–50 (1972, 89): "Deinde est vis aestimationis; quae est vis ordinata in
summo mediae concavitatis cerebri, apprehendens intentiones non sensatas quae sunt in singulis sensibilibus." Cf. Gerard of Berry's analysis, above, lines 6–18.
     5. The sense of the passage seems to require a main clause, which I have supplied.
     6. For Peter's notion of the fantasy, whose essential task is compounding and dividing
images, see SLA, 263–64: "Eius [sc. fantasie] igitur obiecta sunt omnes formes sensibiles que
in sensu communi representate in ymaginatione reponuntur tam proprie quam communes,
omnes etiam *iudicat, distinguit, conponit ac dividit*. Operatio autem eius in harum formarum
conpositione ac divisione consistit, nam ipsa etiam in absentia sensibilium obiectorum has
formas conponit ac dividit et circa ipsarum conpositionem et divisionem *inducit iudicium*.
Quandoque vero eius vigor intenditur et tunc format ymagines conponens ipsas ac dividens

que in re existentiam non habentes nunquam fuerunt exterioribus sensibus presentate. Et hec deviatio ei accidit, cum ad sensus exteriores non inclinatur, nec regimen suscipit intellectus" [emphases mine].

7. The sense seems to require a verb meaning "transfer, transmit" or perhaps "represent." Cf. Version B, line 169: "estimativa . . . mandat desiderium ad memorativam."

8. This passage follows Gerard of Berry's account closely, which in turn depends on Avicenna's chapters on *ilisci* in the *Canon*, lib.3, fen 1, tract. 4, cap. 24–25.

9. Again, I have supplied what the sense seems to demand.

10. Aristotle, *Categoriae vel Praedicamenta* 14a15 (Minuo-Paluello 1961, 37): "Manifestum est autem quoniam circa idem vel specie vel genera nata sunt fieri contraria; aegritudo namque et sanitas circa corpus animalis." On the somatic localization of *amor*, see Version B.61–98 (below) and Egidius (above).

11. Cf. John of St. Amand, *Concordantiae* (Pagel 1894, 65): "Mores sunt sequentes complexionem cordis et ideo a calore cordis procedit virilitas et festinantia (in tegni cap. 4)"; and Aristotle, *De anima* 408b7–8.

12. Aristotle, *De somno et vigilia*, c. 1, 458a. Cf. B.72–73.

13. Peter of Spain, *Commentum in regimine acutorum*, Madrid, BN 1877, fol. 110v: "Nos non distinguimus species morborum nisi per distinctionem humorum. Unde dicimus 'tercianam de colera.'" Cf. B.191–92 and Gerard of Solo, *Determinatio* (Wack 1989b).

14. The sense of this phrase eludes me; the text is possibly defective here.

15. *Viaticum*, above, lines 28–30; cf. Gerard of Berry, lines 1–5 and Peter's version B.5–10.

16. The distinction is between love as one of the *passiones animae*, here termed *passio cordis*, which is not a morbid state, and love that is accompanied by melancholy worry and a damaged estimative faculty, which is both a *passio* and a *morbus* of the brain. This is essentially the same conclusion as that of Egidius. Several decades after Peter, Arnald of Villanova was to declare that "Amor . . . dicitur proprie accidens et non morbus" in the first chapter of the *Tractatus de amore heroico* (McVaugh 1985).

17. On the passions of the soul and the heart, see SLA, 284: "Affective vero virtutis fundamentum primum cor est, sed proximius est cerebrum in quo virtutum sensibilium existit origo et ideo ipso passiones ac perturbationes incurrente affective opera disturbantur, et affectiones prave et inordinate consecuntur. Sed cum ipsa a corde primo procedat et eius in cerebro vigeat ipsius opera ad cordis regionem devolvuntur, ad quorum diversitatem cordis motus suorumque contentorum varietatem agitationemque receptat." Cf. Urso (Creutz 1936, 40): "In cerebro vero per ymaginationem seu cogitationem omnis animae passio sumit exordium, eademque ymaginatione peracta per reductionem spirituum ad cor in corde accipit complementum."

18. See note 14 above and B.179–94.

19. For example, Avicenna, al-Rāzī, and Gerard of Berry (lines 46–8 and notes). Cf. Gerard of Solo, *Determinatio* (Wack 1989b).

20. I have not been able to find in Avicenna's chapter on *ilisci* that sexual stimulation is the greatest cause of lovesickness, unless this is an inference from the prominence Avicenna gives to therapeutic intercourse. Cf. Arnald, *Tractatus*, 47: "Hic autem amor furiosus . . . inter virum et mulierem videtur, imperio subiugato rationis, incendi propter singularem coitus delectationem."

21. Galen, *Tegni*, in *Articella* (Lyons, 1525) fol. cxᵛ: "Calida vero et sicca crasis . . . et citissime ad coitum excitat."

22. Aristotle, *Historia animalium*, 9.1, 608b 11–12: "[Woman] is more prone to despondency and less hopeful than the man."

23. It was a medical commonplace that men were hot and dry and women cold and moist. On lovesickness and gender see B.195–247 and chapter 6.

24. On women's greater libido see Isidore, *Etymologiae* 11.2.24: "Alii Graeca etymologia feminam ab ignea vi dictam putant, quia vehementer concupiscit. Libidinosiores enim viris feminas esse tam in mulieribus quam in animalibus. Unde nimius amor apud antiquos femineus vocabatur." Cf. PSQ B 7 and Bartholomaeus Anglicus, *De proprietatibus rerum* 18.49, trans. John Trevisa (1975, 2:1200).

25. On the differing divisions of the ages of life, see Sears 1986, esp. 25–31. In a common fourfold scheme, the *puer* became a *iuvenis* at 14, a *vir* at 25, and a *senex* at 45. In the *Pantegni* 1.21 theorice, the transitional ages are 30, 40, and 60, and *iuventus* is classified as hot and dry.

26. See note 20 above.

27. On the beginning of intercourse in *pueris*, see PSQ B 9 and B 174.

28. This recommendation is not in the Venice 1507 edition of Avicenna, but al-Rāzī does suggest travel. The question may be more controversial than it seems, since according to William of Saliceto, *Summa conservationis et curationis* (Venice, 1502) fol. 16v, leaving one's country could itself be a cause of melancholy: "Si vero ex desiderio repatriandi contingat [melancolia], hec melancolia vel modus infirmitatis non requirit aliam curam nisi ut inducatur patiens ad repatriandum si possibile fuerit; si non, curetur ut dictum est in cura melancolie ex amore."

29. Cf. Andreas Capellanus, *De amore* 1.1 (Walsh 1982, 32).

30. *Articella* (Lyons, 1525) fol. cxvii r–v, 3.84–87; see also "contraria" in the *Concordanciae* of Jean de St. Amand (Pagel 1894). Cf. Arnald, *Tractatus*, 53: "Forma itaque curationis recte habetur si contrarium huius furie destructivum diligentia procuretur induci. Cum igitur hec furia suique causa formalis sit intensa cogitatio super delectabile, hoc cum confidentia obtinendi, erit illi directe correctivum oppositum, non in hoc delectabili cogitare nec sperare nullo modo eius obtentum. Hec vero perficient competenter quecumque per representationem suarum formarum in virtute fantastica distrahunt in diversam a predicta cogitationem, in toto vel in aliqua parte—saltim veluti forme rerum ducentium rem desideratam in odium, sicut rei turpitudines oculo monstrare vel enarrare sermonibus et cetera."

31. Perhaps the following sentence of the *Canon*, lib. 3, fen 1, tract. 4, cap. 25 is referred to: "Et ex occupationibus predictis [namely cures] est corruptio puellarum et plurimus concubitus ipsarum et renovatio ipsarum et delectatio cum ipsis."

32. *Rhetorica* 2.23, 1397a.

33. *Tegni* 3.91 in *Articella* (Lyons, 1525) fol. cxvii v: "Alteratio quidem est faciens cessare putredinem manente substantia. Evacuatio vero totam a corpore educens substantiam."

34. Peter of Spain, *Glosae super introitum sciencie tegni Galieni*, Madrid, BN 1877, fol. 95r: "Dicit Galienus omne simile augmentat suum similem et facit ipsum furere in commento super afforismos." The reference appears to be to Galen, *Commentary on Hippocrates' Aphorisms* 2.34 (Kühn 17.2:530).

35. See note 31 above.

36. See Egidius' second question.

37. *De diaetis universalibus et particularibus* 2.5 (Basel, 1570) p. 574: "uinum uetustissimum auget calorem naturalem ultra temperamentum, nocetque membraneis cerebri, et mentem percutit."

38. Cf. B.266–81.

39. Al-Rāzī, *Divisiones*, cap. xi (Lyons, 1510) fol. vi v: "Cura eius [sc. amoris] est assiduatio coytus et ieiunium et deambulatio et ebrietas plurima assidue." Avicenna, *Canon*, lib. 3, fen 1, tract. 4, cap. 25: "administra eis . . . nutrimentum ipsorum cum laudabilibus."

40. Avicenna, *ibid.*: "Et etiam vetule ad eum incitentur ut vituperent illud quod diligunt ipsi et rememorentur eius dispositiones et narrent ei res aliquas de ipso vituperationes multas." Cf. Gerard of Berry and Bona Fortuna.

41. Haly appears to be a mistake for al-Rāzī (n. 39 above).

# Peter of Spain, Version B

## Manuscripts

1. Schipperges 1968/9 suggests that Madrid 1877 was written in Siena around 1255. He notes (313) that Cod. Cusanus 307 (14th c.) contains a fragment of Peter's commentary on the *Viaticum* (not remarked by Marx 1905, 296–99). I have not seen this manuscript.

2. Selections from Peter's *De animalibus* commentary in Madrid 1877 and Florence, Fondo Conventi Soppressi, G.4.853 that are printed by da Cruz Pontes 1964, 255–82 show the same types of difference as appear in the Madrid 1877 version of the *Viaticum* commentary and VPA. Alonso 1961, xliv notes that Madrid 1877 holds an abbreviated edition of Peter's commentary on Isaac's *Diaetes universales* as compared to the Lyons 1515 edition. Schipperges 1968, 317 reaches a similar conclusion for the commentary on *De urinis*. See also Alonso 1944, 36–37 and da Cruz Pontes 1981.

3. M lacks many of Peter's characteristic formulae of argumentation (e.g., *Prima ratio*

*talis est*), some citations of authorities, and differs in phrasing at various points from the other 3 mss of the B version (PVA). E.g.:

| M | PVA |
|---|---|
| et habet aspectum ad aliquod membrum particulare | cum in amore sit appetitus rei amate necesse est hoc desiderium et hunc appetitum ad aliquod membrum particulare pertinere |
| est in castratis et in hiis qui non possunt cohire | inest castratis et non potentibus cohire |
| *om.* | ut dicit Philosophus |
| *om.* | per auctoritatem Ovidii |
| extorsio | ereptio |
| representabitur | presentetur |

4. The various forms of the text of Version B may be summarized as follows:
M: no prologue to *Questiones*; no *lectura* on *amor hereos*; earliest version of B?
P: no prologue; no *lectura*; more polished than M
A: prologue (an elaborate *divisio textus*); no *lectura*
V: prologue and *lectura*

## Edition

1. The definition conflates those of Constantine and Avicenna (*Canon medicinae*, lib. III, fen 1, tract. 4, cap. 24) to which is added the difficult last phrase. A marginal gloss in Bethesda, National Library of Medicine MS 12 (*Viaticum*), fol. 17r seems to quote Peter and suggests that V's reading is correct: "Avicenna. hereos est sollicitudo cum profunditate cogitationum in qua figitur mens propter pulchritudinem et dispositionem ad effectum aÍa." *Effectus* can mean *affectus*; given the context, I have translated according to the possibilities suggested in Latham 1975 and Fuchs 1970 under *affectus*.

2. Variants of this definition of love occur in Latin, Old French, and Middle English: see Brown 1932, 14–15; Walther 1963, 681 and 683, nos. 5567 and 5579a; and Speroni 1974, 250. Bernard of Gordon, *Practica dicta Lilium medicine*, quotes this poem in his discussion of *amor hereos* (cap. 20), as does Gerard of Solo, *Determinatio de amore hereos* (Erfurt, Collectio Amploniana F 270, fols. 77v–78v).

3. *Pantegni* IX.8 theorice (1539): "Amor est confidentia animae suspiciosa in re amata, et cogitationis in eadem assiduitas."

4. *De anima* 1 cap. 5 (1972, 89): "Deinde est vis aestimationis; quae est vis ordinata in summo mediae concavitatis cerebri, apprehendens intentiones non sensatas quae sunt in singulis sensibilibus, sicut vis quae est in ove diiudicans quod ab hoc lupo est fugiendum, et quod huius agni est miserendum." Peter devotes a chapter to the estimative faculty in SLA, tract. 7, cap. 5, pp. 265–69, but a passage in the chapter on the *passiones anime* (tract. 8, cap. 4, p. 286) is closer to the process of perception outlined here: "Cum autem passiones ex immutatione obiectorum et inclinatione virtutum anime procedant, quedam inmutatione formarum sensibilium consecuntur, et hee ab exterioribus virtutibus orientes ad primas interiores devolvuntur, quas sensus communis, ymaginatio, et ymaginativa pertractant, sicut delectationes et horrores circa sensibilium formarum apprehensionem; quedam autem sunt altiores que ex intentionibus insensibilibus provenientes ad estimativam spectant, sicut delectatio et tristitia circa amicitias et inimicitias."

5. The definition of *heremis*, though not the word itself, recalls Gerard's gloss *heros*. The unusual term may have arisen from scribal error in the expansion of an abbreviation someplace in the transmission (the word is fully spelled out in V, the unique manuscript for this passage), or was perhaps influenced by the isolation characteristic of melancholia canina.

6. Cf. Constantine, *Liber de coitu*, 16 (ed. Montero Cartelle 1983, 158–60): "Novimus

eciam alia que, si affuerint cum supradictis pocionibus, adaugent libidinem, ut cor ociosum et cotidiana leticia."

7. See below, lines 168–69.

8. See below, lines 197–201. I have not been able to locate a similar passage in the *Pantegni's* chapter on intercourse, V.25. But cf. *De coitu* 1 (Montero Cartelle 1983, 80): "Tria vero sunt in coitu: appetitus ex cogitacione fantastica ortus, spiritus et humor." See also PSQ B 245 and B 6.

9. *Canon*, lib. III, fen 1, tract. 4, cap. 24. Compare Galen's story of the pulse test in *De praecognitione* (Nutton 1979, 100–03).

10. *Canon*, lib. III, fen 1, tract. 4, cap. 24 and 25. Avicenna does not say *expressis verbis* in the chapters on *ilisci* that unsatisfied lovers will become choleric, but does note that excessive burning of humors may be involved, and that patients may require treatment as for melancholy, mania, and *alcutubut* (a type of melancholy). The generation of *cholera nigra* in melancholy (to which *amor hereos* is closely related) does, however, receive lengthier treatment in cap. 19 of the same *tractatus*.

11. *Canon*, lib. III, fen 1, tract. 4, cap. 24.

12. Most of the cures listed can be found in al-Rāzī's chapter on melancholy in the *Liber ad almansorem* IX.13. Gerard of Cremona's gloss on al-Rāzī's *Divisiones* (Lyons, 1510), cap. XI adds travel. Another list of cures appears in the *Liber continens* (Venice, 1509), tract. xx, cap. 2 (flebotomia, cibi humidi, balnea aque dulcis, purgatio, somnus). On travel as a cure, see version A.180–97; on wine, A.232–48 and below, lines 266–81. On baths and food, see A.249–70 and below, 282–89.

13. Compare A.55–107 and Avicenna, *Canon*, lib. I, fen II, cap. 1: "Egritudo est disposicio non naturalis in corpore humano ex qua in operatione essentialiter provenit nocumentum proventu primo."

14. Peter elaborates on universal and particular appetites in his commentary on Galen's *Tegni* (*Ars parva*) in Madrid, Biblioteca nacional, MS 1877, fol. 83r: "Virtus appetitiva duplex est: quedam enim est universalis que toti corpori deservit; quedam vero particularis que insita est omni membro. Sed appetitiva universalis que toti corpori deservit est in stomacho; particularis vero propria est cuilibet membro, per quam appetit cibum sibi conformem et attrahit secundum sui exigentiam. Item appetitiva universalis stomacho componitur ex sensibili et animali, et per sensibilem suam sentit inanitionem et deinde attrahat cibum ut sic repleatur."

15. Aristotle, *De somno et vigilia*, c. 1, 454a8; cf. A.63.

16. *Testiculi* refer to the generative organs of both sexes. This argument is adopted by Gerard of Solo in the *Determinatio de amore hereos* (n. 2 above).

17. The MSS show confusion over the last clause. The origin of sexual desire in the liver was a medical commonplace: *De coitu*, c. 1; *Viaticum* VI.6; and PSQ, B 177: "quare . . . iecore amamus." In SLA, tract. 12, cap. 8, p. 478 Peter lists the components of sexual appetite and their localizations: "cui [sc. virge] spiritus, calor, ventositas, et virtus erectionis a corde, sensus motis animalis appetitus a cerebro et nucha, sanguis et naturalis appetitus ex epate delegatur, licet appetitus origo a corde procedat." Cf. A.117–30.

18. Galen, *Tegni* II.5.4 in *Articella* (Lyons, 1525), fol. cxiiʳ: "Frigidus vero natura venter appetere quidem bonus." The next three questions are raised a number of times in Peter's scientific works and occur in the same order in the fourth book of QSV. Cf. A.117–30.

19. Cf. QSV, Bk. 4, Madrid 1877, fol. 159v: "Quarto queritur propter quid irrigidatio fit a calido. Ad hoc dicendum quod irrigidatio est duobus modis. Uno modo propter corrugationum partium et hoc est a frigido sicut in stomacho. Alia fit irrigidacio per dilatationem parcium et extensionem, et hoc fit a calido dilatante et replente sicut in erectione virge."

20. Johannitius, *Isagoge* (ed. Gracia and Vidal 1974/5, 321): "Nam desiderium uirtute duplici componitur: quarum una est quae appetit, altera quae sentit—stomachus enim suam inanitionem sentit."

21. Cf. QSV, Bk. 4, Madrid 1877, fol. 159v: "Quinto queritur de appetitu matricis que composita <est> ex naturali et animali secundum Constantinum. Et queritur propter quid appetitiva viget per calidum, appetitiva vero stomachi viget per frigidum, ut dictum est. Ad hoc dicendum quod appetitus stomachi est propter coctionem solum; matricis vero non solum appetit recipere sed ea autem expellere secundum Constantinum. Et ideo operatur matrix plus et excitatur ad operationem per calidum."

22. See below, lines 217–19.

23. Mentioned in *Canon*, lib. III, tract. 1, fen xx, cap. 1 and 3, and fen xxi, cap. 1.

24. *Liber pulsuum*, in *Articella* (Venice, 1483), fol. 4v: "Calidum enim velociter mobile."

25. Cf. A.10–54. I have not been able to locate the quotation attributed to Avicenna. Gerard of Solo adduces the same passages from Avicenna (here and next note), with explicit references to the *Canon's* chapter on *ilisci* (*Determinatio*, n. 2 above). Was there a manuscript tradition that differs from the printed editions we have?

26. Again, my search for this in Avicenna has been unsuccessful, but the idea does appear in Gerard of Berry. Cf. Arnald of Villanova, *Tractatus* (McVaugh 1985, 50), lines 9–21.

27. Avicenna, *De anima* IV.1 (1968, 6–7).

28. Avicenna, *De anima* I.5 (1972, 85–89): "Apprehendentium autem quaedam sunt quae apprehendunt et operantur simul, quaedam vero apprehendunt et non operantur . . . Differentia autem quae est inter apprehendere operando et apprehendere non operando haec est: quod de actionibus alicuius virium interiorum est componere aliquas formarum et intentionum comprehensarum cum aliis et separare ab aliquibus : habet ergo apprehendere et operari etiam in eo quod apprehendit. Sed apprehendere non operando, hoc est cum forma aut intentio describitur in vi tantum, ita ut non possit agere in ea aliquid ullo modo. . . . videtur etiam haec vis [aestimatio] operari in imaginatis compositionem et divisionem."

29. On the connection between the estimation and the memory, see Avicenna, *De anima*, I.5; IV.1; and SLA, p. 270: "Est autem memoria virtus insita in posteriori cerebri cellula ordinata ad conservationem impressionum ex intentionibus insensibilium provenientium quas estimatio ex singulis sensibilibus accipit."

30. *album cum rubeo*: The following passage from the *Quinque incitamenta ad Deum amandum ardenter* attributed to Gerard of Liège (Wilmart 1933, 238–39) suggests that "white and red" may be synecdoche for "beauty" or "beautiful face" (lily and rose?), one of the causes of lovesickness: "Unde dicit amica in Canticis, quando queritur ab ea: QUALIS EST DILECTUS TUUS O PULCRA INTER MULIERES—*car a biele amie affiert bias amis*—respondet ipsa et dicit: AMICUS MEUS CANDIDUS EST ET RUBICUNDUS, idest *blans et couloures*. Et hec faciunt pulcritudinem."

31. See A.108–40.

32. See note 1.

33. For convenient summaries of the relations of the four humors to the four ages of man, see Klibansky et al. 1964, 1–11 and Sears 1986, 25–31.

34. Cf. A.66.

35. See above, lines 30–33. QDA, Madrid 1877, fol. 263v raises the same question as here ("Utrum femina magis appetat coitum quam masculus") and arrives at the same conclusion ("Sed masculi sunt calidiores feminis; ergo plus appetit coitum mas quam femina, quod concedo"), though by a slightly different route. The manuscript is damaged at this point, but the last response bears quotation: "plus appetit coitum mas quam femina. Ad tertium dicendum quod quia virtus animalis fortior est in masculis, magis sentiunt delectationem mares quam femine, et propter hoc plus appetunt. Coitus enim, quantum ad expulsionem <est?> a virtute naturali, sed tamen appetitus et sensus delectationis est a virtute animali. Unde Haly: reposuit coytus sub accidentibus anime."

36. *Pantegni* VI.17 theorice: "Delectatio in coitu maior est in mulieribus quam in masculis, quia masculi delectantur tantum in expulsione superfluitatis. Mulieres dupliciter delectantur, et in suo spermate expellendo, et masculi recipiendo ex vulve ardentis desiderio." Cf. PSQ B 7.

37. The source of this remark remains elusive.

38. Al-Rāzī, *Ad almansorem* lib. II cap. lvi (Basel, 1544) fol. 53r: "In omnibus animalium generibus, foeminae magis mortuum habent animum minusque sunt patientes, et citius converti possunt, citiusque irascuntur, et velocius sedantur. . . . Quae in omnibus animalium, ut predictum est, generibus masculis, et timidiores, et deterius inveniuntur morigeratae." Cf. QDA, fol. 284v: "Item queritur propter quid mulier cito decipitur et est sexus fragilis. . . . Ad aliud dicendum quod secundum philosophum quod humidum sicut dicunt est bonum interminabile termino alieno, male autem termino proprio quia igitur mulieres maxime humidum sunt ad quidquid vident se convertunt. unde si vident gaudere, gaudent; si autem tristari, tristantur. Et ex hoc accidit compassio similiter quia est frigida et humida mulier de facili est passibilis et ita de facili fra. .bilis."

39. This seems to have been a common question in the schools: cf. PSQ B 16 and QDA, fol. 264v.

40. Cf. Aristotle, *De gen. animal.* 728a9–14, 31.

41. *De coitu* (ed. Montero Cartelle 1983, 76), prologus: "nullum sit animalium quod non

pernimium delectetur coitu. Nam si animalia coitum odirent, animalium genus pro certo periret."

42. Men have greater sensation because they are hotter and have a stronger *virtus animalis.* See above, note 35 and cf. Galen (Kühn 1821) 1:326: "sensus acres habent, qui temperamento sunt calido simul et sicco." This question is debated in QDA, fol. 263v: "Utrum maior delectatio sit in femina quam in masculo in coitu. Circa secundum principale 5° [?] dicit Philosophus in libro physicorum quod materia appetit formas sicut turpe bonum sive pulchrum et femina masculum. Ergo cum femina appetat masculum plusquam econtro, maior est delectatio in femina quam in viro vel masculo. Preterea Constantinus dicit in pa<n>tegni quod femina delectatur in duo, scilicet in emittendo et recipiendo, masculus autem solum in emittendo. Ergo maior delectatio in femina quam in masculo. Contrarium dicit Galienus quod calida et sicca complexio maxime venerea est. Sed masculus omnis calidus et siccus est respectu femine. Ergo maior est delectatio in masculo quam in femina. Preterea sicut scribitur in libro de coitu: calida complexio stimulat ad coitum. Ergo cum masculi sint calidiores feminis, maior est delectatio in masculis quam in feminis, quod concedo. Ad primum in contrarium dico quod masculus sicut agens et plus habet de calore et spiritibus quam femina. Iterum sperma in masculis est magis digestum et propter hoc maior est delectatio in masculo quam in femina. Ad secundum argumentum dicendum quod licet in pluribus delectetur femina quam masculo, tamen magis intenditur maior delectatio in masculo quam in femina."

The same question is debated in slightly different terms, but with the same conclusion, in Peter's commentary on Johannitius' *Isagoge* (Madrid, Biblioteca Nacional, 1877) fol. 42r: "Consequenter queritur utrum mulieres magis delectentur in coitu quam viri, et videtur quod non, quia viri sunt calidiores quam mulieres. Sed in coitu est delectatio propter reductionem discrasie ad temperamentum. Sed in viro est maior discrasia quam in muliere, ergo etc. Preterea hoc videtur quia quod magis appetitur, magis delectatur. Sed viri magis appetunt quam mulieres cum sint calidiores, et calidi magis appetunt, sicut dicit Galenus in tegni, ergo etc. Contrarium videtur quia qui delectatur .ii. modis delectatur magis quam qui uno modo tantum. Sed mulier in coitu delectatur .ii. modis, scilicet in emissione et receptione; vir autem solum delectatur in emissione, ergo etc. Preterea hoc videtur quia Trotula dampnavit mulierem dicens quod magis concupiscit quam vir; sed si magis concupiscit, magis delectatur, ergo etc. . . . Ad primum dicendum quod viri qualitative magis delectantur ratione maior caliditatis; mulieres autem quantitative magis delectantur."

43. Cf. *Pantegni* VI.17 theorice. I have not located the passage in *De coitu* or *Liber minor de coitu.*

44. *Spiritus*, innate heat, and radical moisture were all thought to be emitted with seed, leading to a diminution of vitality and longevity: "Omne illud per quod consumitur substantialis humiditas corporis et deperditur calor naturalis et spiritus . . . inducit brevem vitam quam longam. Sed coitus est huiusmodi, quia per ipsum dessicatur eo quod per ipsum dessicantur spiritus et calor naturalis et humiditas substantialis. Hec enim omnia cum spermate eo quod per ipsum deperduntur spiritus et calor naturalis et humiditas subtantialis" (Peter of Spain, *Comm. in Tegni*, Madrid 1877, fol. 94v). Cf. Peter's exposition of Aristotle's *De longitudine et brevitate vite* (ed. Alonso 1952, 467), lines 3–5.

45. On the qualitative difference between men's and women's pleasures, see note 41 above and chapter 6.

46. Cf. Aristotle, *De sensu et sensibili*, 438b 28: "Its [the eye's] structure is an offshoot from the brain, because the latter is the moistest and the coldest of all the bodily parts." In QDA, Peter discusses the effect of excessive intercourse, and notes that since the eyes are made of the same substance as the brain and are extremely sensitive, immoderate coitus leads to blindness (Madrid 1877, fol. 270v): "occulos excecat quia oculi ex <e>adem materia sunt cum cerebro." Cf. Jean de St.-Amand, *Concordantiae* (Pagel 1894, 224): "Inter oculos et cerebrum est convenientia plus quam cerebrum et sensus alios (in tegni cap. 8 in fine)."

47. Cf. SLA, p. 226: "oculus igitur naturam habens perspicui aque naturam participat materialiter dominantis . . . oculus igitur et maxime puppilla ex dominio materiali aque constat."

48. *Viaticum* I.20, lines 18–21.

49. *Remedia amoris*, lines 809–10. See version A.232–48 and notes.

50. Al-Rāzī, *Divisiones* (Lyons, 1510), cap. xi: "Cura eius [amoris] est assiduatio coytus et ieiunium et deambulatio et ebrietas plurima assidue." Cf. Egidius, lines 16–37.

51. Cf. A.239–48.

52. Al-Rāzī, *Liber continens* (Lyons, 1509), I.20: "sedeant in aqua dulci . . . humectentur cum . . . balneo." I have not found a corresponding passage in Serapion. Administration of baths was controversial in antiquity: Oribasius, *Synopsis* 8.9 (Bussemaker and Daremberg 1873, 5:413); Paul of Aegina, *Epitome* 3.17 (Heiberg 1921; Heiberg 1912, 38).

53. See A.198–231 and notes.

54. *Viaticum* I.20, lines 38 and 57.

55. A "consimilar" disease "is one affecting the similar members (tissues), and they receive names of like nature to the suffering; such, for instance, as an aching (head)." An "official" disease "is one which occurs in special members, such as the feet, the hands, the tongue, or the teeth." From Johannitius, *Isagoge*, in Grant 1974, 709.

# Bona Fortuna

## Manuscripts

1. The interleaved texts are: 1. Arnald of Villanova, *De sterilitate*, fols. 126r–27v (two leaves added between original fols. 82v and 83r). The text differs significantly in places from the text printed in his *Opera* (Lyons, 1532, fols. 211r–13v). The text corresponds roughly to I.1–II.vii of the printed edition. *Inc.*: "[C]onceptus impeditur ex parte viri ex parte mulieris ex parte utriusque." *Expl.*: "dexter pro masculo sinister pro femina." 2. An unidentified acephalous work on eye diseases, fols. 138r–45v (inserted between fols. 92v and 93r). *Inc.*: "et pone in nase ereo et superinfunde vinum." *Expl.*: "aggregentur cum fece olei(?) de lilio et linet(?) super (illeg). Explicit tractatus oculorum factum a quodam fratre innominato. deo gracias. amen. amen." The author frequently cites Roger Baron's *Practica* (see Wickersheimer 1979 [1936], 720–21 and Jacquart 1979, 263; fl. last third of the 13th c.) and also notes: "dixit mihi magister Galterius cancellarius rothommagus et famosus medicus quod recipiebatur . . ." (fol. 139r). I have not been able to identify Galterius of Rouen.

2. Bernard de Gordon, *Compendium regiminis acutorum*, fol. 162r–v. *Inc.*: "Cum omnis prolixitas sit noverca veritatis." *Expl.*: "non narravi peto veniam de omissis. Explicit"; Anonymous Salernitanus, *De adventu medici ad aegrotum*, fols. 163r–66r. *Inc.*: "Cum igitur o medice ad egrum vocaberis." *Expl.*: "licencia vade in pace. Explicit de visitatione infirmorum." Text printed in De Renzi 1852–59, 2:74–80.

3. See Demaitre 1980, 39–40, 175.

4. Private communication from M.-T. D'Alverny, to whom I am grateful for this information. Cf. Deslisle 1870, 7 and Rouse 1967.

5. Two hands can be distinguished: the first shows northern traits, the second meridional features. The first hand writes an uneven *textualis* that at times shows current features. The second hand is well-controlled, and produces a rounder, more calligraphic *textualis* that holds the line.

6. 1. "Et nota quod ad provocandum urinam cimites optime competit. Et est cimex idem quod pimes in gallico, et est pediculus latus et rufus qui proprie lectos invenitur et in rimis parietum" (R 53v). 2. "alii pisces calida ut kulinge (P: kulenge) qui dicuntur loches in gallico" (R 54v). 3. "Cataplasma et emplastra sunt optima que fiunt de contarius(?) de oleo deben(?) que solet vocari piper album apud parisius" (R 54v). 4. "Unde in caldea lingua sive sclavica scropha interpretatur generatio plurium. Unde aut sunt plures quasi in una sisti, aut si est una tunc tamen habet capita multa sed glandula non habet"(R 71v). 5. R: "Item bedegar hoc frutex que sunt quedam poma habentia interius grana pilosa et hec poma vocantur buᵗtellici theutonice" (66v). P: "Item bedegar .i. quidam fructus habens grana pilosa interius et hec pomula vocantur buthelisi theutonice." 6. R: "[morbilli] vocantur in lumbardico ferre"(66r). P: "vocantur in arabico ssere."

7. Seidler 1967, 60–61 lists BN lat. 15373 among those manuscripts "die zu Anfang des 14. Jahrhunderts als Beitrag zur praktischen Medizin in der Sorbonnebibliothek zur Verfügung standen. Schon der einfache Überblick zeigt, dass dieses Schriftenkorpus keine Sammlung von mehr oder weniger zufällig diesem Bücherfonds zugeflossenen Manusckripten sein kann, sondern dass hier planmässige Aufbauarbeit geleistet worden sein muss. Abgesehen von den offenen Benutzungsmöglichkeiten der Bibliothek war den Sorbonnisten offenbar daran gelegen, auch mit den medizinischen Schriften ein aktives und aktuelles Arbeitsinstrument zu schaffen."

8. I would like to thank Richard Rouse for his opinions on both manuscripts of Bona Fortuna's *Treatise*. Rouen A 176 is written on parchment in two columns, 61–63 lines per column. Citations of Constantine's text are in *textualis formata*. The text of Bona Fortuna's commentary is in a *textualis* showing *anglicana* features—looped ascenders, spikiness, and currency.

9. Nortier 1971, 19–24 and n. 67.

## Edition

1. Cf. Egidius, *Glosule super Viaticum*, 1–16 (above).

2. Cf. Avicenna, *Canon*, lib. 3, fen 1, tract. 4, cap. 24: "Hec egritudo est sollicitudo melancolica similis melancolie in quo homo sibi iam induxit incitationem cogitationis sue super pulchritudine quarundam formarum et figurarum que insunt ei. Deinde adiuvat ipsum ad illud desiderium eius et non consequitur."

3. Roger Bacon uses *species* and *passio* interchangeably to denote the image that is received by the eye from an external object. See Lindberg 1976, 114 and Tachau 1988, 8 n.14.

4. Here Bona Fortuna provides the *propter quid* (cf. line 25), or reasoned cause, for the preoccupation with an individual's image. He shifts causality from an external object to the perceptual process itself by distinguishing the sight of this form (the "extrinsic apprehension") from beauty itself; the perception is the principal cause of *amor hereos*, whereas beauty is a coadjuvant cause. In an extension of the Neoplatonism in Constantine's chapter, Bona Fortuna terms the apprehended form "fitting and congenial" (*conveniens et amicum*). Cf. Jean de St.-Amand, *Concordanciae* (Pagel 1894, 299): "Simile est conveniens et amicum"; Galen, *De inaequali intemperie* (Kühn 1964–65 [1821–33], 7:745–76): "Quod enim simile est, id familiare amicumque est; quod contrarium, id inimicum ac noxium." Cf. Ciavolella 1976, 90 n. 73.

5. The pairing *fantasiam vel intellectum* is unusual. But cf. Peter of Spain, *Expositio libri de anima* (Alonso 1952, 366–71, esp. 366.22–367.24), where the practical intellect operates much as the estimative power does on the data transmitted by the fantasy. See also Bundy 1927, 189–94; Johannitius, *Isagoge* (Maurach 1978, 154, section 15 and notes; Fischer 1983, 223–24).

6. *obvolvunt*: Cf. Arnald of Villanova, *Tractatus de amore heroico*, 50: "tunc quasi motu mixtionis turbate voluntur, [the heated spirits rising to the head] quapropter confundunt virtuale iudicium; et velut ebrii tales iudicant cum fallacia et errore."

7. *In qua*: denotes one of two types of material cause, the other being *ex qua*. Cf. Gerard of Solo, *Commentum super nono Almansoris* (Venice, 1505), fol. 34: "Causa materialis est duplex: quedam est in qua, quedam est ex qua: in qua est materia spermatis stimulantis virtutem estimativam et ymaginativam ad estimandum illud quod non est."

8. In the following sentences Bona Fortuna, like Gerard of Berry, supplements Constantine's account with symptoms taken from Avicenna, including the changes in facial appearance, crying and singing, and alterations in the pulse.

9. The search for solitude is not mentioned by Constantine, Gerard, Peter of Spain, or Avicenna as one of the symptoms of *amor hereos*. But cf. Gerard of Cremona's gloss *In nono almansorem* of al-Rāzī (Lyons, 1510) fol. cxliii v: "neque nominavit solitudinem que ex amoris mulieris vel alicuius rei accidit, cuius cura est ebrietas et mutatio de regione in regionem et coitus cum alia quam cum ea quam diligit." Separation from society is a common symptom of melancholy (Avicenna, *Canon*, lib. 3, fen 1, tract. 4., cap. 20), and Bona Fortuna may have borrowed it from that disease, given his stress (lines 29–32 above) on the similarity of *amor hereos* to melancholy.

10. Something seems to be missing at this point in both mss, which read "hanelitus sive retardant . . ." without any obvious signs of omission. I have supplied the conjectured omission on the basis of this context and lines 88–92 below. The *quando . . . quando* construction may have caused haplography in the archetype.

11. Avicenna describes the pulse test; see also Mesulam and Perry 1972.

12. Although both Constantine and Avicenna remark that all the parts of the body dry out except the eyes, they do not single out the mouth, tongue or throat for particular mention. However, al-Rāzī, *Liber continens* 1.20 (Venice, 1509), "de coturub vel ereos" (a cross between lycanthropy and lovesickness) uses similar language: "dessicatur eorum lingua"; "eorum lingua est sicca"; "multum siciunt"; "dessicantur eorum lingue."

13. Purging is recommended by Avicenna, al-Rāzī and Gerard. William of Brescia, *Prac-*

*tica* (Venice 1508) fol. 24 offers a similar recipe: "venter mollificetur cum prunis, cassiafistula, boragine, et similibus."

14. Exact identification of these herbs is uncertain; the English names given in the translation are tentative. Most or all of them are described in both medieval and modern botanical works as having diuretic and laxative properties that are consistent with the recommendation to purge.

*Caput monachi* is not prominent in medieval herbals or works on medicinal simples; according to two botanical glossaries, it is the same as dandelion: *Alphita* (Mowat 1887, 29): "capud monachi, dens leonis" and *Sinonoma Bartholomei* (Mowat 1882, 16): "Caput monachi, dens leonis idem, herba est." Stuart 1982, 142–43 lists the following uses for dandelion (*Taraxacum officinale*): diuretic, cholagogue, choleretic, laxative, bitter tonic, and stomachic. See also Grieve 1931, 1:249–55.

*Lactucella abbatis* remains elusive; however, Rufinus (Thorndike 1946, 124) identifies *lactuca abbatis* with *endivia agrestis maior*. Since the *Sinonoma Bartholomei* (Mowatt 1882, 27) also claims that "Lactucella, endivia, scariola, sowethistel idem sunt secundum quosdam," I have translated Bona Fortuna's *lactucella abbatis* using Rufinus' equation. Rufinus lists medicinal properties under the third species of *endivia* that he discusses (p. 125); if these are valid for the previous two types (including *endivia agrestis maior*), then Bona Fortuna may have chosen it for the following: Aliquantulam habent amaritudinem, unde diuretice sunt, et ponticitatem, unde virtutem habent confortandi, ex frigiditate alterandi.

Bona Fortuna describes *radix volubilis maioris* in an emetic compound (R 28v): radix volubilis maioris non que facit flores quasi campanulas sed que habet folia quasi folia vitis et valet ad cervisiam. *Alphita* (Mowatt 1887, 29) identifies *volubilis maior* with *caprifolium* and "wodebynde vel honesocles." Cf. Rufinus (Thorndike 1946, 332). Stuart 1982, 88 lists the uses of honeysuckle (*Lonicera periclymenum*) as diuretic, antiseptic, expectorant, emetic, slightly astringent. Cf. Grieve 1931, 2:409–10.

Many types of *basilicon* were familiar in the Middle Ages. According to Dioscorides 2.171, "it is a softner of ye belly, a mover of flatulencies, ureticall, and calling out of milk" (182). Serapion (the Younger), *De temperamentis simplicium* (Venice, 1550) fol. 144v reports a discussion of why basil is both laxative and stiptic (for the latter, see below, note 27). The *Tabula Salerni* considers it a humid diuretic (De Renzi 1859, 5:236), and Ibn Botlan, *Tacuinum sanitatis*, fol. 39v claims that *basilicum curatum* "resoluit superfluitates cerebri."

15. *epithimo*: al-Rāzī quotes Simeon on the cure of "coturub vel hereos" (*Continens* 1.20) as follows: "potare epithimum et odorare est valde iuvativum coturub vel hereos." According to Dioscorides 4.179 (Gunther 1934, 580), dodder (*Cuscuta epithymum*) "purgeth downward phlegm, & black choler. It is properly good for the ye melancholicall." Grieve 1931, 1:261 remarks that the "whole plant, of whatever species, is very bitter, and an infusion acts as a brisk purge." Jean de St. Amand, *Aureolae* (Pagel 1893, 99–100) notes its laxative properties and that it helps "desipientibus, maniacis," and others; cf. PSQ N 50.

16. Cf. R 69v: "postquam morbus magnificatus est tunc non est cura."

17. *Hieras* were compound medicines, often made with aloes, that served as purgatives; see Galen, *De compositione medicamentium secundum locos* (Kühn 13:126–39); Serapion (the Elder), *Practica* (Venice, 1550) fol. 81r. Avicenna recommends purgation with *hieras* for lovesickness: "evacuentur humores eorum predicti cum hieris magnis," as does al-Rāzī, *Continens*, for "coturub vel ereos." The *Antidotarium Nicolai* (in *Opera Mesue* 1541, fol. cclv$^v$) claims that *hiera picra* is good for "diversas capitis passiones" and that "stomachum quoque optime purgat."

*Hiera logodion* and *hiera memphitum* are described sometimes as one compound, sometimes as two in the sources. The *Antidotarium Nicolai* (fol. cclv$^{r-v}$) describes *hieralogodion memphitum*, which "purgat melancholiam et phlegma mirabiliter"; the commentary by Platearius claims that it is efficacious "contra omnes passiones capitis." The *Flos medicinae* (De Renzi 1859, 5:40) describes *memphitum yerologodion*: "Memphito cedunt, quae linguam noxia laedunt, / Phlegma, melancholicus humor, hieranoxa, dolores / Algentis stomachi, vertigo, dolor capitalis." Arnald of Villanova, *Antidotarium* (Lyons, 1531) fol. 259r includes mania and melancholy among the diseases *ieralogodion memphitum* cures.

18. According to Rufinus, *electuarium de suco rosarum* "coleram rubeam purgat et convalescentibus ab infirmitatibus, scilicet tertiana, cottidiana, purgat sine molestia et reliquias malorum humorum qui remanserunt in corpore potenter educit." Cf. *Antidotarium Nicolai*, fol. ccxlij and *Flos sanitatis* (De Renzi 1857, 1:476).

19. *Mel violaceum* and *cassia fistula* were reckoned among the milder purgatives. Rufinus (326) says of *mel violaceum* that "si dederis cum pulvere tartari et parum pulveris masticis, movebit corpus optime et sine periculo." Serapion the Younger, *De temperamentis* (fol. 142v) notes that the violet "laxat cholera a stomacho et intestinis." Stuart 1982, 153 reports that violets are used as emetics, purgatives, and diuretics, among other things. *Cassia fistula*, according to Serapion (fol. 123ᵛ), has the power "purgare choleram adustam, & mollificare ventrem mediocri mollificatione," and Rufinus has a long entry on this herb (66–67). Grieve 1931, 2:734–37 reports of the related species *Cassia acutifolia*: "Its action being chiefly on the lower bowel, it is especially useful in habitual costiveness. It increases the peristaltic movements of the colon by its local action upon the intestinal wall."

20. Avicenna, *Canon*, lib. 3, fen 1, tract. 4, cap. 25: "administra eis somnum et humectationem et nutrimentum ipsorum cum laudabilibus, et fac ipsos balneari secundum conditionem humectationis notam."

21. Cf. Egidius' and Peter of Spain's questions on the usefulness of drunkenness, above.

22. On the general problem of universals in late medieval medicine, see Seidler 1967, 89–91, who summarizes the arguments of Laín Entralgo 1961.

23. Cf. Peter of Spain (above) and Arnald of Villanova, *Tractatus*, 54: "De summe vero iuvantibus et distrahentibus est in partes remotas et etiam peregrinas recedere."

24. The genitive case of *homicidii* and the lack of a complement for *fuit* suggests that something is missing (R has a blank space for 5 or 6 words), perhaps a past participle like "charged with, accused of" (to parallel *compulsus fuit*).

25. The direct discourse is stylistically reminiscent of Bernard de Gordon's section on cures in the *Practica* (or *Lilium*). The objections themselves are traditional: cf. Ovid, *Remedia amoris*, and Andreas Capellanus, *De amore*, Bk. III.

26. This section, which at first sight seems extraneous to the rest of the chapter, in fact contains the "quedam adiutoralia" promised in the introduction. The first section discusses basil as a remedy for problems of the head (*amor hereos* "habet principium a cerebro," lines 3–4), while the second section concentrates on its use in diarrhea, possibly caused by unexpectedly strong purgation earlier in the course of treatment. For the medieval theory of medicinal action, see McVaugh 1975, ch. 1.

27. According to the *Antidotarium Nicolai*, fol. ccxlviʳ⁻ᵛ: "Oleum rosatum virtutem habet frigidam et stipticam et ideo ad dolores capitis et febre seu ex calore solis optimum est." Serapion the Younger, *De temperamentis simplicium* (fol. 144v) reports of *ozimo nongariophilato* (*ocimum basilicum* = basil) that it is both laxative and stiptic, according to whether the expulsive or retentive faculty of the body is stronger. Al-Rāzī, *Liber ad almansorem* 9.13, uses it for melancholy.

28. The seed of *ocymum basilicum*, according to Dioscorides, "causeth also many sneezings, being drawn up by the smell, & the herb doth the like. But the eyes must be shut whilst ye sneesing holds."

29. On violets as purgatives, see above, note 19.

30. Cf. Rocha Pereira 1973, 19, "caputpurgium" and Matthaeus Silvaticus, *Pandectae medicinae* (Lyons, 1541) fol. xlviᵛ: "Caputpurgium .i. liquores qui per nares mittuntur: vel quicquid masticatur vel gargarizatur et apoflegmatismum facit id est a capite flegma deducit."

31. *Antidotarium Nicolai* (fol. ccxlviᵛ): "Oleum camomillinum salubre ad fevorem et dolorem capitis." Cf. Rufinus, "camomilla" (71–72).

32. For a discussion of medieval medical *experimenta*, see McVaugh 1976, 175–80.

33. Elsewhere Bona Fortuna pairs *antiquatus* with *novus* (P 22r *nove vel antiquate*), so that it must refer to a persistent, chronic, or standing symptom or condition.

34. Rufinus (Thorndike 1946, 225) quotes a similar recipe from Alexander: "Herba bassiliconis trita et cum ovis confecta et in sartaginem ad modum crispelle multum confert laborantibus indigestione."

# BIBLIOGRAPHY OF
# WORKS CITED

*Acta sanctorum.* 1866. *Maii tomus tertius,* v. 16. Ed. G. Henschen and D. van Papenbroeck. Paris and Rome: Victor Palmé.

*Aegritudo Perdicae. See* Vollmer.

Agamben, Giorgio. 1977. *Stanze: La parola e il fantasma nella cultura occidentale.* Turin: Einaudi.

Agrimi, Jole and Chiara Crisciani. 1978. *Medicina del corpo e medicina dell'anima.* Milan: Episteme Editrice.

Alexandre-Bidon, Danièle and Monique Closson. 1985. *L'Enfant à l'ombre des cathédrales.* Lyon: Presses Universitaires.

Allen, Prudence. 1985. *The Concept of Woman: The Aristotelian Revolution 750 BC–AD 1250.* Montréal: Eden.

Alonso, Manuel, ed. 1944. *Pedro Hispano: Comentario al* De anima *de Aristoteles.* Obras Filosóficas, 2. Madrid: Instituto de Filosofía Luis Vives.

———, ed. 1952. *Pedro Hispano: Expositio libri de anima. De morte et vita et De causis longitudinis et brevitatis vitae. Liber naturalis de rebus principalibus.* Obras Filosóficas, 3. Madrid: Instituto de Filosofía Luis Vives.

———, ed. 1957. *Exposição sobre os libros do Beato Dionisio Areopagita.* Lisboa: Instituto de alta cultura.

———, ed. 1961. *Pedro Hispano: Scientia libri de anima.* 2nd ed. Obras Filosóficas, 1. Barcelona: Juan Flors.

*Alphita. See* Mowat.

Andreas Capellanus. *See* Walsh 1982.

*Antidotarium Nicolae.* 1541. In *Opera divi Joannis Mesue.* N.p.

Arberry, Arthur J. 1953. *The Ring of the Dove by Ibn Hazm (994–1064): A Treatise on the Art and Practice of Arab Love.* London: Luzac.

Arieti, James A. and John M. Crossett. 1985. *Longinus. On the Sublime.* Texts and Studies in Religion, 21. New York and Toronto: Edwin Mellen Press.

Aristotle. *Categories. See* Minuo-Paluello.

———. In English translation. *See* Barnes.

Arnald of Villanova. 1531. *Opera omnia.* Lyons.

Arnold, Klaus. 1980. *Kind und Gesellschaft in Mittelalter und Renaissance.* Sammlung Zebra, Reihe B, vol. 2. Paderborn: Schöningh.

Arnoul, E. J., ed. 1940. *Le Livre de seyntz medicines.* Anglo-Norman Text Society, 2. Oxford: Blackwell.

*Articella.* 1493. Venice.

———. 1525. Lyons.

Auerbach, Erich. 1941. "Passio als Leidenschaft." *PMLA* 56: 1179–96.

———. 1965. *Literary Language and its Public in Late Latin Antiquity and in the Middle Ages.* Trans. Ralph Manheim. New York: Pantheon.

Avicenna. 1964 [1507]. *Liber Canonis.* Venice; rpt. Hildesheim: Georg Olms.

————. 1972. *Liber de anima seu sextus de naturalibus, I–III*. Ed. Simone van Riet. Leiden: Brill.

Baader, Gerhard. 1967. "Zur Terminologie des Constantinus Africanus." *Medizinhistorisches Journal* 2:36–53.

————. 1974. "Die Entwicklung der medizinischen Fachsprache im hohen und späten Mittelalter." In *Fachprosaforschung: Acht Vorträge zur mittelalterlichen Artesliteratur*. Ed. Gundolf Keil and Peter Assion. Berlin: Erich Schmidt. Pp. 88–123.

————. 1978. "Die Schule von Salerno." *Medizinhistorisches Journal* 13:124–45.

————. 1981. "Galen in mittelalterlichen Abendland." In Nutton, 1981. Pp. 213–328.

Baldwin of Canterbury. *Tractatus quartus decimus seu sermo*. PL 204:359–546.

Baldwin, John W. 1970. *Masters, Princes, and Merchants: The Social Views of Peter the Chanter and His Circle*. 2 vols. Princeton, N. J.: Princeton University Press.

Balsdon, J. P. V. D. 1974. *Roman Women: Their History and Habits*. Rev. ed. London: The Bodley Head.

Barnes, Jonathan, ed. 1984. *The Complete Works of Aristotle*. Revised Oxford Translation. 2 vols. Bollingen Series, 71. Princeton, N. J.: Princeton University Press.

Bazàn, Bernardo, John Wippel, Gérard Fransen, and Danielle Jacquart. 1985. *Les questions disputées et les questions quodlibétiques dans les facultés de théologie, de droit et de médicine*. Typologie des sources du moyen âge occidental, fasc. 44–45. Turnhout: Brepols.

Beccaria, Augusto. 1956. *I codici di medicina del periodo presalernitano*. Rome: Storia e letteratura.

Becker, Gustavus. 1885. *Catalogi bibliothecarum antiqui collegit Gustavus Becker*. Bonn: M. Cohen.

Beecher, Donald. 1988. "The Lover's Body: The Somatogenesis of Love in Renaissance Medical Treatises." *Renaissance and Reformation* n.s. 12, 1:1–11.

Beecher, Donald and Massimo Ciavolella, eds. and trans. 1989. *A Treatise on Lovesickness*, by Jacques Ferrand. Syracuse, N. Y.: Syracuse University Press.

Bell, Joseph Norment. 1979. *Love Theory in Later Hanbalite Islam*. Albany, N.Y.: State University of New York Press.

Benson, Larry D. 1984. "Courtly Love and Chivalry in the Later Middle Ages." In *Fifteenth-Century Studies: Recent Essays*. Ed. Robert F. Yeager. Hamden, Conn.: Archon Books. Pp. 237–57.

————, ed. 1987. *The Riverside Chaucer*. 3rd ed. Boston: Houghton Mifflin.

Benton, John F. 1961. "The Court of Champagne as a Literary Center." *Speculum* 36:551–91.

————. 1970. *Self and Society in Medieval France: The Memoirs of Abbot Guibert of Nogent*. New York: Harper and Row.

————. 1982. "Consciousness of Self and Perceptions of Individuality." In *Renaissance and Renewal in the Twelfth Century*. Ed. Robert L. Benson and Giles Constable. Cambridge, Mass.: Harvard University Press. Pp. 263–95.

Bernard of Gordon. 1574. *Practica dicta Lilium medicinae*. Lyons.

Biesterfeldt, Hans Hinrich and Dimitri Gutas. 1984. "The Malady of Love." *Journal of the American Oriental Society* 104:21–55.

Birchler, Urs Benno. 1975. "Die Rolle der Frau bei der Liebeskrankheit und den Liebestränken." *Sudhoffs Archiv* 59:311–20.

Bird, Otto. 1940, 1941. "The Canzone d'Amore of Cavalcanti according to the Commentary of Dino del Garbo. Text and Commentary." *Mediaeval Studies* 2:150–203 and 3:117–60.

Birkenmajer, Aleksander. 1970 [1930]. "Le rôle joué par les médecins et les naturalistes dans la réception d'Aristote au XIIe et XIIIe siècles." In *Études d'histoire des sciences et de la philosophie du moyen âge.* Studia Copernicana, 1. Wrocław: Ossoliński. Pp. 73–87.

Bloch, Herbert. 1972. "Monte Cassino's Teachers and Library in the High Middle Ages." *La scuola nell'occidente latino dell'alto medioevo.* Settimane di Studio del Centro italiano di studi sull'alto medioevo, 19. Spoleto, 1972. Pp. 563–613.

———. 1986. *Montecassino in the Middle Ages.* 3 vols. Cambridge, Mass.: Harvard University Press.

Bloch, R. Howard. 1977. *Medieval French Literature and Law.* Berkeley: University of California Press.

———. 1983. *Etymologies and Genealogies: A Literary Anthropology of the French Middle Ages.* Chicago: University of Chicago Press.

———. 1987. "Medieval Misogyny." *Representations* 20:1–24.

Blöcker, Monica. 1982. "Frauenzauber—Zauberfrauen." *Zeitschrift für schweitzerische Kirchengeschichte* 76:1–39.

Blonquist, Lawrence B., trans. 1987. *L'Art d'amours (The Art of Love).* New York and London: Garland.

Boase, Roger. 1977. *The Origin and Meaning of Courtly Love.* Totowa, N. J.: Rowman and Littlefield.

Bode, Georg Heinrich. 1968 [1834]. *Scriptores rerum mythicarum Latini tres.* 2 vols. Celle; rpt. Hildesheim: G. Olms.

Bono, James J. 1984. "Medical Spirits and the Medieval Language of Life." *Traditio* 40:91–130.

Bowlby, John. 1969. *Attachment.* New York: Basic Books.

———. 1973. *Separation: Anxiety and Anger.* New York: Basic Books.

———. 1980. *Loss: Sadness and Depression.* New York: Basic Books.

Branca, Vittore, ed. 1964. *Filostrato.* Vol. 2 of Boccaccio, *Tutte le opere.* Milan: Mondadori.

Brereton, Georgine and Janet M. Ferrier, eds. 1981. *Le Ménagier de Paris.* Oxford: Clarendon Press.

Bright, David F. 1987. *The Miniature Epic in Vandal Africa.* Norman, Oklahoma and London: University of Oklahoma Press.

Broomfield, F., ed. 1968. *Thomae de Chobham Summa confessorum.* Louvain: Nauwelaerts.

Brown, Carleton. 1932. *English Lyrics of the Thirteenth Century.* Oxford: Clarendon Press.

Browne, E. G. 1962 [1921]. *Arabian Medicine.* Cambridge: Cambridge University Press.

Brundage, James A. 1987. *Law, Sex, and Christian Society in Medieval Europe.* Chicago: University of Chicago Press.

Bürgel, J. Christoph. 1978. "Islamisches Mittelalter." In *Krankheit, Heilkunst, Heilung.* Ed. Heinrich Schipperges, Eduard Seidler, and Paul U. Unschuld. Historische Anthropologie, 1. Freiburg/Munich: Karl Alber. Pp. 271–302.

Büttner, F. O. 1983. *Imitatio pietatis: Motive der christlichen Ikonographie als Modelle zur Verähnlichung.* Berlin: Mann.

Bullough, Vern L. 1961. "Medical Study at Mediaeval Oxford." *Speculum* 36: 600–12.

———. 1962. "The Medieval Medical School at Cambridge." *Mediaeval Studies* 24:161–68.

———. 1966. *The Development of Medicine as a Profession.* New York: Hafner.

Bullough, Vern L. and James Brundage, eds. 1982. *Sexual Practices and the Medieval Church.* Buffalo, N.Y.: Prometheus.

Bundy, Murray Wright. 1927. *The Theory of Imagination in Classical and Mediaeval Thought.* University of Illinois Studies in Language and Literature, 12. Urbana, Illinois: University of Illinois Press.

Burgess, Glynn and Keith Busby, trans. 1986. *The Lais of Marie de France.* Harmondsworth: Penguin.

Burkhard, C., ed. 1917. *Nemesii Episcopi Premnon Physicon . . . Liber a N. Alfano Archiepiscopo Salerni in Latinum Translatus.* Leipzig: Teubner.

Burns, E. Jane. 1984/5. "The Man Behind the Lady in Troubadour Lyric." *Romance Notes* 25:254–70.

Burton, Robert. 1977. *The Anatomy of Melancholy.* Ed. Holbrook Jackson. New York: Random House.

Bussemaker, Ulco C. and Charles Daremberg, eds. 1851–76. *Oeuvres d'Oribase.* 6 vols. Paris: Imprimérie Nationale.

Bynum, Caroline Walker. 1982. *Jesus as Mother: Studies in the Spirituality of the High Middle Ages.* Berkeley: University of California Press.

———. 1987. *Holy Feast, Holy Fast: The Religious Significance of Food to Medieval Women.* Berkeley, California: University of California Press.

Cadden, Joan. 1984. "It Takes All Kinds: Sexuality and Gender Differences in Hildegard of Bingen's 'Book of Compound Medicine'." *Traditio* 40:149–74.

———. 1986. "Medieval Scientific and Medical Views of Sexuality: Questions of Propriety." *Medievalia and Humanistica* n.s. 14:157–71.

Caelius Aurelianus. *See* Drabkin.

Carley, James P. and John F. R. Coughlan. 1981. "An Edition of the List of Ninety-Nine Books Acquired at Glastonbury Abbey During the Abbacy of Walter de Monington." *Mediaeval Studies* 43:498–514.

Cardoner i Planas, Antoni. 1973. *História de la Medicina a la Corona D'Aragó.* Barcelona: Scientia.

*Cartulaire de l'Université de Montpellier.* 1890. Montpellier.

Castle, Terry. 1987. "The Female Thermometer." *Representations* 17:1–27.

Cavanaugh, Susan. 1980. "A Study of Books Privately Owned in England 1300–1450." Dissertation, University of Pennsylvania.

Chamoux, François. 1962. "Perdiccas." In *Hommages à Albert Grenier.* Ed. Marcel Renard. *Collection Latomus* 58:384–96.

Chaucer, Geoffrey. *See* Benson, Larry, ed.

Chenu, M. D. 1927. "Auctor, actor, autor." *Archivum latinitatis medii aevi* (Bulletin Du Cange) 3:81–86.

———. 1968. *Nature, Man and Society in the Twelfth Century.* Trans. J. Taylor and L. Little. Chicago: University of Chicago Press.

Chodorow, Nancy. 1978. *The Reproduction of Mothering: Psychoanalysis and the Sociology of Mothering.* Berkeley, California: University of California Press.

Choulant, Johann Ludwig, ed. 1826. *Aegidii Corboliensis carmina medica.* Leipzig.

Chrohns, Hjalmar. 1905. "Zur Geschichte der Liebe als 'Krankheit'." *Archiv für Kulturgeschichte* 3:66–86.

Ciavolella, Massimo. 1970. "La Tradizione dell' 'aegritudo amoris' nel 'Decameron'." *Giornale storico della letteratura italiana* 147:496–517.

———. 1976. *La 'malattia d'amore' dall'Antichità al Medioevo*. Strumenti di Ricerca, 12–13. Rome: Bulzoni.

———. 1988. "Métamorphoses sexuelles et sexualité féminine durant la Renaissance." *Renaissance and Reformation* n.s. 12:13–20.

Cogliati Arano, Luisa. 1979. *Tacuinum Sanitatis*, 2nd ed. Milan: Electa.

Constantinus Africanus. *De coitu. See* Montero Cartelle, 1983.

———. *De genecia. See* Green, 1987.

———. *Libri Duo de Melancholia. See* Garbers, 1977; also in *Opera omnia* 1536–39.

———. *Pantegni.* 1515. In *Opera omnia Ysaac*. Lyons.

———. *Opera omnia.* 1536–39. 2 vols. Basel: H. Peter.

Cosman, Madeleine P. 1978. "Machaut's Medical Musical World." In *Machaut's World: Science and Art in the Fourteenth Century*. Ed. Madeleine P. Cosman and Bruce Chandler. *Annals of the New York Academy of Sciences* 314:1–36.

Couliano, Ioan P. 1987. *Eros and Magic in the Renaissance*. Trans. Margaret Cook. Chicago: University of Chicago Press.

Courtenay, William. 1984. "Nature and the Natural in Twelfth-Century Thought." In *Covenant and Causality in Medieval Thought: Studies in Philosophy, Theology, and Economic Practice*. London: Variorum Reprints. Pp. 1–26.

———. 1987. *Schools and Scholars in Fourteenth-Century England*. Princeton, N. J.: Princeton University Press.

Cowdrey, H. E. J. 1983. *The Age of Desiderius: Montecassino, the Papacy, and the Normans in the Eleventh and Early Twelfth Centuries*. Oxford: Clarendon Press.

Crane, Thomas F. 1890. *The Exempla or Illustrative Stories from the Sermones Vulgares of Jacques de Vitry*. London: Folklore Society; rpt. Nendeln/Liechtenstein: Kraus.

Craveiro da Silva, Lucio. 1977. "Pedro Hispano (1277–1977) à luz dos últimos estudos." *Revista Portuguesa de Filosofia* 33:113–23.

Creutz, Rudolf. 1930. "Der Cassinese Johannes Afflacius Saracenus, ein Arzt aus 'Hochsalerno'." *Studien und Mitteilungen zur Geschichte des Benediktiner-Ordens* 48:301–24.

———. 1932. "Additamenta zu Konstantinus Africanus und seinen Schülern Johannes und Atto." *Studien und Mitteilungen zur Geschichte des Benediktiner-Ordens* 50:420–42.

———. 1936. *Die medizinisch-naturphilosophischen Aphorismen und Kommentare des Magister Urso Salernitanus*. Quellen und Studien zur Geschichte der Naturwissenschaften und der Medizin, 5. Berlin: Springer.

Creutz, Rudolf and Walter Creutz. 1932. "Die 'Melancholia' bei Konstantinus Africanus und seinen Quellen." *Archiv für Psychiatrie und Nervenkrankheiten* 97:244–69.

Crisciani, Chiara. 1983. "Valeurs éthiques et savoir médical entre le XIIᵉ et le XIVᵉ siècle." *History and Philosophy of the Life Sciences* 5:33–52.

da Cruz Pontes, J. M. 1964. *Pedro Hispano Portugalense e as controvérsias doutrinais do século XIII: A Origem da alma*. Coimbra: Universidad.

———. 1968. "Para situar Pedro Hispano Portugalense na história da filosofia." *Revista Portuguesa de Filosofia* 24:21–45.

———. 1972. *A obra filosofica de Pedro Hispano Portugalense. Novos problemas textuals.* Coimbra: Universidad.

———. 1981. "Quelques Problèmes sur la voix et la signification dans le commentaire inédit de Petrus Hispanus Portugalensis sur le *De animalibus.*" In *Sprache und Erkenntnis im Mittelalter.* Ed. Jan P. Beckmann, et al. Akten des VI. Internationalen Kongresses für mittelalterliche Philosophie, 29 August-3 September 1977, Bonn. Berlin: De Gruyter. 1:398–402.

D'Alverny, Marie-Thérèse. 1957. "Les traductions d'Avicenne (moyen âge et renaissance)." *Problemi attuali di scienza: Quaderno,* Accademia nazionale dei lincei 40 (April 15): 71–87.

———. 1976. Review of J. M. da Cruz Pontes, *A obra filosofica de Pedro Hispano Portugalense. Novos problemas textuals* (Coimbra: Universidad, 1972). *Scriptorium* 30: 124–26.

———. 1977. "Comment les théologiens et les philosophes voient la femme." *Cahiers de civilisation médiévale* 20: 105–29.

———. 1982. "Translations and Translators." In *Renaissance and Renewal in the Twelfth Century.* Ed. Robert L. Benson and Giles Constable. Cambridge, Mass.: Harvard University Press. Pp. 421–62.

Daremberg, Charles. 1853. *Notices et extraits des manuscrits médicaux grecs, latins et français des principales bibliothèques de l'Europe.* Paris.

Daremberg, Charles and Emile Ruelle, eds. 1879. *Oeuvres de Rufus d'Ephèse.* Paris: Imprimérie nationale.

David of Dinant. *See* Kurdziałek.

de La Roncière, Charles. 1988. "Tuscan Notables on the Eve of the Renaissance." In Duby 1988. Pp. 157–309.

Demaitre, Luke E. 1975. "Theory and Practice in Medical Education at the University of Montpellier in the Thirteenth and Fourteenth Centuries." *Journal of the History of Medicine* 30:103–23.

———. 1976. "Scholasticism in Compendia of Practical Medicine, 1250–1450." *Manuscripta* 20:81–95.

———. 1977. "The Idea of Childhood and Childcare in Medical Writings of the Middle Ages." *Journal of Psychohistory* 4:461–90.

———. 1980. *Doctor Bernard de Gordon: Professor and Practitioner.* Studies and Texts, 51. Toronto: Pontifical Institute of Mediaeval Studies.

———. 1985. "The Description and Diagnosis of Leprosy by Fourteenth-Century Physicians." *Bulletin of the History of Medicine* 59:327–44.

Denifle, H. 1888. "Urkunden zur Geschichte der mittelalterlichen Universitäten: Neue Urkunden zur Universität Lérida." *Archiv für Literatur und Kirchengeschichte* 4:249–62.

Denifle, H. and A. Chatelain, eds. 1889–97. *Chartularium universitatis parisiensis.* Paris.

De Renzi, Salvatore. 1967 [1857]. *Storia documentata della scuola medica di Salerno.* 2nd ed. Naples; rpt. Milan: Ferro Edizioni.

———. 1852–1859. *Collectio Salernitana.* 5 vols. Naples.

Deslisle, Leopold. 1870. "Inventaire des manuscrits latins de la Sorbonne, conservés à la Bibliothèque Impériale sous les nos. 15176–16718 du fonds latins." *Bibliothèque de l'École des Chartes* 31:1–164.

Despars, Jacques. 1498. *Avicennae Canon (liber III) cum Jacobus de Partibus*. Lyons: J. Trechsel.

Diepgen, Paul. 1922. *Die Theologie und der ärztlichen Stand im Mittelalter*. Berlin.

———. 1963. *Frau und Frauenheilkunde in der Kultur des Mittelalters*. Stuttgart: G. Thieme.

Dillon, Myles. 1951. "The Wasting Sickness of Cú Chulainn." *Scottish Gaelic Studies* 7:47–88.

———, ed. 1953. *Serglige Con Culainn*. Dublin: Institute for Advanced Studies.

Dinzelbacher, Peter. 1981. "Über die Entdeckung der Liebe im Hochmittelalter." *Saeculum* 32:185–208.

Dionigi da Borgo San Sepulcro. ca. 1470. *Epistola super declaracione Valerii Maximi*. Strassburg.

Dioscorides. 1934. *The Greek Herbal of Dioscorides, Illustrated by a Byzantine A.D. 512, Englished by John Goodyer A.D.1655, Edited and First Printed A.D. 1933*. Oxford: Oxford University Press.

Dols, Michael, trans. 1984. *Medieval Islamic Medicine: Ibn Ridwān's Treatise "On the Prevention of Bodily Ills in Egypt"*. Berkeley: University of California Press.

Donaldson, E. Talbot. 1970 [1965]. "The Myth of Courtly Love." In *Speaking of Chaucer*. New York: Norton. Pp. 154–63.

Douglas, Mary. 1975. *Implicit Meanings: Essays in Anthropology*. London: Routledge and Kegan Paul.

———. 1982 [1973]. *Natural Symbols: Explorations in Cosmology*. New York: Pantheon.

Drabkin, I. E., ed. and trans. 1950. *On Acute Disease and on Chronic Disease*. Chicago: University of Chicago Press.

Dronke, Peter. 1979. "The Song of Songs and Medieval Love-Lyric." In *The Bible and Medieval Culture*. Ed. W. Lourdaux and D. Verhelst. Louvain: Leuven University Press. Pp. 236–62.

———. 1984. *Women Writers of the Middle Ages*. Cambridge: Cambridge University Press.

Duby, Georges. 1983a. *The Knight, the Lady, and the Priest: The Making of Modern Marriage in Medieval France*. Trans. Barbara Bray and introd. Natalie Zemon Davis. New York: Pantheon.

———. 1983b. *Que sait-on de l'amour en France au xii<sup>e</sup> siècle?* Oxford: Clarendon Press.

———. 1984. *Guillaume le Maréchal ou le meilleur chevalier du monde*. Paris: Fayard.

———, ed. 1988. *A History of Private Life: Revelations of the Medieval World*. Trans. Arthur Goldhammer. Cambridge, Mass.: Belknap Press.

Dugat, Gustav. 1853. "Études sur le traité de médécine d'Abou Djàfar Ah'mad, intitulé Zad al-Moçafir 'La Provision du Voyageur'." *Journal asiatique*, 5th ser., 1:289–353.

Dumeige, Gervais, ed. 1955. *Les quatre degrés de la violente charité*. Textes philosophiques du moyen âge, 3. Paris: J. Vrin.

*The Encyclopedia of Islam*. 1954–79. Ed. H. A. R. Gibb. 2nd ed. 4 vols. Leiden: E. J. Brill.

Ewart, Alfred, ed. 1976. *Marie de France, Lais*. Oxford: Basil Blackwell.

Fackenheim, Emil, trans. 1945. "A Treatise on Love by Ibn Sina." *Mediaeval Studies* 7:208–28.

Falkenhausen, V. von. 1984. "Costantino Africano." *Dizionario biographico degli italiani*. Rome: Istituto della Enciclopedia italiana. 30:320–24.

Faral, Edmond. 1913. *Recherches sur les sources latines des contes et romans courtois du moyen âge*. Paris: H. Champion.

Favati, Guido. 1952. "La glossa latina di Dino Del Garbo a 'Donna me prega' del Cavalcanti." *Annali della r. scuola normale superiore di Pisa*, Lettere, storia, e filosofia, Serie 2, 21:70–103.

———, ed. 1957. *Guido Cavalcanti, Le rime*. Milan: Ricciardi.

Ferrand, Jacques. 1978 [1623]. *De la maladie d'amour ou mélancholie érotique*. Paris. Rpt. Nendeln/Liechtenstein: Kraus Reprint.

Ferreira, Jean, O. F. M. 1960. "L'homme dans la doctrine de Pierre d'Espagne." In *L'homme et son destin d'après les penseurs du moyen âge*. Actes du Premier Congrès International de Philosophie Médiévale, Louvain-Bruxelles, 28 août-4 septembre 1958. Louvain: Nauwelaerts. Pp. 445–61.

Ferreiro Alemparte, Jaime. 1983. "La escuela de nigromancia de Toledo." *Anuario de estudios medievales* 13:205–68.

Filgueira Valverde, José. 1985. *Cantigas de Santa María*. Madrid: Editorial Castalia.

Filthaut, Ephraim, ed. 1955. *Quaestiones super de animalibus*. Opera omnia Alberti Magni, 12. Münster: Aschendorff.

Fischer, Klaus-Dietrich. 1983. "Verbesserungen zur *Isagoge* des Johannicius." *Sudhoffs Archiv* 67:223–24.

Flacelière, Robert and Émile Chambry, ed. and trans. 1977. *Plutarch: Vies*. Vol. 13. Paris: Société d'Édition "Les belles lettres."

Flashar, Helmut. 1966. *Melancholie und Melancholiker in den medizinischen Theorien der Antike*. Berlin: Walter de Gruyter.

Fontaine, M. M. 1985. "La lignée des commentaires à la chanson de Guido Cavalcanti 'Donna me prega'." In *Le Corps et la folie*. Ed. Jean Céard. Paris: Presses Universitaires de France.

Ford, Patrick K., trans. 1977. *The Mabinogi and Other Medieval Welsh Tales*. Berkeley: University of California Press.

———. 1988. "Celtic Women: The Opposing Sex." *Viator* 19:417–38.

Foster, Kenelm and Patrick Boyd. 1967. *Dante's Lyric Poetry*. 2 vols. Oxford: Clarendon Press.

Foucault, Michel. 1973. *Madness and Civilization*. Trans. Richard Howard. New York: Vintage.

———. 1978. *The History of Sexuality: Introduction*. Trans. Robert Hurley. Vol. 1. New York: Pantheon.

———. 1986. *The Care of the Self*. Vol. 3 of *The History of Sexuality*. Trans. Robert Hurley. New York: Pantheon.

Freud, Sigmund. 1957 [1914]. "On Narcissism: An Introduction." In *The Standard Edition of the Complete Psychological Works of Sigmund Freud*. Trans. James Strachey. London: Hogarth Press. 14:67–107.

———. 1957 [1915]. "Instincts and Their Vicissitudes." *Standard Edition* 14:109–40.

———. 1957 [1917]. "Mourning and Melancholia." *Standard Edition* 14:237–60.

Fuchs, J. W. 1970. *Lexicon latinitatis Nederlandicae medii aevi.* Fasc. 1. Amsterdam: Adolf Hakkert.

Furnivall, Frederick J., ed. 1866. *Political, Religious, and Love Poems.* Early English Text Society, old series 15. London: Early English Text Society.

———. 1868. *Hymns to the Virgin and Christ, The Parliament of Devils, and Other Religious Poems.* Early English Text Society, old series, 24. London: Early English Text Society.

Galen. *In Hippocratis Epidemiarum.* See Pfaff.

———. *In Hippocratis prognosticum.* See Heeg.

———. *Quod animi mores.* See Hauke.

———. *Scripta minora.* See Marquardt.

Garbers, Karl, ed. 1977. *Isḥāq ibn ʿImrān, Maqāla Fī L-Mālīhūliyā (Abhandlung über die Melancholie) und Constantini Africani, Libri duo de melancholia.* Hamburg: Helmut Buske.

Geertz, Clifford. 1973. *The Interpretation of Cultures.* New York: Basic Books.

Gerard of Cremona. 1510. *Glossae in nono almansoris.* Lyons.

Gerard of Solo. 1505. *Commentum super nono Almansoris.* Venice.

Geremek, Bronisław. 1987 [1971]. *The Margins of Society in Late Medieval Paris.* Cambridge: Cambridge University Press.

Getz, Faye Marie. 1982. "Gilbertus Anglicus Anglicized." *Medical History* 26: 436–42.

Giedke, Adalheid. 1983. "Die Liebeskrankheit in der Geschichte der Medizin." Dissertation med. Düsseldorf.

Glorieux, P. 1952. *Pour revaloriser Migne, Tables rectificatives.* Lille: Facultés Catholiques.

Goetz, Georg. 1888–1901. *Corpus glossariorum latinorum.* 5 vols. Leipzig: Teubner.

Gold, Penny Schine. 1985. *The Lady and the Virgin: Image, Attitude, and Experience in Twelfth-Century France.* Chicago: University of Chicago Press.

Goldin, Frederick. 1967. *The Mirror of Narcissus in the Courtly Love Lyric.* Ithaca, N.Y.: Cornell University Press.

Goldstein-Préaud, Tamara. 1981. "Albert le Grand et les questions du xiiiᵉ siècle sur le *De animalibus* d'Aristote." *History and Philosophy of the Life Sciences* 3:61–71.

Gourevitch, Danielle. 1984. *Le mal d'être femme: La femme et la médecine dans la Rome antique.* Paris: Société d'Édition "Les Belles Lettres."

Grabmann, Martin. 1979 [1929]. "Mittelalterliche lateinische Aristotelesübersetzungen und Aristoteleskommentare in Handschriften spanischer Bibliotheken." In *Gesammelte Akademieabhandlungen.* Paderborn: Ferdinand Schöningh. 1: 383–496.

———. 1979 [1936]. "Handschriftliche Forschungen und Funde zu den philosophischen Schriften des Petrus Hispanus, des späteren Papstes Johannes XXI († 1277)." In *Gesammelte Akademieabhandlungen.* Paderborn: Ferdinand Schöningh. 2:1123–1254.

Gracia, Diego and Jose-Luis Vidal. 1974–75. "La *Isagoge de Ioannitius*: Introducción, edición, traducción y notas." *Asclepio: Archivo iberoamericano de historia de la medicina y antropologia medica* 26–27:267–382.

Graham, Thomas. 1967. *Medieval Minds: Mental Health in the Middle Ages.* London: Allen & Unwin.

Grant, Edward, ed. 1974. *A Source Book in Medieval Science.* Cambridge, Mass.: Harvard University Press.

Gravdal, Kathryn. 1985. "Camouflaging Rape: The Rhetoric of Sexual Violence in the Medieval Pastourelle." *Romanic Review* 76:361–73.

Green, Monica. 1985. "The Transmission of Ancient Theories of Female Physiology and Disease Through the Early Middle Ages." Ph.D. dissertation. Princeton.

———. 1987. "The *De genecia* Attributed to Constantine the African." *Speculum* 62:299–323.

———. 1989a. "Women's Medical Practice and Health Care in Medieval Europe." *Signs* 14 no.2:434–73.

———. 1989b. "Constantinus Africanus and the Conflict between Religion and Science." In *The Human Embryo: Aristotle and the Arabic and European Traditions.* Ed. Gordon Dunstan. London: Duckworth.

———. Forthcoming. "Essay Review: Female Sexuality in the Medieval West." *Trends in History.*

Green, Richard F. 1988. "Chaucer's Victimized Women." *Studies in the Age of Chaucer* 10:3–21.

Greenblatt, Stephen. 1988. *Shakespearian Negotiations: The Circulation of Social Energy in Renaissance England.* Berkeley: University of California Press.

Gregory, Tullio. 1966. "L'idea di natura nella filosofia medievale prima dell'ingresso della fisica di Aristotele—Il secolo XII." In *La filosofia della natura nel medioevo.* Atti del terzo congresso internazionale di filosofia medioevale. Milan: Società editrice vita e pensiero. Pp. 27–65.

Grieve, Maud. 1931. *A Modern Herbal.* London: J. Cape.

Grotzfeld, Heinz. 1970. *Das Bad im Arabisch-Islamischen Mittelalter: Eine kulturgeschichtliche Studie.* Wiesbaden: Harrassowitz.

Guénon, Anne-Sylvie. 1982. "Gérard de Solo, maître de l'Université de Médecine de Montpellier et practicien du XIVe siècle." *École Nationale des Chartes, Positions des Thèses.* Paris: École des Chartes. Pp. 75–82.

Hamesse, Jacqueline. 1972. *Auctoritates Aristotelis.* Louvain: CETEDOC.

Hansen, Joseph. 1901. *Quellen und Untersuchungen zur Geschichte des Hexenwahns und der Hexenverfolgung im Mittelalter.* Bonn: Carl Georgi.

Häring, Nicolaus. 1982. "Commentary and Hermeneutics." In *Renaissance and Renewal in the Twelfth Century.* Ed. Giles Constable and Robert Benson. Cambridge, Mass.: Harvard University Press. Pp. 173–200.

Harvey, E. Ruth. 1975. *The Inward Wits: Psychological Theory in the Middle Ages and the Renaissance.* London: The Warburg Institute.

Haskins, C. H. 1924. *Studies in the History of Medieval Science.* Cambridge, Mass.: Harvard University Press.

Hatto, A. T., trans. 1967. *Tristan and Isolde.* Harmondsworth: Penguin.

Hauke, Erike. 1937. *Galen: Dass die Vermögen der Seele eine Folge der Mischungen des Körpers sind.* Berlin: Emil Ebering.

Heeg, Joseph, ed. 1915. *Galeni in Hippocratis prognosticum commentum III.* CMG V 9,2. Leipzig: Teubner.

Heiberg, J.L., ed. 1912. *Pauli Aeginetae Libri tertii interpretatio latina antiqua.* Leipzig: Teubner.

———, ed. 1921. *Epitome.* CMG IX, 1. Leipzig: Teubner.

Helm, Rudolph, ed. 1898. *Fabii Planciadis Fulgentii V. C. opera.* Leipzig: Teubner.

Henderson, A. A. R., ed. 1979. *Remedia amoris*. Edinburgh: Scottish Academic Press.

Hendrix, G. 1980a. "Les *Postillae* de Hugues de Saint-Cher et le traité *De doctrina cordis*." *Recherches de théologie ancienne et médiévale* 40:114–30.

———. 1980b. "Hugh of St. Cher O.P., Author of Two Texts Attributed to the Thirteenth-Century Cistercian Gerard of Liège." *Cîteaux* 31:342–56.

Herlihy, David. 1975. "Life Expectancies for Women in Medieval Society." In *The Role of Woman in the Middle Ages*. Ed. Rosemary Thee Morewedge. Albany, N.Y.: State University of New York Press. Pp. 1–20.

———. 1978. "Medieval Children." In *Essays on Medieval Civilization*. Ed. Bede K. Lackner and Kenneth R. Philip. Walter Prescott Webb Memorial Lectures, 12. Austin, Texas: University of Texas Press. Pp. 109–41.

———. 1983. "The Making of the Medieval Family: Symmetry, Structure, and Sentiment." *Journal of Family History* 8:116–30.

———. 1985a. *Medieval Households*. Cambridge, Mass.: Harvard University Press.

———. 1985b. "Did Women Have a Renaissance?: A Reconsideration." *Medievalia et Humanistica* 13:1–22.

Herzlich, Claudine and Janine Pierret. 1987. *Illness and Self in Society*. Trans. Elborg Forster. Baltimore: Johns Hopkins University Press.

Hett, Walter S., ed. 1937. *The Problems of Aristotle*. 2 vols. London: Heinemann; Cambridge, Mass.: Harvard University Press.

Hexter, Ralph J. 1986. *Ovid and Medieval Schooling. Studies in Medieval School Commentaries on Ovid's* Ars Amatoria, Epistulae ex Ponto, *and* Epistulae Heroidum. Münchener Beiträge, 38. Munich: Arbeo-Gesellschaft.

Hicks, R. D., trans. 1937–38. *Diogenes Laertius' Lives of Eminent Philosophers*. 2 vols. Cambridge, Mass.: Harvard University Press.

Hildegard of Bingen. *See* Kaiser.

Holländer, Eugen. 1913. *Die Medizin in der klassischen Malerei*. 2nd ed. Stuttgart: F. Enke.

Howell, Martha C. 1986. *Women, Production, and Patriarchy in Late Medieval Cities*. Chicago: University of Chicago Press.

Hunt, R. W. 1950. "Studies on Priscian in the Twelfth Century." *Mediaeval and Renaissance Studies* 2:1–56.

Hunt, Tony. 1981. "The *Song of Songs* and Courtly Literature." In *Court and Poet*. Ed. Glyn S. Burgess. Liverpool: Francis Cairns. Pp. 189–96.

Ibn Botlan. 1967. *Tacuinum sanitatis in medicina. Codex Vindobonensis series nova 2644 der österreichischen Nationalbibliothek*. Vol. 1: Facsimile. Vol. 2: Commentary by Franz Unterkircher, trans. Heide Saxer and Charles H. Talbot. Graz: Akademische Druck- und Verlagsanstalt.

Ingleby, David. 1982. "The Social Construction of Mental Illness." In *The Problem of Medical Knowledge: Examining the Social Construction of Medicine*. Ed. Peter Wright and Andrew Treacher. Edinburgh: University Press. Pp. 123–43.

Inguanez, M. 1915–41. *Codicum casinensium manuscriptorum catalogus*. 3 vols. Rome: Pontifical Institute.

Isaac Judaeus. 1570. *De diaetis universalibus et particularibus*. Basel.

Isidore of Seville. *See* Lindsay.

Jacoff, Rachel. 1984. "God as Mother: Julian of Norwich's Theology of Love." *Denver Quarterly* 18:134–39.

Jacquart, Danielle. 1979. *Supplément au 'Dictionnaire' d'Ernest Wickersheimer.* Hautes études médiévales et modernes, 35. Geneva: Droz.

———. 1980. "Le Regard d'un médecin sur son temps: Jacques Despars (1380?–1458)." *Bibliothèque de l'École des Chartes* 138:35–86.

———. 1981. *Le milieu médical en France du xiie au xve siècle: En annexe 2e supplément au 'Dictionnaire' d'Ernest Wickersheimer.* Hautes études médiévales et modernes, 46. Geneva: Droz.

———. 1984. "La maladie et le remède d'amour dans quelques écrits médicaux au moyen âge." In *Amour, mariage et transgression au moyen âge.* Université de Picardie, Centre d'Études Médiévales. Actes du Colloque des 24, 25, 26, et 27 mars 1983. Göppingen: Kümmerle. Pp. 93–101.

Jacquart, Danielle and Claude Thomasset. 1981. "Albert le Grand et les problèmes de la sexualité." *History and Philosophy of the Life Sciences* 3:73–93.

———. 1985a. "L'amour 'héroïque' à travers le traité d'Arnaud de Villeneuve." In *La Folie et le corps.* Ed. Jean Céard. Paris: Presses de l'École Normale Supérieure. Pp. 143–58.

———. 1985b. *Sexualité et savoir médical au moyen âge.* Paris: Presses Universitaires de France.

Jacquart, Danielle and Gérard Troupeau, ed. and trans. 1980. *Le Livre des axiomes médicaux (aphorismi).* Hautes études orientales 14. Geneva: Droz; Paris: Champion.

Jaeger, C. Stephen. 1985. *The Origins of Courtliness: Civilizing Trends and the Formation of Courtly Ideals, 939–1210.* Philadelphia: University of Pennsylvania Press.

James, Montague Rhodes. 1909. "The Catalogue of the Library of the Augustinian Friars at York." In *Fasciculus Ioanni Willis Clark dicatus.* Cambridge: Cambridge University Press. Pp. 2–96.

John of Tornamira. 1490. *Clarificatorium super nono almansoris.* Lyons.

Kaeppeli, Thomas. 1970. *Scriptores ordinis praedicatorum medii aevi.* Vol. 1. Rome: S. Sabina.

Kaiser, Paul, ed. 1903. *Hildegardis causae et curae.* Leipzig: Teubner.

Kalinke, Marianne E. 1984. "*Sigurðar saga Jórsalafara*: The Fictionalization of Fact in *Morkinskinna.*" *Scandinavian Studies* 56:152–67.

Karnein, Alfred. 1985. *De amore in volkssprachlicher Literatur: Untersuchungen zur Andreas-Capellanus-Rezeption in Mittelalter und Renaissance.* Heidelberg: Carl Winter.

Kassel, Rudolf. 1958. *Untersuchungen zur griechischen und römischen Konsolationsliteratur.* Munich: Beck.

Keen, Maurice. 1986. "Gadifer de La Salle: A Late Medieval Knight Errant." In *The Ideals and Practice of Medieval Knighthood.* Ed. Christopher Harper-Bill and Ruth Harvey. Woodbridge, Suffolk: The Boydell Press. Pp. 74–85.

Kelly, Henry Ansgar. 1987. "The Varieties of Love in Medieval Literature According to Gaston Paris." *Romance Philology* 40:301–27.

Kelly, Joan Gadol. 1977. "Did Women Have a Renaissance?" In *Becoming Visible: Women in European History.* Ed. Renate Bridenthal and Claudia Koonz. Boston: Houghton Mifflin.

———. 1984. "The Social Relations of the Sexes." In *Women, History, and Theory.* Chicago: University of Chicago Press. Pp. 1–18.

Kenny, Anthony and Jan Pinborg. 1982. "Medieval Philosophical Literature." In

*The Cambridge History of Later Medieval Philosophy*. Ed. Norman Kretzmann, Anthony Kenny, and Jan Pinborg. Cambridge: Cambridge University Press. Pp. 9–42.

Kibre, Pearl. 1939. "Hitherto Unnoted Medical Writings of Domenicus of Ragusa (1424–1425 A.D.)." *Bulletin of the History of Medicine* 7:990–95.

———. 1946. "The Intellectual Interests Reflected in Libraries of the Thirteenth and Fourteenth Centuries." *Journal of the History of Ideas* 7:257–97.

———. 1971. "Dominicus de Ragusa, Bolognese Doctor of Arts and Medicine." *Bulletin of the History of Medicine* 45:383–86.

Kibre, Pearl and Nancy Siraisi. 1978. "The Institutional Setting: The Universities." In *Science in the Middle Ages*. Ed. David C. Lindberg. Chicago: University of Chicago Press. Pp. 120–44.

Kittel, Muriel. 1973. "Humility in Old Provençal and Early Italian Poetry: Resemblances and Contrasts." *Romance Philology* 27:158–71.

Klapisch-Zuber, Christiane. 1985. *Women, Family, and Ritual in Renaissance Italy*. Trans. Lynn Cochrane. Chicago: University of Chicago Press.

Klibansky, Raymond, Erwin Panofsky, and Fritz Saxl. 1964. *Saturn and Melancholy*. London: Thomas Nelson and Sons Ltd.

Koenigsberg, Richard. 1967. "Culture and Unconscious Fantasy: Observations on Courtly Love." *Psychoanalytic Review* 54:36–50.

Könsgen, Ewald, ed. 1974. *Epistolae duorum amantium: Briefe Abaelards und Heloises?* Mittellateinische Studien und Texte, 8. Leiden: Brill.

Kramer, Heinrich and James Sprenger. 1582. *Malleus maleficarum*. Frankfurt.

Kristeller, Paul Oskar. 1956. "The School of Salerno: Its Development and its Contribution to the History of Learning." In *Studies in Renaissance Thought and Letters*. Rome: Storia e Letteratura. Pp. 495–551.

———. 1959. "Beitrag der Schule von Salerno zur Entwicklung der scholastischen Wissenschaft im 12. Jahrhundert." In *Artes Liberales: Von der Antiken Bildung zur Wissenschaft des Mittelalters*. Ed. Josef Koch. Leiden: Brill. Pp. 84–90.

———. 1976. "Bartholomaeus, Musandinus and Maurus of Salerno and Other Early Commentators of the 'Articella', with a Tentative List of Texts and Manuscripts." *Italia medioevale e umanistica* 19:57–87.

———. 1980. *La Scuola Medica di Salerno secondo ricerche e scoperte recenti*. Quaderni del Centro studi e documentazione della Scuola Medica Salernitana 5:1–16.

———. 1986. *Studi sulla Scuola medica salernitana*. Naples: Istituto Italiano per gli Studi Filosofici.

Kristeva, Julia. 1985. *Au commencement était l'amour: Psychanalyse et foi*. Paris: Hachette.

———. 1987. *Tales of Love*. Trans. Leon Roudiez. New York: Columbia University Press.

Kudlien, Fridolf. 1986. *Die Stellung des Arztes in der römischen Gesellschaft. Freigeborene Römer, Eingebürgerte, Peregrine, Sklaven, Freigelassene als Ärzte*. Forschungen zur antiken Sklaverei, 18. Stuttgart: Franz Steiner.

Kühn, C. G., ed. 1964–65 [1821–33]. *Claudii Galeni Opera omnia*. 20 vols. Leipzig. Rpt. Hildesheim: Olms.

Kümmel, Werner F. 1977. *Musik und Medizin: Ihre Wechselbeziehungen in Theorie und Praxis von 800 bis 1800*. Freiburger Beiträge zur Wissenschafts- und Universitätsgeschichte, 2. Freiburg: Karl Alber.

Kulcsár, Péter, ed. 1987. *Mythographi Vaticani I et II*. Corpus Christianorum series latina XCI c. Turnhout: Brepols.

Kurdziałek, Marian, ed. 1963. *Davidis de Dinantó quaternulorum fragmenta*. Studia mediewistyczne, 3. Warsaw: Państwowe Wydawnictwo Naukowe.

Laborde, A. de. 1911–27. *La Bible moralisée illustrée, conservée à Oxford, Paris, et Londres*. 5 vols. Paris.

Laín Entralgo, Pedro. 1961. *La historia clinica*. 2nd ed. Barcelona: Salvat.

Langosch, Karl, ed. and trans. 1975. *Hymnen und Vagantenlieder*. 4th ed. Darmstadt: Wissenschaftliche Buchgesellschaft.

Latham, R. E. 1975. *Dictionary of Medieval Latin from British Sources*. Fasc. 1. London: Oxford University Press.

Lawn, Brian. 1963. *The Salernitan Questions: An Introduction to the History of Medieval and Renaissance Problem Literature*. Oxford: Clarendon Press.

———. 1979. *The Prose Salernitan Questions, Edited from a Bodleian Manuscript (Auct. F.3.10)*. Auctores Britannici Medii Aevi, 5. London: British Academy.

Lawson, R. P., trans. 1957. *Origen: The Song of Songs, Commentary and Homilies*. Ancient Christian Writers, 26. Westminster, Maryland: The Newman Press.

Lawson, Sarah, trans. 1985. *The Treasure of the City of Ladies*. Harmondsworth: Penguin.

Lea, Henry Charles. 1939. *Materials Toward a History of Witchcraft*. Ed. Arthur Howland. Vol. 1. Philadelphia: University of Pennsylvania Press.

Leclercq, Jean. 1979. *Monks and Love in Twelfth-Century France: Psycho-Historical Essays*. Oxford: Clarendon Press.

———. 1982. *The Love of Learning and the Desire for God*. 3rd ed. New York: Fordham University Press.

Le Goff, Jacques. 1980. *Time, Work, and Culture in the Middle Ages*. Trans. Arthur Goldhammer. Chicago: University of Chicago Press.

Lehmann, Hermann. 1930. "Die Arbeitsweise des Constantinus Africanus und des Johannes Afflacius im Verhältnis zueinander." *Archeion* 12:272–81.

Leibbrand, Werner and Annemarie Wettley. 1961. *Der Wahnsinn: Geschichte der abendländischen Psychopathologie*. Freiburg and Munich: Karl Alber.

Lejeune, Rita. 1977. "La femme dans les littératures français et occitane du XIe au XIIIe siècle." *Cahiers de civilisation médiévale* 20:201–17.

Lemay, Helen Rodnite. 1981. "William of Saliceto on Human Sexuality." *Viator* 12:165–81.

———. 1982. "Human Sexuality in Twelfth- Through Fifteenth-Century Scientific Writings." In *Sexual Practices and the Medieval Church*. Ed. Vern Bullough and James Brundage. Buffalo, N.Y.: Prometheus Books. Pp. 187–205.

Leube-Fey, Christiana. 1971. *Bild und Funktion der dompna in der Lyrik des Trobadors*. Heidelberg: Winter.

Liebowitz, Michael R. 1983. *The Chemistry of Love*. New York: Berkley.

Lindberg, David. 1976. *Theories of Vision from Al-Kindi to Kepler*. Chicago: University of Chicago Press.

Lindsay, Wallace M., ed. 1911. *Isidori Hispalensis Episcopi etymologiarum sive originum libri xx*. 2 vols. Oxford: Clarendon Press.

Littré, Émile. 1847. "Géraud du Berri, médecin." *Histoire littéraire de la France* 21:404–08.

Lockwood, Dean. 1951. *Ugo Benzi: Medieval Philosopher and Physician, 1376–1439.* Chicago: University of Chicago Press.

Lowes, John L. 1913/14. "The Loveres Maladye of Hereos." *Modern Philology* 11:491–546.

de Lubac, Henri. 1959. *Exégèse médiévale: les quatre sens de l'Écriture.* Paris: Aubier.

MacDonald, Michael. 1981. *Mystical Bedlam: Anxiety, Madness and Healing in Seventeenth-Century England.* Cambridge: Cambridge University Press.

———. 1983. "Anthropological perspectives on the history of science and medicine." In *Information Sources in the History of Science and Medicine.* Ed. Pietro Corsi and Paul Weindling. London: Butterworth Scientific.

McKeon, Richard. 1961. "Medicine and Philosophy in the Eleventh and Twelfth Centuries: The Problem of Elements." *The Thomist* 24:211–56.

MacKinney, Loren C. 1938. "Medieval Medical Dictionaries and Glossaries." In *Medieval and Historiographical Essays in Honor of J. W. Thompson.* Ed. J. L. Cate and E. N. Anderson. Chicago: University of Chicago Press. Pp. 240–68.

McKnight, George. 1971 [1913]. *Middle English Humorous Tales in Verse.* Rpt. New York: Gordian Press.

McLaughlin, Mary Martin. 1974. "Survivors and Surrogates: Children and Parents from the Ninth to the Thirteenth Centuries." In *The History of Childhood.* Ed. L. DeMause. New York: Psychohistory Press.

Maclean, Ian. 1980. *The Renaissance Notion of Woman.* Cambridge: Cambridge University Press.

Macrobius. 1952. *Commentary on the Dream of Scipio.* Trans. William Harris Stahl. New York: Columbia University Press.

McVaugh, Michael R. 1970. "Constantine the African." DSB 3:393–95.

———, ed. 1975. *Arnaldi de Villanova Aphorismi de gradibus.* Opera medica omnia, 2. Granada and Barcelona: University of Barcelona.

———. 1976. "Two Montpellier Recipe Collections." *Manuscripta* 20:175–80.

———, ed. 1985. *Arnaldi de Villanova liber de amore heroico.* Opera medica omnia, 3. Barcelona: University of Barcelona.

McWilliam, G. H., trans. 1972. *Decameron.* Harmondsworth: Penguin.

Maier, Anneliese. 1968. *Zwei Grundprobleme der scholastischen Naturphilosophie.* 3rd ed. Rome: Storia e letteratura.

Manzaneda, Marcos. 1984. "La ambivalencia afectiva." *Angelicum* 61:404–40.

Marold, Karl and Werner Schröder, eds. 1969. *Tristan.* Berlin: Walter de Gruyter.

Marquardt, J., G. Helmreich, and I. Mueller, eds. 1964 [1891–94]. *Claudii Galeni Pergameni Scripta Minora.* Leipzig: Teubner; rpt. Hildesheim: Olms.

Marx, Friedrich, ed. 1915. *A. Cornelii Celsi quae supersunt.* Corpus medicorum latinorum, 1. Leipzig and Berlin: Teubner.

Marx, J. 1905. *Verzeichnis der Handschriften-Sammlung des Hospitals zu Cues.* Trier: Hospital zu Cues.

Masters, William and Virginia Johnson. 1966. *Human Sexual Response.* Boston: Little, Brown.

Matthaeus Silvaticus. 1541. *Pandectae medicinae.* Lyons.

Maurach, Gregor, ed. 1978. "Johannitius, *Isagoge ad Techne Galieni.*" *Sudhoffs Archiv* 62:148–74.

Maxmen, Jerrold. 1986. *Essential Psychopathology.* New York: W. W. Norton.

Ménagier de Paris. *See* Brereton and Ferrier.

Menocal, María Rosa. 1987. *The Arabic Role in Medieval Literary History*. Philadelphia: University of Pennsylvania Press.

Mesk, Josef. 1913. "Antiochus und Stratonike." *Rheinisches Museum für Philologie* n.s. 68:366–94.

Mesulam, Marek-Marsel and Jon Perry. 1972. "The Diagnosis of Love-Sickness: Experimental Psychophysiology without the Polygraph." *Psychophysiology* 9:546–51.

Meyerhof, Max. 1928. "An Arabic Compendium of Medico-philosophical Definitions." *Isis* 10:340–49.

Micha, Alexandre, ed. 1970. *Chrétien de Troyes: Cligés*. Paris: H. Champion.

Michaud-Quantin, Pierre. 1970. "Les champs sémantiques de *species*: tradition latine et traductions du grec." In *Études sur le vocabulaire philosophique du Moyen Âge*. Rome: Edizioni dell'Ateneo. Pp. 113–50.

Michie, Sarah. 1937. "The Lover's Malady in Early Irish Romance." *Speculum* 12:304–13.

Miles, Margaret. 1985. *Image as Insight: Visual Understanding in Western Christianity and Secular Culture*. Boston: Beacon Press.

———. 1986. "The Virgin's One Bare Breast: Female Nudity and Religious Meaning in Tuscan Early Renaissance Culture." In *The Female Body in Western Culture*. Ed. Susan Rubin Suleiman. Cambridge, Mass.: Harvard University Press. Pp. 193–208.

Minuo-Paluello, L., ed. 1951. *Categoriae vel Praedicamenta*. Aristoteles latinus, I.1–5. Bruges and Paris: Desclée de Brouwer.

Mørland, Henning. 1932. *Die lateinischen Oribasiusübersetzungen*. Symbolae Osloenses fasc. supplet. 5. Oslo: A. W. Brøgger.

———. 1940. *Oribasius latinus. Erster Teil*. Symbolae Osloenses fasc. supplet. 10. Oslo: A. W. Brøgger.

Moi, Toril. 1986. "Desire in Language: Andreas Capellanus and the Controversy of Courtly Love." In *Medieval Literature: Criticism, Ideology, and History*. Ed. David Aers. New York: St. Martin's. Pp. 11–33.

Molinier, A. 1876. "Traductions latines d'Oribase." In Bussemaker and Daremberg, 1851–76, vols. 5 and 6.

Moller, Herbert. 1960. "The Meaning of Courtly Love." *Journal of American Folklore* 73:39–52.

Monter, E. William. 1977. "The Pedestal and the Stake: Courtly Love and Witchcraft." In *Becoming Visible: Women in European History*. Ed. Renate Bridenthal and Claudia Koonz. Boston: Houghton Mifflin. Pp. 119–36.

Montero Cartelle, Enrique, ed. 1983. *Constantini Liber de coitu*. Monografías de la Universidad de Santiago de Compostela, 77. Santiago de Compostela: Universidad.

———, ed. 1987. *Liber minor de coitu*. Valladolid: Universidad.

Moser, Thomas C., Jr. 1986. "Love and Disorder: A Fifteenth-Century Middle English Lyric and Some Literary Antecedents." Paper delivered at the Convention of the Modern Language Association, New York.

———. 1987. "The Latin Love Lyric in English Manuscripts: 1150–1325." Ph.D. dissertation, Stanford University.

Mowat, J. L. G., ed. 1882. *Sinonoma Bartholomei*. Anecdota Oxoniensia, vol. 1, part 1. Oxford.

————, ed. 1887. *Alphita: A Medico-Botanical Glossary from the Bodleian Manuscript, Selden B.35.* Anecdota Oxoniensia, vol. 1, part 2. Oxford.

Müller, I., ed. 1891. *Quod animi mores temperamentum corporis sequuntur.* Claudii Galeni Pergameni scripta minora, vol. 2. Leipzig: Teubner.

Müller, Irmgard. 1984. "Liebestränke, Liebeszauber und Schlafmittel in der mittelalterlichen Literatur." In *Liebe—Ehe—Ehebruch in der Literatur des Mittelalters.* Ed. Xenja von Ertzdorff and Marianne Wynn. Beiträge zur deutschen Philologie, 58. Giessen: Wilhelm Schmitz.

Murdoch, John. 1974. "Philosophy and the Enterprise of Science in the Later Middle Ages." In *The Interaction between Science and Philosophy*, Ed. Y. Elkana. Atlantic Highlands, New Jersey: Humanities Press.

————. 1975. "From Social into Intellectual Factors: An Aspect of the Unitary Character of Late Medieval Learning." In *The Cultural Context of Medieval Learning.* Ed. John Murdoch and Edith Sylla. Boston Studies in the Philosophy of Science, 26. Dordrecht: Reidel. Pp. 271–348.

Nardi, Bruno. 1959. "L'amore e i medici medioevali." In *Studi in onore di Angelo Monteverdi.* Modena: Società Tipografica Editrice Modenese. 2:517–42.

Newton, Francis. 1976. "The Desiderian Scriptorium at Montecassino: The *Chronicle* and some surviving manuscripts." *Dumbarton Oaks Papers* 30:37–53.

Nichols, Stephen G., Jr. 1983. *Romanesque Signs: Early Medieval Narrative and Iconography.* New Haven, Conn.: Yale University Press.

Nider, Johannes. 1569. *Formicarius.* Lyons.

Nortier, Geneviève. 1971. *Les bibliothèques médiévales des abbayes bénédictines de Normandie*, nouvelle éd. Paris: P. Lethielleux.

Nutton, Vivian, ed. 1979. *Galen on Prognosis.* CMG V 8,1. Berlin: Akademie-Verlag.

————, ed. 1981. *Galen: Problems and Prospects.* London: Wellcome Institute.

Offermanns, Winfried. 1970. *Die Wirkung Ovids auf die literarische Sprache der lateinischen Liebesdichtung des 11. und 12. Jahrhunderts.* Beihefte zum Mittellateinischen Jahrbuch, 4. Wuppertal: A. Henn Verlag.

Ogle, Marbury B. and Dorothy Schullian, eds. 1933. *Rodulfi Tortarii carmina.* Papers and Monographs of the American Academy in Rome, 8. Rome: American Academy.

Ohly, Friedrich. 1958. *Hohelied-Studien: Grundzüge einer Geschichte der Hoheliedauslegung des Abendlandes bis um 1200.* Wiesbaden: Franz Steiner.

Olson, Glending. 1982. *Literature as Recreation in the Later Middle Ages.* Ithaca, N.Y.: Cornell University Press.

Oribasius. *See* Bussemaker and Daremberg.

Orofino, Giulia and Carla Casetti Brach. 1984. "Nel nome del bagno." *Kos* 1/3:33–54.

Otis, Leah Lydia. 1985. *Prostitution in Medieval Society: The History of an Urban Institution in Languedoc.* Chicago: University of Chicago Press.

Pagel, Julius L., ed. 1893. *Aureolae.* Berlin: G. Riemer.

————, ed. 1894. *Die Concordanciae des Johannes de Sancto Amando nach einer Berliner und zwei Erfurter Handschriften.* Berlin: G. Riemer.

————. 1896. *Neue literarische Beiträge zur mittelalterlichen Medicin.* Berlin: G. Riemer.

Paravicini Bagliani, Agostini. 1981. "A Proposito dell'insegnamento di medicina allo Studium curiae." In *Studi sul XIV Secolo in Memoria di Anneliese Meyer.* Ed. A. Maierù and A. Paravicini Bagliani. Rome: Storia e Letteratura. Pp. 395–413.

Paris, Paulin. 1868. *Les romans de la table ronde.* Vol. 1. Paris.

Patterson, Lee. 1987. *Negotiating the Past: The Historical Understanding of Medieval Literature.* Madison: University of Wisconsin Press.

Paul of Aegina. *See* Heiberg.

Pellegrin, Elisabeth. 1957. "Les *Remedia amoris* d'Ovide, texte scolaire médiéval." *Bibliothèque de l'École des Chartes,* 115:172–79.

Peters, Edward. 1978. *The Magician, the Witch, and the Law.* Philadelphia: University of Pennsylvania Press.

Petrus Hispanus. *Glosae super introitum sciencie tegni Galieni.* Madrid, Biblioteca Nacional, MS 1877.

————. *Questiones super de animalibus.* Madrid, Biblioteca Nacional, MS 1877.

————. *Super Isagogen Iohannitii.* Madrid, Biblioteca Nacional, MS 1877.

Pfaff, Franz, ed. and trans. 1940. *Galeni in Hippocratis epidemiarum libr. VI comm. VI–VIII.* CMG V 10,2,2. Leipzig: Teubner.

Pietro d'Abano. 1521. *Conciliator differentiarum philosophorum et praecipue medicorum.* Venice.

Pifferi, E., trans. 1962. *Bernardo Provenzale, Commento alle Tavole di Salerno.* Rome: N. pub.

Pigeaud, Jackie. 1981. *La maladie de l'âme: Etude sur la relation de l'âme et du corps dans la tradition médico-philosophique antique.* Paris: Société d'Édition "Les Belles Lettres."

————. 1984. "De la mélancolie et de quelques autres maladies dans les *Etymologies* IV d'Isidore de Séville." *Textes médicaux latins antiques.* Ed. G. Sabbah. Sainte-Étienne: Université. Pp. 87–107.

————. 1987. *Folie et cures de la folie chez les médecins de l'antiquité greco-romaine: la manie.* Collection des études anciennes, 12. Paris: Société d'Édition "Les Belles Lettres."

Pignol, J. 1889. "Géraud du Berry et l'école de médecine de Montpellier au commencement du treizième siècle." *Annales du Midi* 1:395–97.

Pires, Celestino, S.J. 1969. "Logica et Methodus apud Petrum Hispanum." In *Arts libéraux et philosophie au Moyen Âge.* Actes du Quatrième Congrès International de Philosophie Médiévale, Université de Montréal, Canada, 27 août–2 septembre 1967. Montréal: Institut d'Études Médiévales. Pp. 895–900.

Plutarch. *See* Flacelière and Chambry.

Pollmann, Leo. 1966. *Die Liebe in der hochmittelalterlichen Literatur Frankreichs.* Analecta Romanica, 18. Frankfurt: Vittorio Klostermann.

Pouchelle, Marie-Christine. 1983. *Corps et chirurgie à l'apogée du moyen âge: Savoir et imaginaire du corps chez Henri de Mondeville, chirurgien de Philippe le Bel.* Paris: Flammarion.

Powicke, F. M. 1931. *The Medieval Books of Merton College.* Oxford: Clarendon Press.

Raeder, I., ed. 1964 [1926]. *Oribasii Synopsis ad Eustathium.* CMG VI,3. Leipzig and Berlin: Teubner; rpt. Amsterdam: Adolf M. Hakkert.

Rank, Otto. 1926. *Das Inzest-Motiv in Dichtung und Sage.* 2nd ed. Leipzig and Vienna: Franz Deuticke.

al-Rāzī. 1509. *Liber continens.* Venice.

————. 1510. *Divisiones.* Lyons.

————. 1510. *Liber ad almansorem.* Lyons.

————. 1544. *Liber ad almansorem.* Basel.

Régnier-Bohler, Danielle. 1988. "Imagining the Self." In Duby, 1988. Pp. 313–93.

Reichert, Benedictus Maria, ed. 1897. *Vitae fratrum ordinis praedicatorum.* Monumenta ordinis fratrum praedicatorum, 1. Rome: In domino generalitia.

Reynolds, L. D., ed. 1983. *Texts and Transmission: A Survey of the Latin Classics.* Oxford: Clarendon Press.

Ricci, Seymour de. 1935–40. *Census of Medieval and Renaissance Manuscripts in the United States and Canada.* 3 vols. New York: H. W. Wilson.

Rice, Eugene F., Jr. 1980. "Paulus Aegineta." In *Catalogus translationum et commentariorum: Medieval and Renaissance Latin Translations and Commentaries.* Ed. F. Edward Cranz and Paul Oskar Kristeller. Washington, D.C.: The Catholic University of America Press. 4:146–91.

Richard of St. Victor. *See* Dumeige, 1955.

Richards, Earl J., trans. 1982. *The Book of the City of Ladies,* by Christine de Pisan. New York: Persea.

Rijk, L. M. de, ed. 1972. *Tractatus, called afterwards Summule Logicales.* Assen: Van Gorcum.

Robb-Smith, A. H. T. 1971. "Medical Education in Cambridge Before 1600." In *Cambridge and Its Contribution to Medicine.* Proceedings of the 7th British Congress on the History of Medicine, Cambridge, 1969. London: Wellcome Institute. Pp. 1–25.

Robertson, D. W. 1962. *A Preface to Chaucer.* Princeton, N. J.: Princeton University Press.

Rocha Pereira, Maria Helena da, ed. 1959. *Liber de conservanda sanitate. Studium Generale* 6:147–223.

————, ed. 1973. *Obras Médicas de Pedro Hispano.* Coimbra: University.

Rohde, Erwin. 1914. *Der griechische Roman und seine Vorläufer.* 3rd ed. Leipzig: Breitkopf und Härtel.

Rouse, Richard. 1967. "The Early Library of the Sorbonne." *Scriptorium* 21:42–71, 227–51.

Rousselot, Pierre. 1908. *Pour l'histoire du problème de l'amour au moyen âge.* Beiträge zur Geschichte der Philosophie des Mittelalters 6, 6. Münster: Aschendorff.

Roy, Bruno, ed. 1974. *L'Art d'amours.* Leiden: Brill.

Rubió Y Lluch. 1921. *Documents per l'Historia de la Cultura Catalana Mig-eval.* Barcelona: Institut d'Estudis Catalans.

Rufus of Ephesus. *See* Daremberg and Ruelle.

Rupert of Deutz. *Commentum in Matthaeum.* PL 168:1601.

Russell, Jeffrey Burton. 1972. *Witchcraft in the Middle Ages.* Ithaca, N. Y.: Cornell University Press.

Sabra, A. I. 1987. "The Appropriation and Subsequent Naturalization of Greek Science in Medieval Islam: A Preliminary Statement." *History of Science* 25:223–43.

Saffron, Morris Harold. 1972. "Maurus of Salerno: Twelfth-Century 'Optimus

Physicus' With his Commentary on the Prognostics of Hippocrates." *Transactions of the American Philosophical Society*, 62. Philadelphia: The Society.

Sarton, George. 1927. *An Introduction to the History of Science*. Baltimore: Carnegie Institute of Washington.

Scarborough, John. 1969. *Roman Medicine*. Ithaca, N.Y.: Cornell University Press.

Schadewaldt, Hans. 1985. "Der *Morbus amatorius* aus medizinhistorischer Sicht." In *Das Ritterbild in Mittelalter und Renaissance*. Studia humaniora. Düsseldorfer Studien zu Mittelalter und Renaissance, 1. Düsseldorf: Droste. Pp. 87–104.

Schama, Simon. 1979. "The Unruly Realm: Appetite and Restraint in Seventeenth Century Holland." *Daedalus* 108, no. 3:103–23.

———. 1980. "Wives and Wantons: Versions of Womanhood in 17th Century Dutch Art." *The Oxford Art Journal* 3, no. 1: 5–13.

Schipperges, Heinrich. 1961a. "Arzt im Purpur: Leben und Werk des Petrus Hispanus." *Materia Medica Nordmark* XIII/15:591–600.

———. 1961b. "Zur Psychologie und Psychiatrie des Petrus Hispanus." *Confinia Psychiatrica* 4:137–57.

———. 1964. *Die Assimilation der arabischen Medizin durch das lateinische Mittelalter*. Sudhoffs Archiv, Beiheft 3. Wiesbaden: Franz Steiner.

———. 1967a. "Melancholia als ein mittelalterlicher Sammelbegriff für Wahnvorstellungen." *Studium Generale* 20: 723–36.

———. 1967b. "Eine noch nicht veröffentlichte 'Summa medicinae' des Petrus Hispanus in der Biblioteca Nacional zu Madrid." *Sudhoffs Archiv* 51:187–89.

———. 1968. "Handschriftliche Untersuchungen zur Rezeption des Petrus Hispanus in die 'Opera Ysaac' (Lyon 1515)." In *Fachliteratur des Mittelalters*. Ed. Gundolf Keil, et al. Stuttgart: Metzler.

———. 1968/9. "Handschriftenstudien in spanischen Bibliotheken zum Arabismus der lateinischen Mittelalters." *Archiv für Geschichte der Medizin* 52:3–29.

———. 1969. "Grundzüge einer scholastischen Anthropologie bei Petrus Hispanus." *Portugiesische Forschungen der Goerresgesellschaft*, Erste Reihe 7:1–51.

———. 1973. "Petrus Hispanus." *Die Grossen der Weltgeschichte*. Ed. Kurt Fassmann, et al. Zürich: Kindler. 3:679–91.

———. 1978a. "Antike und Mittelalter." In *Krankheit, Heilkunst, Heilung*. Ed. Heinrich Schipperges, Eduard Seidler, and Paul U. Unschuld. Historische Anthropologie, 1. Freiburg/Munich: Karl Alber. Pp. 229–69.

———. 1978b. "Motivation und Legitimation des ärztlichen Handelns." In *Krankheit, Heilkunst, Heilung*. Ed. Heinrich Schipperges, Eduard Seidler, and Paul U. Unschuld. Historische Anthropologie, 1. Freiburg/Munich: Karl Alber. Pp. 447–89.

———. 1982. "Zum topos von 'ratio et experimentum'." In *Fachprosa-Studien: Beiträge zur mittelalterlichen Wissenschafts- und Geistesgeschichte*. Ed. Gundolf Keil. Berlin: Erich Schmidt.

———. 1985. *Der Garten der Gesundheit: Medizin im Mittelalter*. Munich: Artemis.

Schnell, Rüdiger. 1975. "Ovids *Ars amatoria* und die höfische Minnetheorie." *Euphorion* 69:132–59.

———. 1985. *Causa amoris: Liebeskonzeption und Liebesdarstellung in der mittelalterlichen Literatur*. Bibliotheca Germanica, 27. Bern: Francke.

Schullian, Dorothy and Francis Sommer. 1948. *A Catalog of Incunabula and Manuscripts in the Army Medical Library*. New York: H. Schuman.

Schum, Wilhelm. 1887. *Beschreibendes Verzeichniss der amplonianischen Handschriften-Sammlung zu Erfurt*. Berlin.

*Scriptores ordinis praedicatorum*. 1719–21. Ed. J. Quétif and J. Echard. Paris.

Sears, Elizabeth. 1986. *The Ages of Man*. Princeton, N. J.: Princeton University Press.

Seidler, Eduard. 1967. *Die Heilkunde des ausgehenden Mittelalters in Paris: Studien zur Struktur spätscholastischen Medizin*. Sudhoffs Archiv Beihefte, 8. Wiesbaden: Franz Steiner.

Serapion (the Elder). 1550. *Practica*. Venice.

Serapion (the Younger). 1550. *De temperamentis simplicium*. Venice.

Sezgin, Fuat. 1970. *Geschichte des arabischen Schrifttums*. Vol. 3. Leiden: Brill.

Shahar, Shulamith. 1983. *The Fourth Estate: A History of Women in the Middle Ages*. London: Methuen.

Sharpe, William. 1974. "Mental Disease in Paulus Aegineta's *Epitome*." *Transactions and Studies of the College of Physicians of Philadelphia* 41:198–210.

Silverman, Kaja. 1983. *The Subject of Semiotics*. Oxford: Oxford University Press.

Silverstein, Theodore. 1954. "*Elementum*: Its Appearance among the Twelfth-Century Cosmogonists." *Mediaeval Studies* 16: 156–62.

———. 1978. *Salerno and the Development of Theory*. Problemi Attuali di Scienza e di Cultura, Quaderno 240. Rome: Accademia Nazionale dei Lincei.

Singer, Charles. 1917. "A Legend of Salerno: How Constantine the African Brought the Art of Medicine to the Christians." *Johns Hopkins Hospital Bulletin* 28:64–69.

Siraisi, Nancy G. 1981. *Taddeo Alderotti and His Pupils: Two Generations of Italian Medical Learning*. Princeton, N. J.: Princeton University Press.

———. 1982. "Some Recent Work on Western European Medical Learning, ca. 1200–ca. 1500." *History of Universities* 2: 225–38.

———. 1984. "Renaissance Commentaries on Avicenna's *Canon*, Book 1, Part 1, and the Teaching of Medical *Theoria* in the Italian Universities." *History of Universities* 4:47–97.

Smalley, Beryl. 1964. *The Study of the Bible in the Middle Ages*. 2nd ed. Notre Dame, Indiana: University of Notre Dame Press.

Sommer, H. Oskar. 1909. *The Vulgate Version of the Arthurian Romances*. Publications of the Carnegie Institution, 74. Vol. 1. Washington: Carnegie Institution.

Sontag, Susan. 1979. *Illness as Metaphor*. New York: Vintage.

Spargo, John Webster. 1934. *Vergil the Necromancer*. Harvard Studies in Comparative Literature, 10. Cambridge, Mass.: Harvard University Press.

Speroni, G. B., ed. 1974. "Il *Consaus d'amours* di Richard de Fournival." *Medioevo romanzo*, 217–78.

Stapper, Richard. 1898. *Papst Johannes XXI. Eine Monographie*. Kirchengeschichtliche Studien, IV.4. Münster im Westf.

Steadman, John M. 1968. " 'Courtly Love' as a Problem of Style." In Arno Esch, ed. *Chaucer und seine Zeit: Symposion für Walter F. Schirmer*. Tübingen: Niemeyer. Pp. 1–33.

Stechow, Wolfgang. 1945. "'The Love of Antiochus with Faire Stratonica' in Art." *Art Bulletin*, 221–37.

Steenberghen, Fernand van. 1955. *Aristotle in the West: The Origins of Latin Aristotelianism*. Trans. Leonard Johnston. Louvain: Nauwelaerts.

Steinschneider, Moritz. 1866. "Constantinus Africanus und seine arabischen Quellen." *(Virchows) Archiv für pathologische Anatomie und Physiologie und für klinische Medicin* 37:351–410.

Steneck, Nicholas H. 1974. "Albert the Great on the Classification and Localization of the Internal Senses." *Isis* 65:193–211.

Sternberg, Robert and Michael Barnes, eds. 1988. *The Psychology of Love*. New Haven, Conn.: Yale University Press.

Stock, Brian. 1983. *The Implications of Literacy: Written Language and Models of Interpretation in the Eleventh and Twelfth Centuries*. Princeton, N. J.: Princeton University Press.

———. 1984/85. "Medieval Literacy, Linguistic Theory, and Social Organization." *NLH* 16:12–29.

———. 1985. "Literacy and Society in the Twelfth Century." In *The Spirit of the Court*. Ed. Glyn Burgess and Robert Taylor. Cambridge: D. S. Brewer.

Stouck, Mary-Ann. 1987. "'In a valey of þis restles mynde': Contexts and Meaning." *Modern Philology* 85:1–11.

Stuart, Malcolm, ed. 1982. *Van Nostrand Reinhold Color Dictionary of Herbs and Herbalism*. New York: Van Nostrand Reinhold.

Sudhoff, Karl. 1916. "Die medizinischen Schriften, welche Bischof Bruno von Hildesheim 1161 in seiner Bibliothek besass, und die Bedeutung des Konstantins von Afrika im 12. Jahrhundert." *Archiv für Geschichte der Medizin* 9:348–56.

———. 1928. "Salerno, Montpellier und Paris um 1200: Ein Handschriftenfund." *Archiv für Geschichte der Medizin* 20:51–62.

———. 1932. "Constantin, der erste Vermittler muslimischer Wissenschaft ins Abendland, und die beiden Salernitaner Frühscholastiker Maurus und Urso als Exponenten dieser Vermittlung." *Archeion* 14:359–69.

*Summa pulsuum*. *See* Grant 1974.

Summers, Montague, trans. 1971 [1928]. *The Malleus Maleficarum of Heinrich Kramer and James Sprenger*. New York: Dover.

Sutton, Peter. 1984. *Masters of Seventeenth-Century Dutch Genre Painting*. Philadelphia: Philadelphia Museum of Art.

Tachau, Katherine. 1988. *Vision and Certitude in the Age of Ockham: Optics, Epistemology and the Foundations of Semantics*. Studien und Texte zur Geistesgeschichte des Mittelalters, 22. Leiden: Brill.

Talbot, C. H., ed. and trans. 1959. *The Life of Christina of Markyate, a Twelfth-Century Recluse*. Oxford: Oxford University Press.

Talbot, Charles. 1978. "Medicine." In *Science in the Middle Ages*. Ed. David C. Lindberg. Chicago: University of Chicago Press. Pp. 391–428.

Tarbé, Prosper, ed. 1849. *Les oeuvres de Guillaume de Machault*. Paris: Techener.

Tellenbach, Hubertus. 1980. *Melancholy*. Trans. Erling Eng. Duquesne Studies, Psychological Series, 9. Pittsburgh: Duquesne University Press.

Temkin, Owsei. 1973. *Galenism: Rise and Decline of a Medical Philosophy*. Ithaca, N.Y.: Cornell University Press.

Tennov, Dorothy. 1979. *Love and Limerance: The Experience of Being in Love*. New York: Stein and Day.

Thorndike, Lynn. 1923–58. *A History of Magic and Experimental Science*. 8 vols. New York: Macmillan.

———, ed. 1946. *The Herbal of Rufinus*. Chicago: University of Chicago Press.

———. 1965. *Michael Scot*. London: Nelson.

Treggiari, Susan. 1969. *Roman Freedmen During the Late Republic*. Cambridge: Cambridge University Press.

Ullmann, Manfred. 1970. *Die Medizin im Islam*. Leiden and Cologne: E. J. Brill.

Urso of Calabria. *See* Creutz, 1936.

Valerius Maximus. 1966. *Factorum et dictorum memorabilium*. Ed. C. Kempf. Stuttgart: Teubner.

Van Riet, Simone, ed. 1968. *Liber de anima seu sextus de naturalibus IV–V*. Avicenna latinus. Leiden: Brill.

———. 1972. *Liber de anima seu sextus de naturalibus I–III*. Avicenna latinus. Leiden: Brill.

Vazquez Bujan, Manuel Enrique. 1984. "Problemas generales de las antiguas traducciones médicas latinas." *Studi medievali* ser. 3, 25:641–80.

Viarre, Simone. 1966. *La Survie d'Ovide dans la littérature scientifique des XII$^e$ et XIII$^e$ siècles*. Poitiers: Centre d'études supérieures de civilisation médiévale.

Vieillard, Constance. 1909. *Gilles de Corbeil*. Paris: Honoré Champion.

Vollmer, Friedrich, ed. 1914. *Aegritudo Perdicae*. In *Poeti latini minores*. Leipzig: Teubner. 5:238–50.

Wack, Mary F. 1982. "Memory and Love in Chaucer's *Troilus and Criseyde*." Ph.D. dissertation, Cornell University.

———. 1984. "Lovesickness in *Troilus*." *Pacific Coast Philology* 19:55–61.

———. 1986a. "Imagination, Rhetoric, and Medicine in the *De amore* of Andreas Capellanus." In *Magister Regis: Festschrift in Honor of R. E. Kaske*. Ed. Arthur Groos. New York: Fordham University Press. Pp. 101–15.

———. 1986b. "The Measure of Pleasure: Peter of Spain on Men, Women, and Lovesickness." *Viator* 17:173–96.

———. 1986c. "New Medieval Medical Texts on *amor hereos*." In *Zusammenhänge, Einflüsse, Wirkungen: Kongressakten zum Tübinger Symposium des Mediävistenverbandes*. Ed. Karl-Heinz Göller, Joerg Fichte, and Bernhard Schimmelpfennig. Berlin: De Gruyter. Pp. 288–98.

———. 1987. "The *Liber de heros morbo* of Johannes Afflacius and its Implications for Medieval Love Conventions." *Speculum* 62:324–44.

———. 1989a (forthcoming). "From Mental Faculties to Magical Philters: The Entry of Magic into Academic Medical Writing on Lovesickness, 13th-17th Centuries." In *Eros and Anteros: The Medical Traditions of Love in Renaissance Culture*. Ed. Donald Beecher and Massimo Ciavolella. Montréal: McGill-Queen's University Press.

———. 1989b (forthcoming). "Gerard of Solo's *Determinatio de amore hereos*." *Traditio*.

Walsh, P. G. 1982. *Andreas Capellanus on Love*. London: Duckworth.

Walther, Hans. 1963. *Proverbia sententiaeque latinitatis medii aevi*. 7 vols. Göttingen: Vandenhoeck and Ruprecht.

Walzer, Richard. 1962 [1939]. "Aristotle, Galen, and Palladius on Love." In *Greek into Arabic: Essays on Islamic Philosophy*. Oriental Studies, 1. Oxford: B. Cassirer.

Wetherbee, Winthrop. 1972. *Platonism and Poetry in the Twelfth Century*. Princeton, N. J.: Princeton University Press.

Wickersheimer, Ernest. 1979 [1936]. *Dictionnaire biographique des médecins en France au moyen âge*. Hautes études médiévales et modernes, 34/1, 34/2, 35. Geneva: Droz.

Willard, Charity Cannon. 1975. "A Fifteenth-Century View of Women's Role in Medieval Society: Christine de Pizan's *Livre des Trois Vertus*." In *The Role of Woman in Medieval Society*. Ed. Rosemary Thee Morewedge. Albany, N. Y.: State University of New York Press. Pp. 90–120.

William of Auvergne. 1963 [1674]. *De anima*. In *Opera omnia*. Paris; rpt. Frankfurt: Minerva.

William of Auxerre. 1964 [1500]. *Summa aurea in quattuor libros sententiarum*. Paris; rpt. Frankfurt: Minerva. William of Brescia (Corvi). 1508. *Practica*. Venice.

William of Saliceto. 1502. *Summa conservationis et curationis*. Venice.

Williamson, Joan. 1985. "Philippe de Mézières' Book for Married Ladies: A Book from the Entourage of Charles VI." In *The Spirit of the Court*. Ed. Glynn Burgess and Robert Taylor. Woodbridge, Suffolk: D. Brewer. Pp. 393–408.

Wilmart, André, ed. 1933. *Septem remedia contra amorem illicitum valde utile*, by Gérard of Liège. Studi e testi, 59.

Wimsatt, James. 1978. "The Canticle of Canticles, Two Latin Poems, and 'In a valey of þis restles mynde'." *Modern Philology* 75:327–45.

Wingate, Sybil D. 1931. *The Mediaeval Latin Versions of the Aristotelian Scientific Corpus, with Special Reference to the Biological Works*. London: Courier Press.

Winkler, John J. 1982. "The Invention of Romance." *Laetaberis* n.s. 1:1–24.

———. 1989. "The Constraints of Eros." In *The Constraints of Desire: The Anthropology of Sex and Gender in Ancient Greece*. London: Methuen.

Wolf, Ferdinand. 1864. "Über einige altfranzösische Doctrinen und Allegorien von der Minne." *Denkschriften der kaiserlichen Akademie der Wissenschaften*. Philosophisch-historische Klasse, 13. Vienna.

Wolfson, Harry. 1935. "The Internal Senses in Latin, Greek and Hebrew Philosophical Texts." *Harvard Theological Review* 28:69–133.

Woolf, Rosemary. 1962. "The Theme of Christ the Lover-Knight in Medieval English Literature." *Review of English Studies* N.S. 13:1–16.

———. 1968. *The English Religious Lyric in the Middle Ages*. Oxford: Clarendon Press.

Wright, Constance Storey. 1966. "The Influence of the Exegetical Tradition of the Song of Songs on the Secular and Religious Love Lyrics of MS Harley 2253." Ph.D. dissertation, University of California, Berkeley.

Wright, Thomas, ed. 1906. *The Book of the Knight of La Tour-Landry*. Early English Text Society, o.s. 33. London: Kegan Paul.

Wulff, Winifred. 1932. "De Amore Hereos." *Ériu* 11:174–81.

Zola, Irving Kenneth. 1983 [1966]. "Culture and Symptoms—An Analysis of Patients' Presenting Complaints." In *Socio-Medical Inquiries: Recollections, Reflections, and Reconsiderations*. Philadelphia: Temple University Press.

# INDEX

## I. Latin Texts

The index entries for the Latin texts in Part Two are keyed to the text and line number. **CA** = Constantine the African; **GB** = Gerard of Berry; **E** = Giles (Egidius); **PHA** = Peter of Spain, Version A; **PHB** = Peter of Spain, Version B; **BF** = Bona Fortuna.

### Names and Titles

super *Afforismos*, **PHA** 216
De Animalibus, **PHA** 143
Aristoteles, **PHA** 205
Avicenna, **PHA** 80, 266; **PHB** 5, 19, 39, 42, 46, 136, 144, 165, 184, 190; in libro *De Anima*, **PHA** 20; **PHB** 158; in tertio [*Canonis*], **PHA** 119, 125, 171, 181, 203, 220, 250
Constantinus, **PHA** 15; **PHB** 96, 205, 210, 216, 257; in libro *De Coitu*, **PHB** 242; in *Pantegni*, **PHB** 12 Galenus, **CA** 27, 40, 60; **GB** 76; **PHB** 125; in *Tegni*, **PHA** 122; **PHB** 102
Haly, **PHA** 261; **PHB** 30, 198; super *Tegni*, **PHA** 60

Orpheus, **CA** 50
Ovidius, **PHB** 270, 280; in *Remedio amoris*, **E** 25; **PHB** 268
Philaretus, **PHB** 138
Philosophus, **GB** 73; **PHB** 253
*Predicamenta*, **PHA** 56
Rasi(y), **PHA** 249; **PHB** 48, 221, 271, 286
Rufus, **CA** 10, 38, 44
Serapion, **PHB** 286
*Tegni*, **PHA** 199
Ysaac, **PHA** 235; in *Dietis particularis*, **E** 21
Zenon, **CA** 42

### Words

This index contains most Latin words occurring in the texts (forms of *dicere, esse, facere,* and pronouns are not included). In most cases, participles are included under the verb, and adverbs under the corresponding adjective. Where adjectives occur in more than one gender, they are listed as masculine; otherwise they are listed as they occur. *Eriosos, heriosis,* etc. have been listed in oblique forms, since the nominatives are unattested.

a.b.c., **BF** 129
abhominare, **PHB** 236
abhorrere, **CA** 68
ablatio, **PHB** 279
accedere, **CA** 67
acceptabile, **GB** 13
accidens, **GB** 9; **PHA** 59, 60, 61, 95; **PHB** 9, 43, 174, 192, 194
accidentalis, **GB** 72; **PHA** 105
accidere, **PHB** 25, 57, 180, 181, 186, 187, 189, 196; **BF** 61
accipere, **BF** 103, 185
accuere, **E** 22
acquisitus, **GB** 79
actio, **CA** 25, 26; **GB** 70
activa, **BF** 171
actor, **PHA** 109, 113, 136, 252, 257
actus, **PHA** 63; **PHB** 72, 73, 75

addere, **PHA** 218; **BF** 104
adducere, **PHA** 6, 7, 205, 217, 221
adesse, **GB** 37
adipisci, **CA** 16
adiutoralia, **BF** 12
adiuvare, **CA** 33, 49; **BF** 16
administrare, **GB** 48; **E** 18–20, 23, 24, 26; **BF** 139
adustio, **GB** 47; **PHA** 138, 161; **BF** 98
adustus, **PHA** 161, 178; **BF** 98
advenire, **GB** 37; **PHA** 215
aer, **CA** 66
afferre, **E** 37
afflictio, **CA** 4
aggregare, **CA** 57
album, **PHB** 171
alterans, **PHA** 211, 213
alterative, **PHA** 170

amantes, **E** 26
amare, **BF** 71, 75, 78, 91–93, 164
amaritudo, **CA** 42; **BF** 99
amasia, **PHA** 187, 192, 193, 196, 199, 206, 218, 269
amata, **BF** 79, 84
amena, **PHA** 180, 182, 190
amicare, **GB** 84
amicicia, **PHA** 35; **PHB** 19, 158
amicum, **BF** 35
amicus, **CA** 35; **BF** 145
amigdala, **BF** 188
amittere, **PHA** 187, 196
amor, **CA** 1, 2, 8; **GB** 1, 39, 57, 65, 66, 68, 73, 85; **E** 2; **PHA** 1, 12, 56, 58, 64, 84, 91; **PHB** 1–16 *passim*; 55–92 *passim*; 141–92 *passim*; 207–219 *passim*; 249–301 *passim*
amor hereos, **PHA** 2, 5, 6, 8, 11, 14, 17, 22, 24–266 *passim*; **PHB** 20; **BF** 3, 13
amplexata, **BF** 37
amplexus, **GB** 54
ana, **BF** 103
anima, **CA** 15, 17, 19, 25–27, 29, 32, 55, 71; **GB** 12, 15, 17, 31, 69–78 *passim*, 82, 83, 85; **E** 38; **PHA** 59, 60, 95; **PHB** 14, 56; **BF** 11, 95, 123
animalia, **PHB** 236
animalis, **PHB** 93, 274
animare, **CA** 47
animus, **CA** 43, 52, 67, 71; **PHB** 11, 298; **BF** 146
antiquatus, **BF** 182
aperire, **BF** 176
apparentia, **PHB** 262
apparere, **PHB** 262
appetere, **GB** 11; **PHA** 175; **PHB** 125, 126, 129, 130, 135, 211
appetitus, **PHB** 66, 69, 70, 99–139 *passim*, 196, 201, 204, 206
applicare, **PHA** 72
applicatio, **PHA** 106
apponere, **CA** 64; **BF** 106
apprehendere, **GB** 9; **PHA** 19, 36; **PHB** 153, 159, 160, 163, 166, 167; **BF** 36
apprehensio, **GB** 16
apprehensum, **BF** 34
aqua, **CA** 37, 42, 66; **GB** 49; **PHB** 49
aqua rosacea, **BF** 172, 174
aquosa, **PHB** 255
ardere, **PHB** 296
arefactio, **BF** 60
arefieri, **GB** 41
argumentum, **PHA** 10, 107, 131, 176, 195, 210, 228
artifex, **GB** 70
aspectus, **PHA** 104
asperitas, **CA** 43
aspersus, **BF** 174
assiduitas, **PHA** 15; **PHB** 15

assiduus, **GB** 59, 60
assignare, **PHB** 233
assimilare, **PHB** 182, 184
associare, **E** 12; **BF** 165
attenuare, **PHB** 258
auctor, **GB** 2; **E** 3; **PHA** 75, 81; **PHB** 294; **BF** 2, 31, 38, 53, 120, 136
auctoritas, **PHA** 229; **PHB** 270, 271
audacia, **CA** 54
audire, **CA** 35; **GB** 39; **PHB** 49; **BF** 65, 66
auferre, **CA** 29; **PHA** 236; **PHB** 109, 289
augmentare, **PHA** 135, 184; **PHB** 115, 283
auaricia, **CA** 53

balneum, **CA** 46, 47, 66; **GB** 49; **PHB** 49, 282, 284, 285, 288; **BF** 116, 119
basilicon, **CA** 64; **BF** 103, 170, 174, 186
beneficia, **BF** 132
bibere, **CA** 59; **GB** 86; **PHB** 50; **BF** 160, 186
bonitas, **PHB** 157
bonus, **CA** 56; **E** 37; **PHA** 49, 90; **PHB** 50; **BF** 90, 116, 120, 153, 156, 160, 161, 167, 184
bullire, **BF** 105, 107
bullitio, **BF** 107

calefacere, **BF** 173
caliditas, **PHB** 108, 119, 122
calidum, **PHA** 121; **PHB** 111, 114, 128, 134, 136–39
calidus, **PHA** 121, 123, 126, 139, 162; **PHB** 31, 103, 130, 134
calor, **CA** 22; **GB** 26; **PHA** 128; **PHB** 156, 232
caminata, **CA** 63
cantare, **CA** 47; **BF** 61
cantilena, **GB** 40; **PHA** 104; **PHB** 50; **BF** 137
cantus, **BF** 62
capitulum, **PHB** 2, 13, 300; **BF** 5
capud monachi, **BF** 102
caput, **E** 3, 4, 6/7, 15, 16; **PHB** 148; **BF** 2, 174
caputpurgium, **BF** 179
caro, **PHB** 285
cassia fistula, **BF** 113
castrati, **PHB** 85
casus **BF** 56, 113, 114
causa, **CA** 13; **GB** 6, 7, 68; **PHA** 119, 124, 127, 141, 170, 172, 238, 242, 265; **PHB** 3, 23, 26, 33, 36, 99, 217, 224, 226, 229, 231–33; **BF** 7, 19, 24, 31
causa materialis, **PHB** 24
causa principalis, **BF** 33, 40, 45
causare, **PHB** 303
cautela, **BF** 130
cavere, **CA** 65; **BF** 146
caverne, **PHB** 261
celare, **GB** 64; **BF** 71

cerebella, **PHA** 147
cerebrum, **CA** 2; **GB** 59–61; **E** 14; **PHA** 1, 74–100 *passim*, 107, 155–57; **PHB** 44, 67, 79, 82, 86, 87, 91, 94, 251
cessare, **BF** 27
cibum, **PHA** 251, 263, 264, 267; **PHB** 99, 101, 104, 284, 288
circumstancia, **PHA** 86
circumstantionata, **PHA** 86
cito, **CA** 19; **PHA** 151; **PHB** 220
citrinus, **CA** 21; **PHB** 35
clara, **CA** 37
coadiuvans, **GB** 5; **BF** 24, 38, 45
cogitare, **PHA** 196
cogitatio, **CA** 4, 18, 19, 24, 29, 33; **GB** 3, 32; **E** 13, 35–37; **PHA** 15, 41, 78, 87, 100, 132, 164, 169, 184, 191, 208, 224, 226, 236, 270; **PHB** 7, 14, 28, 35, 38, 79, 89, 289; **BF** 14, 21, 22, 36, 43
cogitativa, **PHA** 14, 16, 51, 53
cognitio, **E** 22
cognoscere, **PHB** 18; **BF** 98
coire, **PHA** 98, 173; **PHB** 85; **BF** 141
coitus, **CA** 10; **PHA** 64, 67, 98, 118–21, 124, 128, 130, 153, 171, 174, 175, 232, 259; **PHB** 30, 58, 96, 100, 103, 106, 118, 122, 130, 196–211 *passim*, 223, 233, 237, 245, 283; **BF** 152
colera naturalis, **BF** 114
colerica, **GB** 81
colericus, **PHA** 127, 128; **PHB** 44
colligancia, **PHB** 251
colloqui, **CA** 35, 59, 60
color, **CA** 21; **PHA** 230
comedere, **BF** 100, 159, 187, 189, 190
comitare, **CA** 27; **PHB** 9
commemorare, **GB** 43
commovere, **E** 35
communis, **CA** 72; **GB** 86
comparare, **GB** 83
compati, **PHB** 252, 256
competere, **E** 38; **PHA** 5, 8, 70, 180–93 *passim*, 201, 226, 232–59 *passim*, 263; **PHB** 51, 267–87 *passim*, 290; **BF** 114
complementum, **PHB** 177
complexio, **CA** 28; **GB** 24, 71, 77, 78; **PHA** 3, 110–12, 116, 117, 121, 123, 126, 139, 229; **PHB** 31, 101, 103, 199
compositio, **BF** 97
comprehendens, **PHB** 172
comprehensio, **PHB** 171
comprimere, **PHB** 107, 110
compulsus, **BF** 155
computandus, **CA** 41
concavare, **BF** 53
concavitas, **GB** 25, 27
concavus, **CA** 19
concedere, **PHA** 50, 91, 107, 124, 168, 203, 222

concubitus, **GB** 54
concupiscentia, **CA** 3; **BF** 16, 25
concupiscere, **GB** 19
concupiscibilis, **GB** 18–20, 29
concurrere, **PHB** 30, 198, 200
condelector, **CA** 51
conferre, **PHA** 23, 27, 28; **PHB** 274, 275; **BF** 138
confidencia, **PHB** 14
confirmare, **GB** 47
confricatio, **PHB** 231
coniunctio, **GB** 44
consensus, **BF** 154
consequens, **PHA** 191, 225; **PHB** 301
consequenter, **PHB** 173
consequi, **CA** 22; **E** 12; **PHA** 60; **PHB** 157
conservare, **GB** 74
considerare, **CA** 14; **GB** 47
consilium, **GB** 52; **BF** 154
consimilis, **CA** 14; **GB** 13, 43, 68; **PHB** 194, 302
consistere, **PHB** 78, 131; **BF** 94, 96
consocii, **CA** 57
consorcium, **GB** 54
conspicere, **CA** 14
consumere, **PHA** 260; **PHB** 245
contentio, **BF** 151, 162
contiguus, **CA** 2; **GB** 59
contingere, **BF** 44
continuus, **GB** 38
contractio, **PHB** 123
contrahere, **BF** 54
contrariare, **PHA** 199
contrarium, **E** 9; **PHA** 57, 198, 211, 213; **PHB** 103, 214, 242, 257, 286, 292, 294
contrarius, **PHA** 212, 251
contristare, **GB** 75
conveniens, **GB** 14, 22; **BF** 35
conversi, **BF** 167
convictus, **GB** 80
conuiuia, **CA** 50
copia, **PHB** 33, 200
cor, **E** 9; **PHA** 44, 58, 60, 62, 79, 80, 84, 91, 96
corpus, **CA** 25, 26, 28, 31, 49, 71; **GB** 31, 34, 46, 61, 70, 74, 75, 78, 84–6; **PHA** 261; **PHB** 26; **BF** 11, 50, 52, 59, 63, 95, 96, 118
corrigibilis, **BF** 125, 142
corrumpere, **CA** 25; **PHB** 144
corrupcio, **PHA** 88, 92, 132, 246
crebris, **PHB** 11
credere, **GB** 10; **PHB** 214, 243; **BF** 74, 77, 92
crescere, **PHB** 259
cura, **E** 17; **PHA** 70, 71, 102–4, 137, 154, 193, 198, 210; **PHB** 4, 47, 60, 266, 269, 272, 274, 276, 279; **BF** 6, 9, 72, 94, 118, 140, 165

curare, **GB** 44; **PHA** 103, 105; **PHB** 53; **BF** 29
curatio, **PHB** 291; **BF** 19
currens, **CA** 37; **GB** 35

dampna, **BF** 145
dare, **CA** 34; **BF** 111, 186, 187, 189, 191
debere, **E** 6, 8, 19, 20, 23, 26; **PHA** 52, 252, 266; **PHB** 253, 292, 295; **BF** 100, 106, 130, 143, 145, 146
debilis, **PHA** 142; **PHB** 38
debilitas, **PHA** 141, 152; **BF** 183
decoctio, **BF** 103, 104, 115
decrescere, **PHB** 261
deducere, **CA** 38
defectus, **PHA** 17, 24, 34, 92, 99, 169, 177
deficere, **PHB** 236
defixus, **GB** 3, 17
deformis, **PHB** 41
delectabilis, **PHA** 174; **PHB** 230
delectare, **CA** 51, 66; **GB** 64, 83; **PHB** 59, 134, 218, 227, 228, 237, 285; **BF** 133
delectatio, **CA** 5, 7, 59; **GB** 64; **PHB** 154, 173, 197, 203, 205, 216, 222, 233, 235, 240, 241, 244, 246
delicia, **PHB** 26
denominare, **PHA** 66, 68; **PHB** 191
depauperare, **BF** 159
deponenda, **GB** 66
deserviens, **PHB** 147
desiccare, **GB** 27; **PHB** 149
desiderare, **CA** 20; **PHB** 105, 106
desiderium, **CA** 3; **GB** 4; **PHB** 27, 69, 96, 169, 299; **BF** 16, 24
designativum, **CA** 5
determinare, **GB** 29; **E** 3, 6, 8; **PHA** 81; **PHB** 2; **BF** 2, 4, 43
deus, **PHB** 234
dieta, **BF** 117
difficilis, **GB** 7; **PHA** 154, 156, 158
diffinire, **PHB** 10, 13
diffinitio, **PHB** 2, 6; **BF** 7, 18
dilatare, **CA** 23; **PHB** 108
dilectio, **CA** 6; **PHB** 278
dilectissimus, **CA** 35
diligere, **CA** 12; **GB** 51, 62; **PHA** 146, 155, 165, 188, 226; **PHB** 37, 214, 292; **BF** 56, 88
diminuere, **PHB** 256
dinoscere, **CA** 56
discernere, **BF** 42
discretio, **PHA** 244; **PHB** 32; **BF** 125, 126
discursus, **PHB** 229
dispositio, **GB** 28, 46, 53; **PHB** 8, 52, 225
dissolvere, **PHB** 111, 256
distancia, **PHB** 288
distemperare, **BF** 115
distendere, **PHB** 264

diversus, **GB** 50, 55, 56, 71, 72; **BF** 69, 77, 142
diuertere, **GB** 51
diuicia, **GB** 58
divisus, **PHB** 68
divortium, **BF** 55
docere, **GB** 85; **E** 18; **PHA** 113, 136; **BF** 128
documenta, **BF** 135, 149
dolores, **PHB** 11
dominari, **CA** 11
dormire, **CA** 65
ducere, **BF** 43, 91, 116
dulcedo, **CA** 44
dulcis, **GB** 50; **PHB** 49
duplex, **PHA** 102, 239; **PHB** 66, 92, 95, 246
dupliciter, **PHA** 83
durus, **PHB** 37

ebibitum, **CA** 43, 45
ebrietas, **CA** 65; **PHA** 8, 233–45 *passim*; **PHB** 266, 269, 272, 274, 279; **BF** 121
ebriosus, **PHA** 233
educere, **CA** 40
effective, **BF** 23
effectus, **PHB** 8
efficere, **PHB** 44, 299
egritudo, **E** 3, 15, 17, 19, 20; **BF** 8, 9, 49, 120, 124
eicere, **CA** 60
electuarium, **BF** 111
elevare, **PHB** 32, 40, 200, 262, 264
elucescere, **PHA** 204
emissio, **PHB** 246
emittere, **PHB** 113, 218, 219, 245
emplastrum, **PHA** 70, 72, 106; **BF** 173
epar, **PHB** 96, 97
epithimum, **BF** 104, 106
eradiatio, **PHA** 158
erectio, **PHA** 265
ereos, **PHB** 80
ereptio, **PHB** 279
eriosis, -os, **CA** 28, 33, 40, 72
eripere, **PHB** 269
eros, **CA** 1, 2, 6, 13
error, **GB** 7
essentia, **BF** 29
estimare, **GB** 13; **PHA** 37
estimatio, **PHA** 201, 241, 244
estimativa, **GB** 15–36 *passim*; **PHA** 21, 47, 48, 53, 88, 92, 99, 133, 177
estuans, **BF** 67
etas, **PHA** 4
evacuare, **GB** 48; **PHA** 113, 136, 212, 214; **PHB** 106; **BF** 100, 109
evacuatio, **BF** 116
excoriatio, **BF** 176, 182, 184, 185
exercenda, **CA** 72
exhiberi, **PHA** 267
exhonorare, **PHB** 112

exire, **PHA** 5, 181, 182, 186, 189; **PHB** 49
existens, **PHA** 44, 261
exitus, **PHA** 190
expellere, **CA** 9; **BF** 32, 39, 46
expendere, **BF** 160
experimentum, **BF** 172, 181
expertus, **BF** 162, 183, 185
explere, **CA** 15; **BF** 17, 26
expulsio, **PHB** 132
exsiccare, **BF** 54
extensio, **PHB** 121
extollere, **BF** 75
extrahi, **PHB** 6
extreme, **GB** 65
extremitas, **CA** 7; **GB** 64
extrinsecum, **BF** 34
exulare, **BF** 156

fabula, **PHB** 48
facies, **PHB** 35, 259, 261; **BF** 56, 57
facilis, **GB** 38
fallere, **PHB** 220
falsa, **PHA** 195
fantasia, **PHA** 22, 27, 29, 51, 54; **PHB** 17; **BF** 41
farcire, **BF** 190
febricitantes, **E** 30
febris, **PHA** 66
feditas, **BF** 143
femina, **CA** 38; **PHB** 201, 202, 206, 207, 213, 216–18, 244, 245
femineus, **PHB** 209, 211
femininus, **PHB** 58
ferre, **CA** 70
fetida, **GB** 53
fetus, **PHB** 228
fidelitas, **CA** 6; **GB** 62
fides, **GB** 45
figere, **GB** 23; **PHA** 191; **PHB** 7, 97
figura, **GB** 4; **BF** 14
finis, **PHB** 234; **BF** 104
firmiter, **BF** 36
flectere, **CA** 52
flere, **GB** 39; **BF** 61
fletus, **GB** 37, 39; **BF** 62
fluere, **PHB** 95, 112
fluxibilis, **PHB** 255
fluxus, **BF** 181, 185
forma, **CA** 14; **GB** 4; **PHA** 17, 19, 34, 36, 40, 104, 155, 156, 165, 169, 208; **PHB** 153, 160, 161, 171, 291–93; **BF** 14, 18, 19, 20, 35, 49, 52, 62
formale, **PHB** 91
formositas, **CA** 13
forte, **GB** 9
fortificare, **PHB** 41
fortis, **CA** 17, 39; **PHA** 132, 145, 146, 155; **PHB** 93, 296
fortiter, **GB** 26; **PHA** 153; **BF** 36

fovere, **PHB** 285
frequencia, **PHB** 28
frequens, **GB** 42; **PHA** 151, 153
frequenter, **PHB** 48; **BF** 68
frigiditas, **PHB** 118
frigidum, **PHB** 107, 110, 115, 123, 128, 139
frigidus, **GB** 24; **PHA** 139; **PHB** 101, 131, 135
frixa, **BF** 186
frixatum, **BF** 191
fructiferus, **CA** 37, 62
furere, **PHA** 216

gaudere, **GB** 74; **BF** 86
gaudia, **PHB** 12
genera, **CA** 35
generare, **PHA** 4, 109, 138, 151, 160, 264; **PHB** 108
generatio, **PHA** 178; **PHB** 236
gradus, **BF** 170
gratia, **E** 12; **BF** 97
gratum, **GB** 12
grauis, **CA** 21, 69
guttur, **BF** 99

habere, **CA** 17, 20, 37; **GB** 17; **PHA** 111, 115, 117, 120, 122, 126, 143, 147, 150, 157, 163, 166; **PHB** 84, 204, 250, 288; **BF** 3, 43, 67, 69, 90, 164, 166
habitudo, **PHA** 262
habundancia, **PHB** 24
habundare, **PHA** 110, 115, 139
hanelare, **BF** 68
hanelitus, **BF** 52, 65, 67, 86, 88–90
herba, **BF** 101
heremis, **PHB** 21
hereos, **GB** 67; **E** 7; **PHA** 1; **PHB** 1; **BF** 1, 17
herios, **CA** 12
heriosis, **E** 38
heroes, **GB** 57
heros, **GB** 1, 57; **E** 2, 11
herosis, **E** 23, 35
homicidium, **BF** 155
homo, **CA** 69, 70; **PHA** 173; **BF** 124–26
honestas, **BF** 76
honestus, **BF** 167
honores, **BF** 132
horribilis, **CA** 69, 70
humana, **BF** 14
humectare, **GB** 87
humectatio, **GB** 49
humiditas, **PHB** 229
humidum, **PHA** 149, 159
humidus, **BF** 54
humor, **CA** 9; **GB** 47; **PHA** 161, 178, 264; **PHB** 51; **BF** 97, 98, 183

iacere, **PHB** 47
ieiunium, **PHA** 250, 260

ieiunus, **E** 34
iera, **BF** 110
iera logodion, **BF** 110
iera memphitum, **BF** 110
iera pigra, **BF** 110
ignis, **BF** 176
imaginatio, **GB** 17
immatura, **BF** 100
immediate, **PHA** 32, 33, 47, 51
immundicia, **PHB** 235
impedire, **GB** 6; **PHA** 240, 243; **PHB** 143; **BF** 157
imperare, **GB** 17; **PHA** 39, 44, 45
imperatores, **CA** 50
imperium, **GB** 21
impinguare, **PHB** 260
impossibile, **BF** 84
impotentia, **PHB** 74, 75
inania, **PHB** 11
inanire, **PHB** 107
inanitio, **PHB** 105, 124, 126
incidere, **CA** 30, 31; **PHB** 4, 55
incipere, **PHA** 173
incitata, **BF** 21
incitatio, **BF** 13, 20
inclinare, **GB** 21
incorporare, **BF** 175
incorrigibiles, **BF** 126
incurrere, **PHB** 22
individualis, **BF** 15
inducere, **GB** 8; **E** 27; **PHB** 109, 230; **BF** 122, 157
indurare, **CA** 23
industria, **BF** 139
inesse, **PHB** 85
inexpletus, **BF** 17, 26
inferre, **PHA** 11, 31, 33, 48, 50
infirmitas, **CA** 17
infixa, **GB** 15
influere, **E** 33
infrigidare, **GB** 27; **PHB** 44; **BF** 172, 174
infundere, **CA** 43
ingredi, **CA** 47
inicialis, **PHB** 172, 176
inicium, **PHB** 176
inimicicia, **PHA** 35; **PHB** 19
innaturalis, **PHA** 138
innatus, **GB** 26, 73
inordinatio, **PHB** 78, 89
inordinatus, **GB** 42; **PHB** 41
inpressio, **PHA** 145, 146, 154, 156, 158; **PHB** 93
inprimere, **PHA** 148, 149
insania, **PHB** 11; **BF** 26, 134, 146
insanire, **CA** 15; **GB** 69; **BF** 135
insensata, **GB** 9; **PHA** 18, 19, 34, 36
instillatus, **BF** 177, 178
instrumentum, **GB** 70; **BF** 138
intellectus, **PHB** 221; **BF** 41

intelligere, **GB** 33; **E** 29; **PHA** 37, 229, 261, 266
intendere, **PHB** 101
intensior, **PHB** 207, 215
intentio, **GB** 3, 8, 15; **PHA** 208, 224; **PHB** 161
interior, **CA** 61; **PHB** 17
interrogatus, **C** 68
intersectio, **BF** 69
intersectus, **BF** 89
intime, **GB** 62
intrare, **PHB** 16, 49
introducenda, **PHB** 137
intuitus, **GB** 18
invenire, **CA** 20; **BF** 85
inuitare, **CA** 50
iocundus, **CA** 62; **BF** 58
ira, **CA** 52; **GB** 81
irascibilis, **PHA** 43
irradiacio, **PHA** 156
irrigidare, **PHB** 117, 119, 120
irrigidatio, **PHB** 121, 123, 124
irrorare, **BF** 172, 173
iudex, **GB** 16
iudicare, **GB** 22; **PHA** 25, 88, 92; **PHB** 174
iudicium, **PHA** 17, 24, 34; **BF** 44
iungere, **BF** 131
iuvare, **PHB** 139
iuvenis, **PHA** 162, 163, 179; **PHB** 187

labor, **CA** 31, 32, 60
laborare, **GB** 58
laboriosa, **CA** 31
lacrima, **GB** 36
lacrimare, **BF** 56
lacrimosi, **BF** 54
lactucella abbatis, **BF** 102
largitas, **CA** 54
latus, **BF** 79, 86
laudabilis, **GB** 49; **PHA** 264; **PHB** 284, 288
laudare, **BF** 75, 82
ledere, **GB** 85; **PHB** 143
leticia, **CA** 53; **E** 27
letificare, **E** 38
letus, **PHB** 50
leuigare, **CA** 29
lex, **GB** 45
liber, **BF** 90
licet, **GB** 22; **PHA** 153
lingua, **BF** 99
litigiosa, **BF** 150, 162
littera, **PHA** 9, 75, 109, 252
locus, **GB** 35; **PHA** 180, 182, 190
longus, **GB** 48
loqui, **C** 12; **GB** 33; **PHA** 83, 85, 213
lucens, **CA** 61
lucidus, **CA** 64, 67
luciferus, **CA** 36

ludus, **GB** 56
lupinus, **CA** 42

macilenta, **PHA** 262
magis, **GB** 11, 69; **E** 15; **PHA** 118, 143, 146, 161, 204, 207; **PHB** 57, 86, 179–89 *passim*, 195, 200, 209, 211, 251, 254, 255; **BF** 135
magnificare, **PHB** 258, 265; **BF** 109
magnus, **CA** 3; **PHB** 234; **BF** 72, 119
maior, **PHB** 196, 201, 203–7, 216, 239, 240, 243, 251, 262; **BF** 80, 87
malicia, **PHB** 157
malus, **GB** 23; **E** 37; **PHA** 185, 209; **PHB** 31, 199
mandare, **PHB** 169
mania, **CA** 11
manicus, **BF** 30
manifestare, **BF** 71
mansuetudo, **CA** 53; **BF** 128
mas, **CA** 38; **PHB** 197, 214, 215, 240, 244
masculinus, **PHB** 58, 211, 212, 238, 239
masculus, **PHB** 201, 202
materia, **PHA** 66, 67, 129, 258; **PHB** 52, 192, 193
matrix, **PHB** 128–30, 134, 136
maturus, **BF** 167
maximus, **CA** 5, 58; **GB** 83; **PHA** 3, 109–126 *passim*, 139, 150, 165–80 *passim*, 193; **PHB** 21, 181, 186, 187
media, **GB** 25
mediate, **E** 28; **PHA** 51
medicina, **CA** 39, 72; **PHB** 51
medicus, **BF** 139
medietas, **BF** 105
mel violaceum, **BF** 112
melancolia, **CA** 32; **GB** 3; **PHA** 75, 76, 110, 113, 114, 135, 137, 138, 140; **PHB** 10, 13, 52, 194
melancolicus (sb.), **PHA** 115; **PHB** 181–84, 189; **BF** 29
melancolicus, **CA** 30; **GB** 2, 28; **PHA** 77, 87, 108, 111, 112, 116, 133; **PHB** 6, 9, 42, 45, 51, 81, 185, 188–90, 193, 289; **BF** 15, 27
melior, **CA** 33; **GB** 10; **PHA** 26, 38; **PHB** 47
membrum, **CA** 61; **GB** 41, 61; **PHA** 3, 46, 71; **PHB** 56, 61, 63, 68, 70, 98, 105, 106, 119, 147, 225, 229, 231, 238, 250, 257; **BF** 183
memorativa, **PHB** 169
memoria, **BF** 55
mens, **E** 18, 29, 31, 32; **PHA** 269; **PHB** 6, 7, 10
mentio, **GB** 40
minime, **PHB** 188
minor (sb.), **PHA** 195; **PHB** 164
minor, **PHB** 180; **BF** 89

minuere, **PHB** 114, 260
minuus, **PHB** 260
mirabiliter, **BF** 188
mirta, **CA** 64
miser, **BF** 161
mobilis, **CA** 19; **PHB** 36, 138
moderatus, **GB** 86; **BF** 147
modica, **BF** 121
molestatio, **CA** 11
molitus, **CA** 41
mollitia, **GB** 58
moralis, **BF** 50, 63
morbus, **CA** 2; **GB** 44; **E** 2, 3, 5, 11; **PHA** 1, 10, 31, 66, 70, 71, 85, 90, 92, 94, 99; **PHB** 52, 191, 267, 301; **BF** 5, 6, 18–20, 27, 109
mos, **CA** 58; **GB** 79; **BF** 169
motiva, **PHA** 43, 45
motus, **CA** 22; **GB** 37; **PHB** 176, 230
movere, **GB** 34, 39, 69, 72, 78, 81; **PHA** 46; **PHB** 124, 136, 137, 149; **BF** 41, 42
mulier, **PHA** 6, 7, 25, 38, 72, 106, 142–57 *passim*, 199–221 *passim*; **PHB** 220, 295, 296, 298; **BF** 32, 35, 39, 46, 74, 77, 81, 141, 152
multus, **CA** 9; **GB** 51, 52; **PHA** 233; **PHB** 25, 263; **BF** 75, 83, 92
munda, **CA** 63
musicus, **CA** 35, 55; **GB** 82; **BF** 138
mutare, **CA** 44; **BF** 79, 85
mutatio, **BF** 150, 153

nares, **BF** 177, 178
narrare, **GB** 52; **BF** 74, 88, 143, 144
nata, **PHA** 55, 57
natura, **CA** 8; **PHB** 112
naturalis, **GB** 46, 71; **PHA** 137; **PHB** 95, 97
naturaliter, **CA** 23; **GB** 79
necessarius, **BF** 72, 151, 157
necesse, **CA** 30; **PHB** 69
necessitas, **CA** 8, 9; **BF** 32, 39, 46
nervosa, **PHB** 226, 231
nervus, **PHA** 45
nigra colera, **CA** 10
nimius, **CA** 3, 8, 18, 31, 34; **PHB** 32
nobiles, **GB** 57
nobilior, **GB** 10, 16
nobiliores, **PHB** 21
nocumentum, **GB** 61; **PHA** 11, 12, 31, 33, 50
nomen, **CA** 5
nominare, **PHB** 40
notare, **PHB** 16; **BF** 5–13 *passim*, 18–20, 48, 64, 70, 94, 105, 118–20, 123, 149, 181
novella, **BF** 100
nuces, **BF** 129
nutrimentum, **GB** 49

obedire, **GB** 20
obicere, **PHA** 230
obiectum, **PHA** 23, 24, 26, 28
oblivio, **PHA** 238, 242
oblivisci, **PHA** 193
obvolvere, **BF** 42
occium, **PHB** 25
occultare, **GB** 14
occupatio, **GB** 60; **PHA** 170; **BF** 150, 151, 157, 162
occupatus, **GB** 50
occurrere, **GB** 12
oculi, **CA** 18; **GB** 35, 36; **PHB** 36, 249, 252–55, 258, 260–62, 264; **BF** 53
odium, **E** 9; **PHA** 56, 57; **BF** 145
odor, **PHB** 156
odoratum, **BF** 177
odoriferus, **CA** 34, 36, 62
officialis, **PHB** 302
oleum camomillinum, **BF** 179, 180
oleum rosatum, **BF** 175, 186
oleum violaceum, **BF** 178
operari, **GB** 26, 78; **PHB** 103, 163, 166, 167
operatio, **GB** 72, 77; **PHA** 240; **PHB** 64, 143, 226–28, 273; **BF** 50, 51, 63–65
opilatio, **BF** 177
oportet, **CA** 24, 65
oppositus, **PHA** 55, 204; **PHB** 77, 152, 203, 273
optimus, **CA** 62; **BF** 85, 93, 101, 141, 165, 175, 178, 181, 191
opus, **PHB** 235
ordinata, **PHB** 278
ordinatio, **CA** 54
organicus, **CA** 55
organum, **GB** 24, 82; **PHB** 147, 150
ortus, **CA** 36, 61
os, **BF** 99
ostendere, **PHB** 62, 141, 180, 186, 197, 249, 267, 282, 291
ova, **BF** 108, 191

palpebre, **CA** 21; **GB** 38; **BF** 58
parentes, **BF** 154
pares, **BF** 132
pars, **GB** 16, 30, 31, 34, 37; **PHB** 27, 148, 149, 206, 215, 217, 226, 234, 245; **BF** 10, 11, 44, 64, 72, 95, 96, 123, 170
particularis, **PHB** 67, 68, 70; **BF** 136
particulariter, **E** 30
parvitas, **PHB** 221
parvus, **BF** 58, 69
passibilis, **PHB** 254
passio, **CA** 27, 30, 31; **GB** 1, 6, 7, 30, 59, 76; **E** 6–10, 15; **PHA** 2, 3, 10–31 *passim*, 53–108 *passim*, 133, 134, 172, 187; **PHB** 20, 22, 24, 35, 42, 56–90 *passim*, 141–89 *passim*, 252, 299; **BF** 2–4, 12, 23
patella, **BF** 186

patere, **PHA** 46, 49, 52, 66, 159, 185, 209, 247, 248, 256; **PHB** 102, 165, 184, 244; **BF** 24
pati, **PHB** 148, 168, 249, 253; **BF** 25, 124
patiens, **PHA** 186, 191, 192, 200–22 *passim*, 253, 254, 268, 270; **PHB** 290; **BF** 37, 74, 142, 144, 163, 187
patria, **PHA** 5, 181, 182, 186, 189; **PHB** 49; **BF** 156
peccatum, **BF** 166
peiores, **E** 34
penitus, **PHA** 240, 243
percussio, **CA** 23
percutere, **E** 19, 29
perfecte, **GB** 44
perfectissimum, **CA** 56
periculum, **BF** 166
perire, **BF** 160
permiscens, **PHB** 12
permissio, **GB** 45
permutatio, **GB** 55
persimilis, **BF** 16, 27
persona, **CA** 38; **GB** 10, 18, 21
pertinere, **PHB** 70
perturbacio, **PHA** 246
perturbare, **PHA** 244; **PHB** 274
philosophia, **GB** 80
philosophus, **CA** 4, 48, 68
placare, **PHB** 298
placere, **BF** 37, 66
plenus, **PHB** 106
plurimum, **GB** 2, 54
plus, **PHB** 183, 213, 219, 244, 245; **BF** 77
pocius, **GB** 58
poma, **BF** 129
pondus, **CA** 69–71
ponere, **PHB** 96, 234; **BF** 31, 38, 136
posita, **PHA** 204
potentes, **PHB** 85
potentia, **PHA** 63, 64, 98; **PHB** 73, 74
potissime, **GB** 65
potus, **E** 33
precedentes, **PHB** 300
precipere, **PHB** 47
precipitare, **PHB** 210
precipue, **GB** 40
predictus, **PHA** 246; **BF** 105, 115
preferre, **PHB** 90
presentare, **PHB** 295, 297
prevalere, **PHA** 89, 93
primitus, **CA** 40
principium, **PHA** 96; **PHB** 91; **BF** 3
prior, **GB** 27; **PHA** 208, 226; **BF** 80, 81
priuatio, **GB** 36
probantia, **PHA** 107
procedere, **PHB** 5, 23, 34, 46, 54, 61, 140, 179, 195, 248, 280; **BF** 130
processus, **BF** 112
prodesse, **GB** 55; **BF** 153, 163, 188

profundatio, **GB** 34; **E** 13, 14; **PHA** 41, 78, 87, 100, 132, 164, 168, 184; **PHB** 89
profundere, **CA** 25, 34; **E** 22, 31, 36; **PHA** 40, 207, 223; **PHB** 38
profunditas, **PHB** 78
profunditatio, **PHB** 7
profundus, **GB** 32; **PHA** 236; **PHB** 35–37; **BF** 58
prohibere, **PHB** 110; **BF** 120
promittere, **BF** 129, 131, 132
proponere, **BF** 145
propria, **PHB** 227
prosecucio, **PHA** 46
provenire, **PHA** 246; **PHB** 75, 144, 232; **BF** 146
pruna, **BF** 100
puella, **GB** 54; **PHB** 39; **BF** 91
puer, **PHA** 166–68, 172, 177; **BF** 127
puericia, **PHA** 173
pulchra, **CA** 13, 38; **PHA** 7, 25, 39, 104, 190, 200–25 *passim*; **PHB** 292, 296–98
pulchritudo, **CA** 57; **GB** 4; **PHB** 8; **BF** 32, 39, 46, 76
pulli, **BF** 190
pulsus, **CA** 22; **GB** 42; **PHB** 37, 39–41; **BF** 51, 68, 74, 79, 85, 87, 89
purgare, **PHB** 50
putare, **BF** 34

radix volubilis maioris, **BF** 102
ratio, **PHA** 49, 90, 93, 101, 159, 248; **PHB** 62–98 *passim*, 142–81 *passim*, 209, 238, 250, 267, 271, 273, 283; **BF** 42
recedere, **BF** 134
receptio, **PHB** 132, 246
recipiendum, **PHB** 218
recitatio, **CA** 36
rectitudo, **PHB** 277
reddere, **CA** 11
redire, **GB** 45; **BF** 80, 81
reducere, **BF** 96, 116
reductio, **PHB** 277
remanere, **GB** 27
remedia, **GB** 86
rememorari, **PHA** 255, 269
remissior, **PHB** 298
remittere, **PHB** 102, 299
remotissimum, **PHA** 96
reperire, **PHA** 118, 166
replere, **PHA** 129, 234; **PHB** 105, 126, 129, 133, 134
repletio, **PHA** 130; **PHB** 109
representare, **PHB** 293
repudio, **GB** 40
res, **GB** 43, 50; **PHA** 18, 34–46 *passim*, 63, 88, 190, 197, 223, 225, 226; **PHB** 20, 90, 204; **BF** 9, 71, 143
res amata, **PHB** 14, 43, 69; **BF** 70, 73, 86, 144

res delectabilis, **PHB** 239
res desiderata, **GB** 37, 53, 68; **PHB** 27
res dilecta, **GB** 41, 43, 60; **PHA** 223, 243, 252, 255, 270; **PHB** 31, 47, 93, 199
respectu, **PHB** 74
respicere, **BF** 118
respondere, **PHB** 88
retardare, **BF** 66, 88
retrahere, **PHA** 192, 225, 269
reuelare, **GB** 63
ridere, **GB** 38; **BF** 57
risus, **GB** 39
rosa, **CA** 64
rubeum, **PHB** 172

sagacia, **PHB** 48
salices, **CA** 64
sana, **E** 32
sanatus, **BF** 156
sanguineus, **PHA** 127, 128
sanitas, **CA** 55
sapientes, **CA** 59; **E** 32
sapientissimus, **CA** 41
scientia, **CA** 58
scire, **BF** 72, 73, 93, 121, 171
scolares, **BF** 133
scribere, **PHA** 56, 142, 198, 216
se amantes, **CA** 60
secreta, **GB** 63
sedere, **CA** 63
semen, **BF** 185
senciens, **PHB** 126
senes, **PHB** 186, 188
sensatus, **GB** 8, 12–15; **PHB** 154
sensibilis, **GB** 17; **PHA** 11; **PHB** 160, 161, 171, 225
sensitiva, **PHA** 240
sensus, **CA** 11; **PHB** 16, 239
sensus communis, **PHA** 240, 241
separare, **GB** 75
separatio, **GB** 41; **BF** 55
sequi, **CA** 26, 28; **GB** 35, 69, 77; **E** 13; **PHB** 43, 154, 173
sermo, **BF** 78
sexus, **PHA** 4; **PHB** 57, 195, 196, 209, 211, 212, 237, 238
siccitas, **GB** 36; **BF** 99
siccum, **PHA** 148, 158
siccus, **GB** 24; **PHA** 148, 157, 162; **BF** 170
signare, **BF** 8, 9, 48
signum, **GB** 30, 34; **PHB** 3, 34, 59, 248; **BF** 6, 7, 48, 49, 52, 62, 70, 73, 85, 93
simile, **PHA** 215, 217, 218, 229, 230
similis, **CA** 46, 65; **GB** 2; **PHA** 75; **BF** 28, 57
similiter, **CA** 43
singularis, **BF** 15
sita, **GB** 29
socius, **BF** 131

solere, **PHB** 22; **BF** 108
solitudo, **BF** 60
sollicitudo, **CA** 20; **GB** 2, 28, 32; **PHA** 77, 87; **PHB** 6, 42, 185, 190, 193, 280, 289; **BF** 15, 27
sollicitus, **BF** 158
solus, **CA** 71; **GB** 19; **PHB** 131, 218; **BF** 60
solutio, **E** 27; **PHA** 49, 159, 248
solvere, **PHA** 90, 101; **PHB** 98, 177
somnus, **CA** 66; **GB** 48; **BF** 58, 61, 119, 122
sonitus, **CA** 48; **GB** 81, 82
sonus, **BF** 138
sopita, **E** 35, 36
spatiari, **CA** 37
species, **GB** 56; **BF** 14, 22, 23
spectare, **PHB** 63, 64
sperma, **PHA** 67, 68; **PHB** 25, 33, 110, 111, 200
spermatica, **PHA** 129, 259; **PHB** 229
spes, **PHA** 141, 142, 152
spiritus, **CA** 48; **GB** 25, 35, 82
statim, **GB** 33
stimulacio, **PHA** 118, 120, 124, 126, 171; **PHB** 92
stimulare, **PHA** 121, 128, 130, 153, 232, 259; **PHB** 31, 112, 199; **BF** 147
stomachus, **PHB** 100–17 *passim*, 125, 127, 129
suadere, **BF** 168
subsequentia, **CA** 17
substantia, **PHB** 147, 255
subtilis, **PHA** 264
successive, **BF** 76, 82, 91
succurrere, **CA** 29
sucus, **BF** 178
sucus rosarum, **BF** 111
sufficere, **PHA** 129; **BF** 112
sumere, **GB** 30; **E** 28; **PHB** 26; **BF** 49, 52, 187
summa, **BF** 165
superflua, **PHB** 133
superfluitas, **CA** 9; **GB** 67; **PHA** 234, 261, 265; **BF** 33, 39, 47
superius, **BF** 1
superuenientes, **GB** 76
suppositum, **PHA** 195
suspecte, **PHB** 39
suspendere, **BF** 89
suspicio, **PHA** 185; **PHB** 14
suspirium, **PHB** 36; **BF** 68

tamarindi, **BF** 113
tangere, **GB** 66, 67; **PHB** 43 **BF** 23, 53
temperamentum, **BF** 171
temperatus, **CA** 34, 45, 46, 67; **PHA** 251, 263, 267; **PHB** 232
tenere, **PHB** 39; **BF** 73
tenuis, **PHA** 262

testiculus, **PHA** 64–80 *passim*, 101, 106, 130, 234; **PHB** 62–88 *passim*, 98, 100
timere, **PHA** 187, 196
timidus, **CA** 39
titillatio, **PHB** 230
tollere, **CA** 12, 42; **BF** 17
tortella, **BF** 189
totus, **GB** 3
trahere, **GB** 25
transferre, **GB** 62, 84
transire, **BF** 106
tristari, **BF** 87
tristicia, **CA** 45, 53; **PHB** 36, 154, 158, 173
tristis, **CA** 39
tumidus, **BF** 59
turpis, **PHA** 6, 199, 201, 212; **PHB** 291, 293, 296; **BF** 83, 87
turpitudo, **BF** 143

ultimitas, **CA** 6
ultimo, **BF** 106
universalis, **PHB** 67; **BF** 136, 137, 139, 148, 149
universaliter, **E** 29
ustio, **BF** 176
usus, **BF** 180

vagare, **PHB** 11
valde, **GB** 12; **PHA** 209; **PHB** 225; **BF** 153
valere, **CA** 10, 57; **GB** 51, 53; **PHA** 176, 177, 228; **BF** 122, 140, 175
vapores, **PHB** 263
uegetandum, **GB** 73
uehementer, **GB** 15
velle, **CA** 52; **PHB** 210, 216; **BF** 57, 71
velociter, **PHB** 138
velox, **GB** 42; **PHB** 38; **BF** 80
uenatio, **GB** 55
venire, **PHB** 97, 111; **BF** 78, 84, 123, 161
venter, **BF** 181
ventositas, **PHB** 32, 199
verba, **PHB** 48
verbera, **BF** 128
vereri, **BF** 168
versus, **CA** 36; **E** 33
verus, **GB** 66, 67
vestitus, **BF** 158
uetula, **GB** 52
uia, **CA** 72
vicinum, **BF** 171
vicium, **BF** 144, 183
victus, **BF** 158
videre, **CA** 10, 36; **GB** 7, 68; **E** 14; **PHA** 14, 22, 26, 65, 74, 180, 182, 190, 197, 206, 222; **PHB** 84, 187, 188, 238, 260, 270, 291, 297; **BF** 140, 153
vigere, **PHB** 79, 113, 114, 116, 127, 128, 135, 219
vigilia, **CA** 22; **PHB** 263; **BF** 59

vilia, **BF** 83, 87
villus, **PHB** 116, 118
vincere, **PHB** 220
vinum, **CA** 34, 39, 40, 43, 44, 48, 55, 59;
    **GB** 86; **E** 18–34 passim, 37; **PHB** 50; **BF**
    173
vir, **GB** 57; **PHA** 142, 144, 147, 150, 154,
    155, 157; **PHB** 206, 208, 218
virga, **PHA** 265; **PHB** 32, 110, 111, 114,
    121, 133, 136
virtus, **CA** 27; **GB** 6, 45, 76, 77; **PHA** 2, 10,
    23, 27, 31, 43, 44, 49, 247; **PHB** 17, 56,
    140, 142, 146, 153, 163, 172, 227; **BF** 168
virtus cogitativa, **PHA** 40
virtus concupiscibilis, **PHA** 43
virtus irascibilis, **PHA** 43
virtus estimativa, **GB** 8; **PHA** 18, 30, 33,
    36, 37; **PHB** 18, 28, 94, 155–77 passim,
    277
virtus expulsiva, **PHB** 228
virtus memorativa, **PHB** 28

virtus motiva, **PHA** 45
virtus spiritualis, **BF** 51, 64
virtus ymaginativa, **GB** 23; **PHA** 12, 42;
    **PHB** 141, 145, 150, 151, 165, 175
visus, **PHA** 201
uita, **GB** 58
uitis, **CA** 41
vituperare, **PHA** 253; **BF** 82
uituperatio, **GB** 52
vituperium, **PHA** 254, 268
vivere, **PHB** 25; **BF** 160
vocare, **PHB** 21, 39
uoluptas, **CA** 15

ymaginacio, **PHA** 165, 169, 192, 224; **PHB**
    31, 79, 145, 159, 198
ymaginari, **PHA** 42
ymaginativa, **GB** 18, 20; **PHA** 12, 50, 53,
    146
ymago, **PHA** 132

## II. Subject Index

Also included here are manuscripts and names of scholars cited in the text.

Aegidius Portugalensis. See Giles
Affective piety, 25
Alain de Lille, 53, 58
Albert the Great, Quaestiones super De ani-
    malibus, 85, 118–19
Alexander, 54
Alfonso X, "The Wise," 154
ʿAli ibn al-ʿAbbās al-Majūsī (Haly Abbas),
    Kitāb al-Malakī (Pantegni), 34, 35
Alonso, Manuel, 231
Alphanus, archbishop of Salerno, 31, 34
Ambiguity: of amor, 22, 94–95, 107–8, 122;
    of maior, 122; of passio, 79
Ambivalence, 21, 72–73, 152, 155–62. See
    also Anger; Melancholy
Amnon and Thamar, 19–21
Amor hereos, 38, 60, 88–89, 182–85. See also
    ʿIshk; Lovesickness
Andreas Capellanus: and Gerard of Berry,
    61–62; and signa amoris, 65–66; De amore,
    51, 64, 96, 112, 159, 167
Anger: and lovesickness, 20–21, 27–28,
    152–53, 158, 162, 176; and melancholy,
    12–13, 162. See also Ambivalence
Anorexia (wasting), 40, 151
Antiochus and Stratonice, 15–18, 136, 154
Anxiety: displaced as lovesickness, 171; sci-
    entific discourse as mastery of, 173–74
Appetite, 58, 97–98, 107; sexual, 116–17
Archpoet, 31–32
Aristotle, 78, 85; Categories, 94; De anima 98,

105, 134; De animalibus, 76, 114; Nichoma-
    chaean Ethics, 105; Physics, 117, 119
Arnald of Villanova, 125, 151; Flebotomia,
    206; Parabolae aphorismi, 206; Tractatus
    (Liber) de amore heroico, 63, 102, 106–7,
    133
L'Art d'amours, 15, 63, 109, 110; on anger
    and melancholy, 162; on love service,
    70–71, 146; on pleasure, 111–12
Atto, 34, 47
Aurelius, 13
Averroes, 49
Avicenna, 35, 46, 54, 85, 100–101; Canon
    medicinae, xiii, 48–49, 53, 55, 63, 136;
    cures in, 66–68, 89, 103; Liber de anima,
    53, 55, 56

Baader, Gerhard, 182
Baldwin of Canterbury, 21, 22
Baltimore, Johns Hopkins University, Wil-
    liam H. Welch Medical Library, MS lat.
    13.1, 194
Bartholomaeus, 53
Bartholomaeus Anglicus, 111
Basel, Universitätsbibliothek, D.III.6, 194,
    195
Basil as remedy, 45, 140, 141
Baths, 44–45, 70, 89, 105
Bazán, Bernardo, 78
Beauty as cause of lovesickness, 12, 39, 59,
    132–34

Bern, Burgerbibliothek A 94 (10), 180, 184
Bernard of Clairvaux, 32
Bernard of Gordon, 70, 112, 142; *Compendium regiminis acutorum*, 252; *Practica dicta Lilium medicinae*, 88, 106, 120
Bernardus Provincialis, 53, 54; *Commentarium super tabulas Salerni*, 52, 112
Bethesda, National Library of Medicine, MS 11, 194, 195–96; MS 12, 181, 194
Bible, 5–6, 18–24
*Bible moralisée*, 21
Bloch, R. Howard, 59, 70
Boase, Roger, 157
Boccaccio, 65, 83; *Decameron*, 69, 109, 176
Body: interaction with soul, 39–40, 58–59, 78–79, 93–94; site of lovesickness in, 78–79, 81–82, 93–98. *See also* Materialism; Somaticism; Unity, psychosomatic
Bona Fortuna: identity, 127–29; *Treatise on the Viaticum (Tractatus super Viaticum)*, 126–45, 254–65; and scholastic medicine, 129–30; manuscripts of, 127, 128, 252–53; outlined, 131–32
Bona Hora, Bernard de, 129, 252
Bowlby, John, 160
Brain: as site of lovesickness, 38, 78–79, 95–96, 97, 150; physiology of, 114–15
Breathing as symptom, 64, 135, 151
Bredon, Simon, 48
Burton, Robert, 101, 102
Business as cure, 142
Bynum, Caroline W., 151

Caelius Aurelianus, *On Acute and Chronic Diseases*, 11–13
Cambridge, 48
Cambridge, Gonville and Caius College, MS 97, 194, 196; MS 117/186, 194, 195; MS 411/415, 180; St. John's College, MS D.24 (99), 194; Trinity College, MS O.1.40 (1064), 181, 194; MS R.14.35 (907), 194, 196
Cassiodorus, 11
Causality, material, 98
Causes of lovesickness, xii, 39–40, 56–59, 89, 90–92, 132–35. *See also* Beauty; Humors; Mental faculties; *Species*
Cavalcanti, Guido, "Donna me prega," 83
Chaucer, Geoffrey, 6, 73, 169, 174
Chrétien de Troyes, *Cligés*, 110
Christ, 153; as lover, 24, 171–73; as model, 24–25
Christina of Markyate, 27
Christine de Pisan, 146, 167; *Epistre au dieu d'amours*, 154
*Chronicle of Montecassino*, 32
Clerks, 72, 113, 173–74
Cogitative faculty (*virtus cogitativa*), 91
Color as symptom, 40

*Commentary on* De secretis mulierum, 119–20
Complexion, role of, in lovesickness, 98–101. *See also* Humors
*Concordantiae*, 48–49
*Consilia*, 122
Constantine the African, 65, 81; biographical legends, 32–34; *De coitu*, 41, 61; *De melancholia*, 40, 61, 101; *De stomacho*, 34; *Pantegni*, 34, 40, 88, 111, 182; *Viaticum*, 12, 23, 31–50, 51, 100, 145, 186–93; commentaries on, xiii-xiv, xv (*see* Bona Fortuna; Gerard of Berry; Giles; Peter of Spain); influence of, 30, 32, 47–50; manuscripts of, 47–48, 179–82
Contraries, cure by, 103
Control: lovesickness as form of, 30, 169–71, 173–74; loss of, in lovesickness, 63–64, 72
Couliano, Ioan, 36
"Courtly love": and excess, 174; and lovesickness, 30, 166–73; as social practice, 147. *See also* Love conventions
daCruz Pontes, J. M., 231
Crying as symptom, 63–64
Cú Chulainn, wasting sickness of, 27–29
Cures of lovesickness, xii, 10, 41–46, 66–70, 89–90, 102–5, 139–45. *See also* Basil; Baths; Business; Games; Gardens; Herbs; Hunting; Intercourse; Litigation; Purgation; Sleep; Travel; Vituperation; Wine

D'Alverny, Marie-Thérèse, 252
Damian, Peter, 160
Dante, 83, 162; "Amor, da che convien," 157–58; *Rime*, 126, 158
Daremberg, Charles, 183
David of Dinant, *Quaternuli*, 12–13, 61, 78–79
*De adventu medici ad aegrotum*, 252
Demaitre, Luke, 129
Depression (depressed thoughts), xii, 40, 81, 151, 160
De Renzi, Salvatore, 52
Desiderius, abbot of Montecassino, 21–22, 32, 34
Desire: incestuous, 5, 15–18; for the maternal, 154; psychophysiology of, 58–59; sexual, 96–97, 116
Despars, Jacques, 64, 65, 68, 112, 121–22, 150
Determinism, 39–40, 90
Diagnosis, 137–38, 144–45. *See also* Eyes; Pulse Test; Secrecy
Dialectic, 94, 97–98, 122
*Dialogue between a Rustic and a Noble*, 166
Dionigi da Borgo San Sepulcro, 18
Disputed questions, 76–77, 85–88
"The Doctor's Visit," 124, 138, 139, 175

Domenico da Ragusa, 89
Dowry system, 160
Duby, Georges, 160
Dugat, Gustav, 181
Duplicity, 72, 169
Durham, Dean and Chapter Library, MS
   C.IV.4, 181

Elements, 55, 59
Emotional lability as symptom, 63–64
Emotions, location in body of, 78, 94–98
   *See also* Body; Brain; Heart; Passions of
   the soul
*Epistolae duorum amantium*, 110–11
Erfurt, Wissenschaftliche Allgemeinbib-
   liothek, CA 212, 212; CA F 221, 194, 196,
   230; CA F 266, 181, 194, 196
*Esculapius*, 13
Estimative faculty (*virtus estimativa*), 56, 91,
   93. *See also* Mental faculties
*L'Estoire del Saint Graal*, 163–64
*Experimenta*, 52, 129, 139–40
Eyes as symptom, 40, 63, 101–2

Faculty psychology. *See* Mental faculties
*Fantasia (virtus fantastica)*, 91–92, 134
Fasting as cure, 104–5
Fear somaticized as illness, 28–29, 166
Feminine: love defined as, 13; symptoms as,
   65, 151–52
Ferrand, Jacques, 122, 142
Ferreiro Alemparte, J., 76
Food as cure, 70, 104–5
Foucault, Michel, 68
Frenzy, Platonic, 10, 36, 39
Freud, Sigmund, 21, 160, 162
Fulgentius, 18

Gadifer de la Salle, 146, 166, 171
Galen, 7–9, 35, 40, 41; commentary on Hip-
   pocrates' *Epidemics*, 8–9; commentary on
   Hippocrates' *Prognostics*, 7–8; *Prognostics*,
   9, 136
Games, 70
Garbo, Dino del, 83, 134, 151
Gardens as cure, 41–45
Geertz, Clifford, xiv
Gender and lovesickness, 109–25. *See also*
   Men; Women
Gerard, *De modo medendi*, 206
Gerard of Berry, 39, 89, 112–13, 121, 150,
   151; *Glosses on the Viaticum (Glosule super
   Viaticum)*, 51–73, 198–205; and Andreas
   Capellanus, 61–62; date of composition,
   52–53; influence, 52; manuscripts, 194–97;
   prologue, 54–55, 196–97
Gerard of Cremona, 38
Gerard of Solo, 142; commentary on al-
   Rāzī's *Liber ad almansorem*, 101, 105, 121,

150; *Determinatio de amore hereos*, 93, 98,
   105–6, 120–21, 135
Gerona, Archivo Capitular, Codex (78)
   20,e,11, 206–7
Gentile da Foligno, 185
Giles (Egidius): identity, 74–76; *Gloss on the
   Viaticum (Glose super Viaticum)*, 74–82,
   208–11; manuscript of, 206–7; relation to
   Peter of Spain's *Questions*, 75–76
Giles of Santarem. *See* Giles
Gilles de Corbeil, 53, 54
*Glose dietarum universalium ysaaci*, 206
*Glose super librum de febribus Isaac*, 206
Gottfried von Strassburg, 25, 64, 73
Gourevitch, Danielle, 9
Guibert of Nogent, 27, 159, 160
Guillaume de Machaut, 167

Hartmann von Aue, *Gregorius*, 154
Heart, as site of lovesickness, 78–79, 93–94
Henry of Lancaster, 147
Herbs, 45, 139–40
"Heroic" love, 46–47
Hierarchy: and lovesickness, 123–25,
   150–52; of mental faculties, 58–59;
   sexual, 123, 167; threatened by lovesick-
   ness, 72. *See also* Love service; Nobility
Hildegard of Bingen, 146, 162
Hippocrates, 163–64
Hugh of St. Cher, 51, 52, 75; *De doctrina cor-
   dis*, 24, 66, 123
Hukbert of Sens, 29
Humectation, 70
Humors, xii, 39–40, 58–59, 98–101, 104
Hunting as cure, 70

Ibn al-Jawzi, 36
Ibn Jazlah, *Tacuini aegritudinum et morborum*,
   126
Ibn al-Jazzār, *Zad al-musāfir*, 11, 34–35,
   36, 46
Idealization, 70, 151, 167–69
Identification with desired object, 152
*Iera*, 140
*Ilisci*, 49, 150. See also ʿ*Ishk*
Illness: anxiety somaticized as, 164–71; fear
   somaticized as, 28–29
Imagination, 58
Imaginative faculty (*virtus imaginativa*), 58,
   90, 92–93. *See also* Mental faculties
*Imitatio Christi*, 25
"In the valley of restless mind," 153
Incest, 154. *See also* Desire, incestuous
Infantile, symptoms of lovesickness as,
   64–65, 151–52. *See also* Object relations,
   childlike
Insomnia, 40
Intension and remission, language of, 118.
   *See also* Quantification of qualities

Intensity of sexual pleasure, 115–17
Intercourse, therapeutic, 10, 11–12, 41, 66–70, 79, 89, 142
Internal senses. *See* Mental faculties
Inward wits. *See* Mental faculties
Isḥāq ibn ʿImran, 35, 40
Isḥāq ibn Sulaymān al-Isrāʾīlī (Isaac Judaeus), 35, 81
ʿIshk, 35–38, 46–47, 49, 182–83. See also *amor hereos*
Isidore of Seville, *Etymologies*, 13, 65

Jacquart, Danielle, 68, 183
Jacques de Vitry, 162
Jean de St. Amand, 48; *Glose super librum regimen acutorum ypocratis*, 206
Johannes Afflacius, 34, 46–47. See also *Liber de heros morbo*
John of Gaddesden, 101
John of Tornamira, 101, 118
Johnson, Virginia, 121
Julian of Mt. Cornillon, 25, 111
Julian of Norwich, 153
Justus' wife, 7, 9

Karnein, Alfred, 62, 65
al-Kindi, 35
Klapisch-Zuber, Christiane, 159
Knight of the Tour Landry, 166
Krakow, Biblioteka Jagiellońska, Rps BJ 781, 212
Kristeva, Julia, 3

Laín Entralgo, Pedro, 133
Lecherometers, 121
Leclercq, Jean, 18, 20
*Liber de heros morbo*, 34, 47, 51, 60–61, 150, 181. See also Ibn al-Jazzār; Johannes Afflacius
Limerance, xii
Litigation as cure, 142
London, British Library, Egerton 2900, 180
Longinus, 14
Love: as divine illness, 7–8; as psychological or social threat, 6, 65, 73, 136–39; incestuous, 21. *See also* Ambivalence; Desire; Lovesickness
Love conventions: and lovesickness, xiv, 50; in art, 147, 148; in literature, 51. *See also* "Courtly love"
Love potions, 11, 27. *See also* Magic, erotic
Love service, as source of conflict, 70–72, 151, 167–71. *See also* "Courtly love"; Hierarchy
Lovesickness: as cultural symptom, 173–74; as marriage strategy, 176; as social practice, 50, 147, 174; contemporary views of, xii; definitions of, 55–56, 88–89, 132–33; in antiquity, 3–18; in classical literature,

14–18; in Christianity, 18–27, 171–73; reality of, 143–45, 148–49. *See also* Causes; "Courtly love"; Cures; Love; Melancholy; Symptoms
Loyalty, 47, 65
Lucretius, 70

McVaugh, Michael, 118
Madrid, Biblioteca Nacional, MS 1877, 230, 231
Magic, erotic, 27, 29, 162–66. *See also* Love potions
*Malleus Maleficarum*, 164–66
Mania, 6–7, 10–11, 112. *See also* Melancholy
Marie de France, *Guigemar*, 63
Marriage as cure, 66–68, 175, 176
Mary Magdalen, 25
Masters, William, 121
Materiality, 49; of human organism, 32, 55
Materialism, 39–40, 59–61, 95, 98
Maternal, desire for, 154. *See also* Incest; Mother
Maurus, 54; commentary on Johannitius' *Isagoge*, 98
Medicine: and literature, 5, 125; and philosophy, 83–84, 98, 118; and theology, 7–8, 68–70, 79, 131; as science, 54–55; relation to other discourses, 7, 30, 72–73. *See also* Practical medicine, lovesickness as part of
Melancholy (melancholia), 12, 160; and ambivalence, 21; and anger, 12–13, 162; and lovesickness, xii, 6–7, 10, 35, 40, 56, 61, 100–101
Men: and fear of women, 28–29, 164–66; and lovesickness, 108, 112–13, 175; and sexual vengeance, 162–64; associated with form, 117
Menagier of Paris, 154
Menocal, María Rosa, 37
Mental faculties, 56–59, 90–93. *See also* the names of individual faculties
Mesue, John, *Book of Medical Aphorisms*, 75
Montecassino, 10, 34, 47, 184
Montpellier, 48, 54, 105, 128–29
Montpellier, MS 161, 194
Mother: desire for, 15–18, 154; God as, 153
Mourning, 160. *See also* Melancholy; Separation
Munich, Bayerische Staatsbibliothek, Clm 3512, 194, 196; Clm 13033, 194, 195
Murdoch, John, 109
Music as cure, 45–46, 89–90, 142
*Muwashshaha*, 37

Narcissism, 72, 151, 152
Neckham, Alexander, 14, 48
Nemesius, *On the Nature of Man*, 31
Nobility and lovesickness, 46–47, 60–61,

62, 70–73, 112, 150. See also "Courtly love"; Hierarchy; Social class
Non-naturals, 41, 94

Object relations, childlike, 152, 155. See also Infantile, symptoms as
Odo of Cluny, Collations, 29
On True Love, 167
Optics, 93
Oribasius, Synopsis, 10
Origen, 22, 64
Ovid, 14–15, 51, 70; Ars Amatoria 110 (see also L'Art d'amours); Heroides, 110; Remedia amoris (Remedies for Love), 15, 81, 110, 126, 139
Oxford, 48
Oxford, Bodleian Library, MS Bodl. 489, 181; MS Laud 106, 182; MS Laud misc. 567, 180, 184; Corpus Christi College, MS 189, 180, 184, 185

Paris, 48, 54, 128–29
Paris, Bibliothèque Nationale, lat. 6951, 181; lat. 15373, 129, 252
Passions of the soul, 6–7, 8, 59, 79
Patients of lovesickness, 60–61; 98–101, 115–16; female, 112, 114–15, 122–25; male, 112
Patterson, Lee, 66
Paul of Aegina, 14
Penitentials, 29
Perdica's Malady (Aegritudo Perdicae), 3–5, 15; in art, 4, 18
Peter the Deacon, Illustrious Men of Montecassino, 32–34
Peter of Spain: biography, 84–85; commentary on Galen's Tegni, 85; commentary on Isaac's De dietis universalibus et particularibus, 85; commentary on Isaac's De urinis 85, 231; commentary on Johannitius' Isagoge, 85; Expositio libri de anima, 85, 134, 231; influence, 120–25; Questiones super De animalibus, 85, 97, 98, 114, 116–17, 231; Questions on the Viaticum (Questiones super Viaticum), 83–108, 214–29, 232–51; influence of, 105–7; manuscripts, 105, 212–13, 230–31; outlined, 86–87; two versions, 85–88; Scientia libri de anima, 85, 90, 91–92, 94; Summule logicales, 84, 94
Philippe de Mézières, 166–67
Pierre de St. Flour, 49, 119–20
Pietà, 171, 172
Pietro d'Abano, Conciliator, 120
Pigeaud, J., 7
Pleasure: and lovesickness, 38–39, 49, 109–25; as final cause of lovesickness, 118; measurement of, 115–21
Plutarch, 15
Poetry as cure, 41, 46. See also Music

Popular lore, 27–30
Power and lovesickness, 27–28, 72, 152, 164–66
Practical medicine, lovesickness as part of, 9, 14, 35, 55, 129, 145, 149
Preoccupation, 64
Prose Salernitan Questions, 53, 58, 75, 98, 100
Pseudo-Aristotle, Problem 30, 12, 61
Pseudo-Hippocrates, Astrologia ypocratis, 206
Psychotherapy, Bona Fortuna's, 142–43. See also Cures
Puissance d'amour, La, 167
Pulse test, 9, 48, 89, 135–39; in art, 138, 139
Purgation, 90, 139–40

Quantification of qualities, 117–20
"Queritur de fluxu et refluxu maris," 206
"Queritur de cibo per quam virtutem nutriat," 206
"Questio est que complexio est longioris vitae," 206

Rapture, mystical, and lovesickness, 23–24, 113, 152–57; and signa amoris, 66
Ratinck, Amplonius, 48, 52, 105, 212
al-Rāzī, 35, 49, 54; cures in, 89–90, 102; De secretis in medicina, 75; Liber continens, 126, 144–45
Reportationes, 77–78, 127
Richard de Bury, 38
Richard de Fournival, 48, 63, 71, 72, 169; Consaus d'amours, 66
Richard of St. Victor, 213, 157; Four Degrees of Violent Charity, 152–53
Rodulphus Tortarius, 18
Roman d'Eneas, 110
Romance of the Rose, 102, 113
Rouen, Bibliothèque Municipale, A 176 (983), 253
Rufus of Ephesus, 10, 35, 41
Rupert of Deutz, 24

Salernitan questions, 77, 111–12
Salerno, 47, 54
Sappho, 14
Sarton, George, 48
Schipperges, Heinrich, 231
Scientific discourse, 55, 174–75
Scot, Michael, 76
Secrecy: and pulse test, 136–37; as sign of love, 65
Separation and ambivalence, 159–62
Sexuality and lovesickness, xii, 109–25. See also Desire; Pleasure
Signa amoris, 22–23, 62–66, 135. See also Symptoms
Silence as symptom, 64, 151
Similarity as cause of love, 133–34
Sleep as cure, 45, 70

Social class, xi, 9, 59–60, 166. *See also* Nobility
Social context: of cures, 142; of lovesickness, 123, 146–74
Solitude as symptom, 135
Somaticism, 85. *See also* Body; Materialism
"A Song of great sweetness from Christ to his daintiest dam," 155
Song of Songs, 21–24, 110–11
Soranus, 11
*Species* as cause of lovesickness, 132–35
*Spiritus*, 56, 58, 63, 64
Steen, Jan, "The Doctor's Visit," 124, 138, 139
Stock, Brian, 49
Subject: causes of, 55; human body as, 55
Subjectivity, 59–60, 70–73, 171
Suffering, 24–27, 171
Symptoms, xi, 10, 40, 63–66, 101–2, 135–39, 144–45; social meaning of, xiii. *See also* Anorexia; Breathing; Color; Crying; Depression; Feminine, symptoms as; Infantile, symptoms as; Preoccupation; *Signa amoris*; Silence

*Tacuinum sanitatis*, xvi
Testicles, 94–97
*Thesaurus pauperum*, 61, 84
Thomas of Chobham, 29
Thomasset, Claude, 68, 183
Toledo, 76
Travel as cure, 102–3, 142
*Twelve Signs of True Love*, 65

Unity, psychosomatic, 79, 82, 93–94, 97. *See also* Body, interaction with soul
Urso of Calabria, 54; *Glosses on Aphorisms*, 58

Valerius Maximus, 15, 18, 136
Van Foreest, Pieter, 136, 175
Vatican Mythographers, 18
Vatican, Biblioteca Apostolica, lat. 4425, 181; lat. 4432, 194; pal. lat. 1085, 230; pal. lat. 1149, 194, 196; pal. lat. 1158, 182; pal. lat. 1161, 194; pal. lat. 1163, 181, 184; pal. lat. 1165, 181, 194, 196; pal. lat. 1166, 88, 122, 230; reg. lat. 1304, 194, 196
Vergil, 164
*Virtus affectiva*, 94
*Virtus appetitiva*, 94
*Virtus estimativa* and other *virtutes*. *See* Estimative faculty, etc.
Vituperation as cure, 70, 104–5, 143

Wetnursing, 160
Wife of the Knight of the Tour Landry, 146–47
William of Auvergne, 23–24, 113
William of Auxerre, 24, 113
William of Corvi (or Brescia), 89, 135, 150, 151
William of Saliceto, 102–3
Wine as cure, 41–45, 63, 79–81, 90, 104
Witchcraft, 164–66
Womb, suffocation of, 131
Women: absence from medical accounts of love, 111–13, 174; and lovesickness, 7, 9, 114–15, 121–25, 174–76; and lovesickness, in art, 124, 138–39, 175; and lovesickness, in literature, 110–11; and lovesickness, in the Renaissance, 123–25, 175–76; and sexual vengeance, 165–66; associated with matter, 117; fear of, 28–29, 164–66

Zeno, 35, 41

University of Pennsylvania Press
MIDDLE AGES SERIES
Edward Peters, General Editor

Edward Peters, ed. *Christian Society and the Crusades, 1198–1229*. Sources in Translation, including The Capture of Damietta by Oliver of Paderborn. 1971

Edward Peters, ed. *The First Crusade: The Chronicle of Fulcher of Chartres and Other Source Materials*. 1971

Katherine Fischer Drew, trans. *The Burgundian Code: The Book of Constitutions or Law of Gundobad and Additional Enactments*. 1972

G. G. Coulton. *From St. Francis to Dante: Translations from the Chronicle of the Franciscan Salimbene (1221–1288)*. 1972

Alan C. Kors and Edward Peters, eds. *Witchcraft in Europe, 1110–1700: A Documentary History*. 1972

Richard C. Dales. *The Scientific Achievement of the Middle Ages*. 1973

Katherine Fischer Drew, trans. *The Lombard Laws*. 1973

Edward Peters, ed. *Monks, Bishops, and Pagans: Christian Culture in Gaul and Italy, 500–700*. 1975

Jeanne Krochalis and Edward Peters, ed. and trans. *The World of Piers Plowman*. 1975

Julius Goebel, Jr. *Felony and Misdemeanor: A Study in the History of Criminal Law*. 1976

Susan Mosher Stuard, ed. *Women in Medieval Society*. 1976

Clifford Peterson. *Saint Erkenwald*. 1977

Robert Somerville and Kenneth Pennington, eds. *Law, Church, and Society: Essays in Honor of Stephen Kuttner*. 1977

Donald E. Queller. *The Fourth Crusade: The Conquest of Constantinople, 1201–1204*. 1977

Pierre Riché (Jo Ann McNamara, trans.). *Daily Life in the World of Charlemagne*. 1978

Edward Peters, ed. *Heresy and Authority in Medieval Europe*. 1980

Suzanne Fonay Wemple. *Women in Frankish Society: Marriage and the Cloister, 500–900*. 1981

Edward Peters. *The Magician, the Witch, and the Law*. 1982

Barbara H. Rosenwein. *Rhinoceros Bound: Cluny in the Tenth Century*. 1982

Steven D. Sargent, ed. and trans. *On the Threshold of Exact Science: Selected Writings of Anneliese Maier on Late Medieval Natural Philosophy*. 1982

Benedicta Ward. *Miracles and the Medieval Mind: Theory, Record, and Event, 1000–1215*. 1982

Harry Turtledove, trans. *The Chronicle of Theophanes: An English Translation of anni mundi 6095–6305 (A.D. 602–813)*. 1982

Leonard Cantor, ed. *The English Medieval Landscape*. 1982

Charles T. Davis. *Dante's Italy and Other Essays*. 1984

George T. Dennis, trans. *Maurice's Strategikon: Handbook of Byzantine Military Strategy*. 1984

Thomas F. X. Noble. *The Republic of St. Peter: The Birth of the Papal State, 680–825*. 1984

Kenneth Pennington. *Pope and Bishops: The Papal Monarchy in the Twelfth and Thirteenth Centuries*. 1984

Patrick J. Geary. *Aristocracy in Provence: The Rhône Basin at the Dawn of the Carolingian Age*. 1985

C. Stephen Jaeger. *The Origins of Courtliness: Civilizing Trends and the Formation of Courtly Ideals, 939–1210*. 1985

J. N. Hillgarth, ed. *Christianity and Paganism, 350–750: The Conversion of Western Europe*. 1986

William Chester Jordan. *From Servitude to Freedom: Manumission in the Sénonais in the Thirteenth Century*. 1986

James William Brodman. *Ransoming Captives in Crusader Spain: The Order of Merced on the Christian-Islamic Frontier*. 1986

Frank Tobin. *Meister Eckhart: Thought and Language*. 1986

Daniel Bornstein, trans. *Dino Compagni's Chronicle of Florence*. 1986

James M. Powell. *Anatomy of a Crusade, 1213–1221*. 1986

Jonathan Riley-Smith. *The First Crusade and the Idea of Crusading*. 1986

Susan Mosher Stuard, ed. *Women in Medieval History and Historiography*. 1987

Avril Henry, ed. *The Mirour of Mans Saluacioune*. 1987

María Rosa Menocal. *The Arabic Role in Medieval Literary History*. 1987

Margaret J. Ehrhart. *The Judgment of the Trojan Prince Paris in Medieval Literature*. 1987

Betsy Bowden. *Chaucer Aloud: The Varieties of Textual Interpretation*. 1987

Michael Resler, trans. *EREC by Hartmann von Aue*. 1987

A. J. Minnis. *Medieval Theory of Authorship*. 1988

Uta-Renate Blumenthal. *The Investiture Controversy: Church and Monarchy from the Ninth to the Twelfth Century*. 1988

Robert Hollander. *Boccaccio's Last Fiction: "Il Corbaccio."* 1988

Ralph Turner. *Men Raised from the Dust: Administrative Service and Upward Mobility in Angevin England*. 1988

David Anderson. *Before the Knight's Tale: Imitation of Classical Epic in Boccaccio's Teseida*. 1988

Charlotte A. Newman. *The Anglo-Norman Nobility in the Reign of Henry I: The Second Generation*. 1988

Joseph F. O'Callaghan. *The Cortes of Castile-León, 1188–1350*. 1989

William D. Paden. *The Voice of the Trobairitz: Essays on the Women Troubadours*. 1989

William Chester Jordan. *The French Monarchy and the Jews: From Philip Augustus to the Last Capetians*. 1989

Edward B. Irving, Jr. *Rereading* Beowulf. 1989

David Burr. *Olivi and Franciscan Poverty: The Origins of the Usus Paper Controversy*. 1989

Willene B. Clark and Meradith T. McMunn, eds. *Beasts and Birds of the Middle Ages: The Bestiary and Its Legacy*. 1989

Richard C. Hoffmann. *Land, Liberties, and Lordship in a Late Medieval Countryside: Agrarian Structures and Change in the Duchy of Wrocław*. 1989

J. M. W. Bean. *From Lord to Patron: Lordship in Late Medieval England*. 1989

Mary F. Wack. *Lovesickness in the Middle Ages: The* Viaticum *and Its Commentaries*. 1989

Robert I. Burns, S. J., ed. *Emperor of Culture: Alfonso X the Learned of Castile and His Thirteenth-Century Renaissance*. 1990

E. Ann Matter. *The Voice of My Beloved: The Song of Songs in Western Medieval Christianity*. 1990

Patricia Terry. *Poems of the Elder Edda*. 1990

Ronald Surtz. *The Guitar of God: Gender, Power, and Authority in the Visionary World of Mother Juana de la Cruz (1481–1534)*. 1990